**This book is to be returned on or before
the last date stamped below.**

Sexual Attitudes and Lifestyles

Sexual Attitudes and Lifestyles

ANNE M. JOHNSON

BA, MA, MSc, MBBS, MRCGP, FFPHM, MD
Senior Lecturer in Epidemiology
Academic Department of Genitourinary Medicine
University College Medical School, London

JANE WADSWORTH

BSc, MSc
Senior Lecturer in Medical Statistics
Academic Department of Public Health
St Mary's Hospital Medical School, London

KAYE WELLINGS

BA, MA, MSc
Senior Research Fellow
Academic Department of Public Health
St Mary's Hospital Medical School, London;
London School of Hygiene and Tropical Medicine

JULIA FIELD

BA
Research Director
Social and Community Planning Research
Northampton Square, London

WITH ## SALLY BRADSHAW

BSc, MSc
Academic Department of Genitourinary Medicine
University College Medical School, London

FOREWORD BY **SIR DONALD ACHESON**

OXFORD
BLACKWELL SCIENTIFIC PUBLICATIONS
LONDON EDINBURGH BOSTON
MELBOURNE PARIS BERLIN VIENNA

© 1994 A.M. Johnson, J. Wadsworth
K. Wellings, and J. Field
Published by
Blackwell Scientific Publications
Editorial Offices:
Osney Mead, Oxford OX2 0EL
25 John Street, London WC1N 2BL
23 Ainslie Place, Edinburgh EH3 6AJ
238 Main Street, Cambridge
    Massachusetts 02142, USA
54 University Street, Carlton
    Victoria 3053, Australia

Other Editorial Offices:
Librairie Arnette SA
1, rue de Lille
75007 Paris
France

Blackwell Wissenschafts-Verlag GmbH
Düsseldorfer Strasse 38
D-10707 Berlin
Germany

Blackwell MZV
Feldgasse 13
A-1238 Wien
Austria

First published 1994

Set by Excel Typesetters Co., Hong Kong
Printed and bound in Great Britain by
Hartnolls Ltd, Bodmin, Cornwall

DISTRIBUTORS

Marston Book Services Ltd
PO Box 87
Oxford OX2 0DT
(*Orders*: Tel: 0865 791155
        Fax: 0865 791927
        Telex: 837515)

USA
Blackwell Scientific Publications, Inc.
238 Main Street
Cambridge, MA 02142
(*Orders*: Tel: 800 759-6102
        617 876-7000)

Canada
Times Mirror Professional Publishing, Ltd
130 Flaska Drive
Markham, Ontario L6G 1B8
(*Orders*: Tel: 800 268-4178
        416 470-6739)

Australia
Blackwell Scientific Publications Pty Ltd
54 University Street
Carlton, Victoria 3053
(*Orders*: Tel: 03 347-5552)

A catalogue record for this title
is available from the British Library

ISBN 0-632-03343-6

Library of Congress
Cataloging-in-Publication Data.
Sexual attitudes and lifestyles /
Anne M. Johnson . . . [et al.].
        p.   cm.
    Includes bibliographical references
and index.
    ISBN 0-632-03343-6
    1. Sex customs – Great Britain.
    2. Sexual behavior surveys – Great
Britain.   I. Johnson, Anne M.
HQ18.G7S46   1994
306.7′0941 – dc20

Contents

Foreword, vii
SIR DONALD ACHESON

Preface, ix

Acknowledgements, xi

1 Studying Sexual Lifestyles, 1
ANNE JOHNSON & KAYE WELLINGS

2 Designing the Survey, 19
KAYE WELLINGS & JULIA FIELD

3 Survey Methods and Sample Characteristics, 42
JULIA FIELD, JANE WADSWORTH & SALLY BRADSHAW

4 First Intercourse between Men and Women, 68
KAYE WELLINGS & SALLY BRADSHAW

5 Heterosexual Partnerships, 110
ANNE JOHNSON & JANE WADSWORTH

6 Heterosexual Practices, 145
ANNE JOHNSON & JANE WADSWORTH

7 Sexual Diversity and Homosexual Behaviour, 183
KAYE WELLINGS, JANE WADSWORTH & ANNE JOHNSON

8 Sexual Attitudes, 225
KAYE WELLINGS, JULIA FIELD & LUKE WHITAKER

9 Physical Health and Sexual Behaviour, 259
JANE WADSWORTH & ANNE JOHNSON

10   Risk Reduction Strategies, 296
     JANE WADSWORTH & KAYE WELLINGS

     Appendices

1   Survey Questionnaires, 345

2   Technical Details of the Survey, 423

3   Appendix Tables, 427

     Index, 495

Foreword

SIR DONALD ACHESON

I regard it as a privilege to have been invited to write the foreword to this crucial book, and I commend the courage and determination of the pioneers who have brought it to a successful conclusion.

As the authors point out, the emergence in the 1980s of a lethal epidemic of sexually transmitted infection focused attention on our profound ignorance about many aspects of sexual behaviour. Not only was there no reliable baseline against which the success of efforts to reduce risky behaviour could be judged, but we lacked a firm base from which to predict the future course of the epidemic. The results of this survey have gone a long way towards filling these gaps.

However, the importance of *Sexual Attitudes and Lifestyles* goes beyond HIV and AIDS. The high response rate shows beyond a peradventure that most members of the public will accept and cooperate with the efforts of responsible people working to protect and improve their health in the sensitive area of sex. This was also the experience of my predecessor as Chief Medical Officer, Sir Wilson Jamieson, who during World War II first used the mass media (BBC National Radio News) to give advice on 'venereal disease', and later of myself. Neither of us received complaints or criticisms for discussing frankly in public, subjects previously regarded as taboo.

It is well known that the Government declined to finance the survey and that the Wellcome Trust speedily came to the rescue. Ironically, according to my notes written at the time, the Government's door was still ajar when on 10 September 1989 an article entitled 'Thatcher halts survey on sex' hit the front page of *The Sunday Times*. It certainly closed with a bang the following week!

However, time moves on and attitudes change. In the Government's *'The Health of the Nation': A Strategy for Health in England*, published in 1992, the nettle has been grasped in no uncertain way. HIV/AIDS and sexual health figure in it as one of only five areas selected as key priorities for action, and targets have been set to reduce the frequency of risky behaviours. The work described in this book will form the basis for monitoring progress in this area, and will encourage others abroad to do likewise.

Preface

This detailed account of the British National Survey of Sexual Attitudes and Lifestyles is the culmination of nearly 8 years' work. In this period, lessons have been learnt, friendships formed and alliances forged. We have each gained experience of one another's disciplines and have drawn strength from this multidisciplinary approach.

Without question, the HIV epidemic has provided the impetus, the rationale and the legitimation for the survey. Some will say it also created the funding opportunities. The emergence of the HIV pandemic, and attendant concern to assess and control its spread, have heralded a new era of sexual research throughout the world. In many important respects, this has been beneficial. The AIDS epidemic has led to greater openness in public discussion of sexual matters. Yet because of the heightened profile of work in this area, constraints have been too often political rather than scientific.

The study has been a challenge intellectually, scientifically and politically. We have tried to broaden out the scope of enquiry to include a range of aspects of sexual attitudes and lifestyle of interest to all those concerned with social, epidemiological and health aspects of the field. This also reflects our varied interests and training, in the fields of epidemiology, sociology, social survey research and statistics. Deciding how to draw boundaries around the scope of the survey, recognizing that public acceptability was likely to be limited to questions relevant to public health, and how to maximize response, understanding, consistency and validity has taught us all a great deal about the problems and limitations of large-scale survey research into sensitive topics.

Once the scientific and political hurdles were overcome, through the generous financial support of the Wellcome Trust, the main survey was completed without major problems in the course of the fieldwork, despite the concerns of many about attempting an enquiry of such a sensitive nature among a random population sample.

This book provides an account of the process of the research and of some of the major findings. The study has generated a rich and complex data set, and even in a full-length book there is space to present only a broad overview of the major results. The data set lends itself to almost limitless enquiry, and it is our hope that it will provide a major resource for many different types of scientific analysis. The results presented provide an account of sexual lifestyle in Britain at the end of the 20th century. A total of 18 876 men and women aged 16–59 participated in the survey in an enquiry that ranged across early education and experience, the extent of homosexual experience, patterns of sexual partnership formation, sexual practices and attitudes to sexual expression.

The survey is, as much as any previous research in the field, a product of its time. Probably as many questions remain unanswered as were asked, and certainly many areas of sexual expression remain unexplored. In compiling this account of the largest representative sample survey of sexual lifestyle ever undertaken in the British population, we hope we are at the starting point rather than the finishing post, and that the study opens the field to other avenues of enquiry.

Acknowledgements

The preparation, execution and completion of the survey has been a genuinely collaborative venture, and we wish to thank a large number of people.

For financial support, we are indebted to the Wellcome Trust, especially for their speedy processing of our application when public funding was declined. In particular, we thank David Gordon for support and encouragement over the years. We also wish to thank the ESRC and HEA for financial support of the development work.

At SCPR, many people were involved in all stages of the survey. Special thanks are due to Liz Spencer and Jill Keegan, the principal actors in the qualitative work for the questionnaire design; to Peter Lynn, for sample design and statistical advice; to Margaret Weatherby, field controller for the survey; to Sally Harford, one of the senior interviewers who came to play a key role in briefing interviewers; to over 500 members of the SCPR fieldforce of specially trained interviewers, whose commitment to the project ensured the quality of the data; to Ann Palmer, who masterminded the clerical editing and coding, and her team; and to Jo Periam, the computer programmer responsible for the final editing of the data. Because of its size and high public profile, the survey tended to dominate the life of SCPR for a long time and few staff escaped some involvement. Our thanks go to them all.

Carol Morgan had sole responsibility for all graphical material presented throughout the book. Kay Stratton prepared a substantial part of the manuscript. We thank them for their diligence and patience in the seemingly endless redrafts prepared.

Many people have provided practical help, encouragement and intellectual advice, particularly when the project looked close to being moth-balled. In particular, we thank the project's advisory group: Mike Adler, Roy Anderson, Roger Jowell and David Miller. In addition, we are very grateful to the following people for their helpful contributions: Sir Donald Acheson, Valerie Beral, Toni Belfield, Graham Bird, Mildred Blaxter, Lindsay Brook, Manuel Carballo, Margaret Chekvi, Tony Coxon, Sir David Cox, Nicholas Day, Caroline Gardner, Graham Hart,

Keith Hatfield, Lord Kilmarnock and the All-Party Parliamentary Group on AIDS, Peter Linthwaite, John McEwan, Sally MacIntyre, Klim McPherson, Phil Strong, Charles Turner, John Watson, Jeffrey Weeks, Luke Whitaker and Daniel Wight. We wish also to thank Stuart Taylor, our editor at Blackwell Scientific Publications, for his tolerance and patience with missed and ever tighter deadlines.

Our greatest debt is to the 18 876 participants in the survey who gave freely of their time, and allowed us to enquire into one of the most intimate areas of their lives.

Chapter 1
Studying Sexual Lifestyles

ANNE JOHNSON & KAYE WELLINGS

The amount of speculation and discussion of sexual behaviour stands in stark contrast to the lack of reliable empirical evidence. Despite the apparent trend towards greater openness in sexual matters, this remains one of the most underdeveloped fields in the human sciences. Scholars from many disciplines have contributed to the understanding of sexuality and its expression, but their insights have often been limited by the difficulty of investigative work in the area. Research has seldom been conducted without controversy, and researchers who have ventured into the area have rarely avoided suspicion and constraint. As a result, important questions have gone largely unanswered. What proportion of people have homosexual experience, have exclusive relationships, are celibate or have visited prostitutes? When do men and women first become sexually active? What factors influence the range and regularity of sexual practices? How are attitudes to sex and sexuality changing, and how are they associated with behaviour? What evidence is there for generational trends in behaviour, and what are the social and demographic correlates of variability in sexual lifestyle?

The emergence in the 1980s of a worldwide epidemic of a sexually acquired infection, human immunodeficiency virus (HIV), sharply focused these gaps in knowledge, and served to demonstrate the need for research into sexual lifestyles. Efforts to mount effective public health education campaigns, to predict the likely extent and pattern of spread of HIV and to plan services for those affected by HIV were all impeded by the absence of reliable data on sexual behaviour.

In fact, although the HIV epidemic highlighted the dearth of information on sexual lifestyles, the need for robust research had been recognized for some time. The lack of sound information on the subject, based on modern survey methods and random samples, has long handicapped those specializing in the fields of sexual and reproductive health, as well as those in the broader disciplines of education and medicine. Reliable quantitative data are essential for understanding fertility patterns, contraceptive use and the epidemiology of sexually transmitted diseases (STDs), for example, and are fundamental to informed debate about the timing and content of sex education.

Information is needed not only about current behaviour, but also about the dynamics of change and its possible explanations. In addition to fundamental biological imperatives, the forces which fashion human sexual behaviour are as yet imperfectly understood, but contributory factors include technological and demographic changes, population mobility, advances in the control of fertility and sexually transmitted diseases, the emergence of new diseases and revisions of theories of sexuality, in addition to changes in the moral climate and legislative framework.

Examples of such forces in the recent past are easily instanced. In the past 30 years, reliable contraception has increasingly separated sex from its procreative function and diminished the fear of unwanted pregnancy. Modern medicine has improved control of the traditional venereal diseases such as syphilis and gonorrhoea, reducing further the negative consequences of sexual expression. Studies of the physiology of sexual intercourse and sexual satisfaction, as well as wider discussion of such topics, may have increased expectations of sexual performance and pleasure (Masters & Johnson, 1966, 1970). The Kinsey studies of the 1930s and 1940s (Kinsey *et al.*, 1948, 1953) emphasized the wide variation in human sexual expression. Successive acts of legislative and statutory reform have liberalized aspects of sexual behaviour: for example, the legalization of homosexuality and abortion, and the provision of contraceptive advice and supplies to single women. More recently, with the emerging HIV epidemic and concerns about other sexually acquired conditions resistant to cure such as genital herpes and invasive cervical cancer, new forces may be affecting sexual behaviour. The influence of these factors on patterns of behaviour has gone largely uncharted.

In particular, little reliable information has been available on basic population parameters of sexual behaviour using probability samples. Whilst the acquired immune deficiency syndrome (AIDS) epidemic has given rise to a large number of focused studies of sexual behaviour amongst those at particularly high risk of HIV infection – homosexual men, injecting drug users and prostitutes, for example (Winkelstein *et al.*, 1987; Johnson, 1988; Wodak & Moss, 1990) – these studies have generally been based on clinic and volunteer samples of individuals, selected on the basis of a particular lifestyle.

Valuable as these surveys undoubtedly are in identifying features of interest in particular groups, they cannot be used to assess the extent of that behaviour in the whole population. Estimates of behaviours in a national representative sample are necessary to set other studies in context, as well as to assess whether purposive samples typify accurately the wider populations they are chosen to represent.

Absence of existing data

The study of sex in the last century can be traced from the psycho-pathology of sexual behaviour in the late 19th century, the psychological work of Havelock Ellis and the interpretative work of the psychoanalysts in the early 20th century, through the recurrent concerns of social hygienists and early feminists for the control of the syphilis and gonorrhoea epidemics, and the growing concerns with population growth reflected in the eugenics movement (Weeks, 1981).

In terms of quantification, though, the most renowned attempts to explore and measure human sexual behaviour in the 20th century are undoubtedly those of Kinsey and Pomeroy, carried out primarily in the 1930s and 1940s in the USA (Kinsey *et al.*, 1948, 1953). Their studies represented a landmark in research into sexual behaviour. Recording for the first time the variety of human sexual experience in thousands of men and women, they created an uproar when they were first published.

The methodological drawbacks of Kinsey's studies have been well documented (Cochran *et al.*, 1953). The samples consisted of volunteers recruited from a variety of sources without a strictly formalized sampling procedure, as used in modern survey research. The overwhelming majority were white, middle class, young, college-educated men and women embarking on their sexual careers. Forty-five per cent were in college at the time of interview. In addition, 'delinquent' samples were recruited from penitentiaries amongst criminals and sex offenders, and informal networks were used to recruit subjects. Since the sample was not representative of the US population, the findings could not be generalized to that wider population. Yet they have frequently been treated as if they could. That this is so, even in the AIDS era, testifies to the lack of reliable, relevant, contemporary data on sexual behaviour.

Sexual behaviour research in the USA achieved little to improve upon the methodology of Kinsey in the decades following the publication of their reports, although there was no absence of interest in the subject. A review of the field abounds with 'surveys' conducted through magazine readerships. (For a chronological review of these studies, see Reinisch *et al.*, 1990.) Evaluating these approaches, the US Committee on AIDS Research and the Behavioral, Social and Statistical Sciences in its 1989 report issued the following, damning indictment (p. 87): 'Research quackery abounds. Surveys have been conducted by journalists, women's and men's magazines, and enterprising professionals using invalid and unreliable questionnaires and collections of respondents whose population characteristics and response rates are unspecified . . . Individually, such "reports" are transient sources of fun, fantasy and profit – a short flash in the media pan'.

The application of modern survey methods to the study of human sexual behaviour began to gather momentum in the 1960s and 1970s, but studies undertaken in that period were often small or limited to specific subsets of the population (Reinisch *et al.*, 1990). On occasions their utility was restricted by other mishaps. Data from a US survey of over 3000 adults carried out in 1970 by the National Opinion Research Centre, using a combination of random and quota sampling, was not published for nearly 20 years because of a dispute between the investigators – a cautionary tale for all involved in such enterprises (Fay *et al.*, 1989).

In Britain, too, there has been a similar lack of quantitative data gathered from surveys that use probability sampling methods. The Mass Observation studies of the 1930s and 1940s (England, 1950) represent an early attempt to study sexual attitudes and behaviour in the British population, but very few data were ever published from the study. Chesser's (1956) study of the sexual, marital and family relationships of English women was based on responses from 6500 respondents recruited through general practitioners, but did not attempt a true random sample. Gorer's (1955) survey, based on a random sample of nearly 2000 English men and women aged under 45 selected through the electoral register (ER), provides some limited data on first intercourse, sex before marriage, frequency of intercourse and number of partners, but does not contain the detail required to answer questions of relevance to the HIV epidemic.

Work using quota samples was carried out in Britain in the 1980s in response to the need for data in the context of AIDS/HIV prevention, most notably through research funded by the Health Education Authority (HEA) concerned primarily with tracking changes in knowledge and attitudes in response to AIDS education campaigns, rather than detailed behavioural surveys (British Market Research Bureau (BMRB), 1987). However, little was known about the acceptability of carrying out more detailed work on behaviour, using a random sample.

Studies have often been undertaken in response to a particular social or health problem, investigation being seen to be legitimized by the policy relevance of the findings. British studies have been motivated by contemporary concerns relating to social and health 'problems' – those of teenage sexuality in the 1960s, and the rising incidence of teenage pregnancy in the next decade, for example. The apparent increase in sexual activity amongst young people prompted the Health Education Council to sponsor the first national survey of teenage sexual behaviour (Schofield, 1965, 1973), which in turn was to form a useful benchmark a decade later for Farrell's (1978) study of young people's experience of sex education and knowledge of birth control in the 1970s. These studies provided useful data on the sexual behaviour of teenagers, but none on other age groups.

Material relevant to sexual behaviour has been collected in large-scale studies of family formation and family planning (Bone, 1978, 1986; Dunnell, 1979; Office of Population Censuses and Surveys (OPCS), 1985), but this has again been confined to women of reproductive age and to what was relevant in the context of those studies.

Specific contemporary problems addressed by research limit the applicability of findings to other social and health issues and to other points in historical time. Because sexual research has frequently been undertaken in response to a perceived moral or health problem, this area of human behaviour is often seen in pathological terms. This applies equally to research undertaken in response to the AIDS epidemic. Behaviours which are of concern epidemiologically (such as sex between men, anal intercourse and injecting drug use) are those which are also morally and, on occasions, legally censured in many societies.

The possible disadvantages in linking scientific surveys with specific contemporary social and health issues are clear. If the research tools are finely tuned to one issue, they provide data of limited value in other contexts and are too narrow in focus to be of general applicability. Nevertheless, despite attempts to broaden the focus of studies, the scope of research may in turn be limited by what is deemed acceptable and justifiable by the concerns of the era. Viewed in this light, our own work is probably no exception.

The rationale for the survey

Without doubt the emergence of the HIV epidemic provided the impetus, the legitimation and the funding opportunities for this study, and the public health implications of the growing epidemic guided the direction of the research. Two of the main purposes of the survey were to provide data that would increase understanding of the transmission patterns of HIV and other sexually transmitted infections, and that would aid the selection of appropriate and effective health education strategies for epidemic control. The theoretical framework of the survey, the size of the sample and the content of the questionnaire necessarily reflect the aims of the survey and the uses to which the data are to be put.

When AIDS was first described in the USA in 1981, the disease was thought to be confined to a small group of highly sexually active homosexual men. In the course of the next few years, it became clear that the magnitude of the epidemic was greater than originally supposed. Contemporary evidence pointed to a primarily homosexual epidemic in the developed world and a primarily heterosexual epidemic of major proportions in sub-Saharan Africa. This realization prompted public concern in every part of the globe to assess the magnitude of the epidemic and to mount control efforts through education programmes.

Both these objectives required information on patterns of sexual behaviour in the population. Epidemiological evidence indicated that the virus behaved like many other sexually acquired infections. Once it was introduced into a community, the likelihood of an individual becoming infected in the early stages of the epidemic increased with the number of sexual partners (homosexual or heterosexual) with whom unprotected intercourse had taken place (Johnson, 1988). The spread outside the populations initially affected was likely to depend on the proportion of the population engaging in high-risk activities, the pattern and frequency of partner change in the population and the extent of mixing between higher- and lower-activity groups (Anderson *et al.*, 1986; Potts *et al.*, 1991; Johnson, 1992), as well as mixing between bisexual men and their female partners and between injecting drug users and their non-injecting partners.

A series of studies aimed at estimating the potential spread of HIV in England and Wales was commissioned through the Department of Health (Report of Working Group, 1989, 1990), employing both direct approaches based on surveillance and behavioural data as well as more theoretical approaches from mathematical models. Some attempt was made to assess the prevalence of risk behaviours from available data sources, but it became evident that little was known about key behavioural variables that could determine current prevalence or future transmission.

There were, for example, no estimates of the proportion of men who had homosexual partners. Available studies were limited to homosexual men attending STD clinics (particularly in London) or to volunteer samples (often recruited through gay networks or through magazines) of self-identified homosexual men (McManus & McEvoy, 1987; Coxon, 1988). No one knew how representative these men were of all homosexual men, how homosexuality should be defined or what was the extent of same-gender contact in the population. Furthermore, within the range of homosexual experience, it was unclear what proportion engaged in practices which were risky for the transmission of HIV (primarily anal intercourse).

Similar concerns arose in relation to the heterosexual population. Little was known about the overall pattern of sexual behaviours. A key consideration in assessing the likelihood of a purely heterosexual epidemic in the non-drug-using population was to assess the pattern of heterosexual partner change in the population, as well as the frequency and prevalence of different sexual practices. Those using techniques of mathematical modelling were concerned with assessing the likely value of the 'case reproduction number' (R_o). This describes the average number of new infections propagated by an infected individual. Where its value exceeds 1, theoretically an epidemic will develop. Its estimate required much greater quantitative detail on the population distribution of reported numbers of partners. Preliminary studies (BMRB, 1987; Johnson *et al.*, 1989) indicated that there is great heterogeneity in the reported numbers of partners (Anderson *et al.*, 1986); many people have few partners and a minority have many. Some of the highest-risk practices (such as drug use and homosexual anal intercourse) involved only a small minority of the population.

A large sample size was required in order to represent and characterize these patterns adequately, and to obtain sufficient representation of rarer kinds of behaviour. The relatively small proportion of the population with very large numbers of sexual partners may contribute disproportionately to transmission of STDs in a population because they change partners sufficiently rapidly to maintain sexually acquired infections in the population (these are sometimes termed a 'core' group) (Hethcote & Yorke, 1984).

Reliable data on sexual behaviour were also essential for those concerned with developing an effective policy for prevention. In particular, it was necessary to describe the sociodemographic and attitudinal characteristics of those with different sexual lifestyles. Success in limiting further spread of the virus is currently dependent on the ability of educational and other interventions to establish norms of safer sex. Advice on risk reduction practices must be acceptable to sexually active populations. A sound understanding of patterns of human sexuality in a specific population is a necessary prerequisite for the design of such interventions, since it is extremely difficult to focus them or to monitor their impact over time in the absence of such data. This survey sought to collect data which could help to define target populations for specific interventions, to identify those risk reduction messages which are most likely to meet with acceptance, to discover preferred educational agencies, to identify needs for information and to provide baseline data for monitoring and evaluating the impact of interventions.

While public health concerns both legitimized and limited the scope of the survey within the constraints of what is deemed appropriate to the era, the survey has potentially wider application than health policy alone. The focus on the spread of HIV and its prevention may place too strong an emphasis on the adverse effects of particular sexual lifestyles. The many positive and pleasurable aspects of sexual behaviour are, of course, very important. Sexual expression is a fundamental human need, a near-universal experience, a keystone of intimate human relationships and a prerequisite of procreation. Social, legal and technological changes of the 20th century have done much to diminish the negative social and health consequences of sexual lifestyles.

The description of the wide variety of human sexual experience is of importance to many disciplines: to social historians documenting the generational changes in sexual behaviour; to anthropologists concerned with cross-cultural comparisons; to schoolteachers who require a more realistic understanding of contemporary teenage sexual experience in order to design effective sex education programmes; to demographers concerned with changing patterns of family formation; to health workers in many fields; and to the general public, for despite the taboos, censure and sanction, there may be few subjects of greater fascination to most people.

The limitations of problem-specific research were apparent in the development of the survey. As a result, the protocol was designed to include a range of enquiries sufficiently durable and broadly based for it to be relevant to a number of disciplines concerned with sexuality, sexual health and reproduction. While the need for data for use in the context of the AIDS epidemic remained high on the research agenda, we were very conscious of the need to provide data for use in other contexts. These concerns led us to endeavour to employ a sufficiently durable methodology for the survey (or parts of it) to be replicated, and for the data to have a broad application in order to shed light on a wider variety of health and social issues than are relevant simply to AIDS and HIV.

This said, the desire to provide data of broad interest had to be balanced against a concern to maximize response on the key issues of the era, rather than risk reducing the acceptability of the survey by widening its scope too far. Future historians may wonder at the absence of information on the psychological and pleasurable nature of sexual relationships and at the descriptive rather than explanatory nature of the enquiry. In our defence, the acceptability of detailed enquiry into sexual behaviour in the general population was largely unknown when this work began, while the sensitivities of funding bodies spending Government money were made clear at a relatively early stage. The omissions at this stage of enquiry must remain the responsibility of the researchers, but in seeking to provide material of interest to many disciplines, the methodology may provide a first step in developing more detailed enquiry into many new areas.

Theoretical framework for the study

The theoretical perspective of the survey, reflecting its aims, is social and epidemiological. In the past, the notion of sex as a predominantly biological instinct tended to dominate the study of sexuality. The belief at the heart of much writing on the subject, that the determinants of sexual expression are to be found in instinct – as Weeks (1985) points out – has a long provenance, going back to Plato and Aristotle and reappearing in the Middle Ages in the concept of natural law. The concept of sex as a natural urge is a recurrent theme in the writing of the sexologists of the late 19th century; Havelock Ellis (1948), for example, described it as an 'impulse', and Freud as a 'drive' (Freud, 1953). The biological imperative is hinted at in the choice of terms used in the accounts of Kinsey's research, in the term 'outlet' for example (Kinsey *et al.*, 1948, 1953), and certainly the attempt to develop a taxonomy of human sexual behaviours, carefully categorized in a manner characteristic of the natural sciences, very much reflected Kinsey's disciplinary base in biology.

Biological determinants of sexual behaviour cannot be ignored. Any theory of sexuality will have recourse to an understanding of anatomical and biological potential and limits that provide the preconditions for human sexuality (Weeks, 1985). But while the biological human sexual drive is universal, its expression is influenced by sociocultural forces (Carballo *et al.*, 1989). Sexuality is defined, regulated and given meaning through cultural norms. Whilst biological and psychological causes may be central when comparing individuals, they are not of the first importance when comparing societies. Biology explains little of the variation between population groups. If sexuality were solely biologically determined, then forms of sexual expression would vary little cross-culturally or historically; however, evidence suggests that they do (Ford & Beach, 1952). Narrowly biological explanations are inadequate when research questions concern social trends and variations between different populations and subgroups.

It is in this potential of sexuality for diversity rather than uniformity that the seeds of hope may be found in the selection of sexual health strategies. If sexual expression were immutably fixed in nature, there would be no possibility for change or choice. In the context of the search for healthy sexual lifestyles, a perspective that sees potential for change, choice and diversity may be of greater value than one that sees sexual behaviour as simply biologically determined. Human relationships offer a range of choices in terms of sexual expression. Kinsey is owed a debt for demonstrating this to be so.

The approach taken here is one that accepts the influence of social factors and the importance of human agency in sexual expression and changing sexual lifestyles, but which at the same time recognizes the potentially harmful effects of repressive social engineering, which has characterized historical attempts to 'control' sexual behaviour (Weeks, 1981). By the same token, our theoretical framework recognizes the constraints of contemporary concerns, which in turn have influenced the approach taken.

Sexual behaviour studies of the AIDS era: progress and politics

Some 4 years elapsed between the first mooting of a national survey of sexual lifestyles and the launch of the main stage of the British study. Much of this time was taken up with essential development work, including careful qualitative work aimed at designing the questionnaire, smaller-scale pilots to test it and feasibility studies carried out to assess reliability and validity (Spencer *et al.*, 1988; Johnson *et al.*, 1989; Wellings *et al.*, 1990). However, the factors involved in the delay were political as well as practical. These were perhaps made most public in a front page article in *The Sunday Times* on 10 September 1989, with the headline 'Thatcher halts survey on sex'.

The political sensitivity about research into this area of human behaviour is by no means a problem unique to late 20th century Britain. Examples of hindrance, obstruction and discouragement are legion in the history of sex research. Questionnaires have been seized as pornographic and researchers slanderously attacked and their findings suppressed. Kinsey, for example, faced hostility from colleagues and threats of dismissal from his college (Kinsey *et al.*, 1953), whilst Lanval, a Belgian researcher working in the 1930s, was forced to work at night to avoid police raids on his data. In the Preface to the 1950 version of his book he writes: 'The research work for this book was hindered and discouraged in all possible ways. Press campaigns in political papers, denunciations on the grounds of public indecency were formulated to the Police. Slanderous rumours were put out on the author's professional honour, etc . . . .' (Lanval, 1950).

This sentiment was expressed succinctly by Kinsey (1953): '. . . human sexual behaviour represents one of the least explored segments of biology, psychology and sociology. Scientifically, more has been known about the sexual behaviour of some farm and laboratory animals. It is obvious that the failure to learn more about human sexual activity is the outcome of the influence which the custom and the law have had upon scientists as individuals, and of the not immaterial restrictions which have been imposed upon scientific investigations in this field'.

In the design of the British protocol, the researchers were repeatedly at pains to justify the legitimacy of every question in terms of its public health and educational relevance. By demonstrating the clear need for data, the HIV epidemic has in many senses legitimized scientific research in the area and this may have softened both public and political attitudes to such endeavours. Research proceeded apace in parallel with the British work, particularly in Europe (Sundet *et al.*, 1988; Wadsworth & Johnson, 1991; ACSF Investigators, 1992; Melbye & Biggar, 1992). Surveys have now been conducted in several European countries – in Norway, The

Netherlands, France and Finland, for example – and a Concerted Action has been established by the Commission of the European Community to coordinate the findings of these surveys. A research protocol for surveying sexual lifestyles developed by the World Health Organization is being used in several developing countries (Carballo *et al.*, 1989).

Despite this obvious progress and the urgent need for data, the British experience finds close parallels in several other countries. Researchers in many countries have been frustrated in their attempts to commence studies. US efforts to launch a national survey of sexual behaviour foundered on opposition from the Bush administration and from conservative law-makers, which resulted in both the House of Representatives Appropriations Committee and the Office of Management and Budget withdrawing funding (Aldhous, 1992). The US research teams finally achieved some success in attracting alternative funding, but the research currently under way is a greatly scaled down version of the original project.

In Sweden, too, widely regarded as one of the most sexually tolerant societies, plans for a national survey were thwarted. In 1991, the Swedish Board of Statistics approached one of the country's leading sexologists to develop a feasibility survey for a national survey, but retracted when the time came to make these plans public. The publicity given to the decision on the British survey had an adverse effect on the Swedish decision since it drew attention to the political sensitivities surrounding the subject (Lewin, personal communication, 1992). In Switzerland, a country with one of the highest AIDS incidence rates in Europe, a proposal in 1991 for a survey of sexual behaviour to be conducted by the Institute for Social and Preventive Medicine in Lausanne failed to receive financial support. Even the French team encountered some testing hurdles as the proposal went through appropriate ethical committees.

It might seem surprising that political reservations have persisted in the face of such a serious health problem. The nature of the demand for data might have been expected to confer legitimacy on investigation in this area. AIDS is a public health issue and sex research has traditionally achieved respectability through its association with the medical profession: '. . . the findings of sex research . . . have been allowable when they have been compatible with an acceptable discourse, usually that of medicine' (Weeks, 1985). Kinsey, for example, was strongly urged by the Indiana University President to publish his findings through a medical publisher, on the grounds that the book would be circulated only amongst those who needed the data for scientific purposes and consequently that it would not be misinterpreted (it sold 200 000 copies in the first 2 months).

While scientific endeavour *per se* is generally concerned with improving the understanding of patterns of behaviour, and not with sexual ethics (Reiss, 1986), it would nevertheless be naïve to ignore or under-estimate the political impact of data on sexual behaviour. As Weeks (1985) points out, 'The production in sexological discourse of a body of knowledge that is apparently scientifically neutral . . . can become a resource for utilization in the production of normative definitions that limit and demarcate erotic behaviour'.

The impact of Kinsey's data testifies to this. The exposure of sexual diversity in the USA in the mid-20th century had major implications for sexual ethics. Most people at the time understood that the official version of sexuality did not concur with practice in US society, but also that such sexual conduct that did not conform to the official 'norms' was judged harshly. The publication of the Kinsey volumes exposed an entire society to the difference between official dogma and the actuality of people's experience (Gagnon, 1988). Some of the political disquiet about surveys of sexual behaviour may be associated with the power of survey infor-mation to change moral norms, and the difficulty of maintaining ethical values in the face of evidence that considerable proportions of the popu-lace feel or behave differently.

The emergence of the main study

The format of the British study can be traced back to two major but overlapping strands of academic interest, epidemiological and socio-logical; and to two separate groups initially working independently, but with common interests. Late in 1986, a group of epidemiologists and statisticians from University College and Middlesex School of Medicine (UCMSM), St Mary's Hospital Medical School and Imperial College (including Anne Johnson and Jane Wadsworth) met to consider the possibility of undertaking a large random sample survey in Britain with the prime interest of measuring sexual behaviour in the population, and particularly patterns of partner change, in order to assist in measuring the current and future magnitude of the HIV epidemic. Their focus was almost entirely behavioural.

In September 1987, Gallup International, funded by a private dona-tion, was commissioned by the epidemiology group to carry out a random sample survey of 783 men and women aged 16–64 in Britain, using households in the electoral register as the sampling frame. The survey used a combination of face-to-face interview with a self-completion module. The outcomes of this pilot study were mixed. On the one hand, the study demonstrated that the method was acceptable to the majority invited to take part (61% of those contacted and invited to participate agreed), but the overall response rate to the study was low (48%) due in part to the failure to contact the selected individual in over 20% of eligible households (Johnson *et al.*, 1989). Despite their sensitivity, there was little objection to the nature of the questions, while key questions on numbers of partners in different time intervals were completed logically. The study results showed great heterogeneity in numbers of partners reported and a low incidence of high-risk behaviours such as injecting drug use and male homosexual experience. Thus, very large samples would be required in any national study in order for adequate subsamples of those with higher-risk lifestyles to be available for analysis. Similarly, large numbers would be required to reduce the standard errors of prevalence estimates of rare behaviours.

The scope of the questionnaire was fairly limited. Although data were collected on demographic variables, little information was gathered either on key sexual practices of relevance to the spread of sexually acquired infections, or on attitudes to sex and sexuality that might help to inform public education strategies. An implausibly low proportion of men reported any same-gender sexual experience in their lifetime (0.5%) and it was evident that further work was needed on question design, wording and layout if the quality of information were to be improved. Plans were made to improve the methodology with the intention of seeking funding for a major national survey. In particular, the group met with staff of the Economic and Social Research Council (ESRC) to discuss the possibility of further feasibility work, with a view to a larger national survey of 20 000 individuals in the longer term. Throughout 1987, in parallel with the work undertaken by the epidemiology group, the HEA was also involved in discussions with the Department of Health and Social Security (DHSS) about carrying out a national survey.

In response to a meeting of the Chief Scientists Group at the Department of Health on 30 June 1987, an internal discussion paper was prepared on a possible national study of sexual behaviour for consideration by the Behavioural Research Group set up by the DHSS. This paper suggested that a study should be established with the dual objectives of facilitating the development of a well targeted and effective educational campaign, and enabling more accurate estimates of the possible future spread of HIV.

This paper was discussed at the meeting of the DHSS Behavioural Change Group in September 1987, and it was decided that the HEA should take forward the survey. With a predominant emphasis on the first of the two aims, the HEA set in progress plans for a study involving 5000 respondents, with a particular focus on the social determinants of attitudes and behaviour. Early in 1987, Kaye Wellings (then at the Family Planning Association) and Julia Field at the research institute, Social and Community Planning Research (SCPR) had drawn up proposals for a national study of sexual behaviour and submitted them to the HEA for funding. A protocol based on this earlier document was drafted by Kaye Wellings, then Senior Research Officer at the HEA, and Peter Linthwaite, Director of Research. The project was approved by the DHSS in the HEA's Operational Plan in October 1987.

Development work on the HEA survey began in January 1988 when SCPR was commissioned to carry out a three-stage development programme. This was to begin with a qualitative phase, consisting of a series of unstructured, exploratory interviews aimed at guiding the design of a structured questionnaire, followed by a period of testing the structured questionnaire through small-scale piloting and culminating in a large-scale feasibility study with a random sample large enough to give reasonably accurate measures of response rates and the prevalence of particular behaviours within the population. Funding for the main stage would depend on the success of the feasibility work.

The merger of common interests

The shared interests of the HEA and epidemiological groups became evident to senior research management at the DHSS, and in December 1987 a meeting was organized by the Medical Research Council (MRC), under the chairmanship of Sir Richard Doll, to discuss the possibility of a large scale random sample survey of sexual lifestyles in Britain. Present at this meeting were scientists involved in the pilot study undertaken by Gallup, and representatives from the MRC, ESRC, HEA and DHSS. It was also agreed that any Government funding for such a study should be channelled through the ESRC, and that any monies awarded through the DHSS would be subject to ministerial approval.

The common interests of the health education and the epidemiological groups were evident and collaboration began in earnest. There were sound reasons for the merger of the projects, not least among them a concern for economies of human and financial resources and a desire to pool expertise and share experience. The two research teams began to work on one joint project. The two studies were grappling with identical methodological problems, such as the most appropriate sampling frame to employ, methods of maximizing response rates, the issue of self-completion versus interviewer-administered questionnaires and the special difficulties of interviewer training for a study of this kind. This meant addressing such practical problems as how to introduce the survey, what age groups to include or exclude, how to cope with sexual terminology and how to assess reliability of response.

A research proposal was submitted to the ESRC in May 1988 for a further feasibility study of 1000 individuals to provide 'solid evidence' that a large-scale survey was achievable. By this time, the outline of a combined design for a major survey had been defined. The final sample would comprise 20 000 individuals, all of whom would provide behavioural data, and of these 5000 would be invited to complete a longer questionnaire, including a substantial attitudinal module. It was agreed that funding should be shared by the ESRC and HEA.

The feasibility survey took place in the autumn of 1988. In all, 977 interviews were completed with men and women aged 16–59 in Great Britain, based on a systematic probability sample of addresses selected from the Post Office Postcode Address File (PAF). The hoped-for improvement in response rate (to 65%), as well as greatly diminished rates of item non-response and high levels of internal consistency, were achieved (Wellings et al., 1990) (see Chapter 2).

A report on the feasibility stage of the study, and an application for the main phase of the study, was submitted to the ESRC in mid-December 1988 and sent out to scientific referees. The ESRC AIDS Steering Group reported being 'satisfied with the scientific standard' and the proposal (amended only in administrative detail) went forward to the ESRC full Council at the end of January 1989. It in turn approved the study and correspondence from that era repeatedly attests to the scientific merits of the protocol. The proposal was sent forward to the DHSS with the suggestion that the larger sample necessary to meet the epidemiological objectives should be financed by the DHSS with funding channelled through the ESRC, and that the cost of the rest should be met by a separate contract with the HEA. In the same month, the HEA's Project Review Committee sanctioned the release of funds for the survey for the years 1988–9 and 1989–90. The study was discussed with senior members of Research Management of the DHSS and the scientific merits of the study again endorsed, and the team promised a rapid decision on funding. The research team was poised for a project start date of February 1989.

By the end of February, no decision had been reached. In March, the research team was warned in a letter from the ESRC (3 March 1989) of the 'need for extreme caution in giving information' about the survey because of the 'present delicate stage reached in the negotiations to fund the study, and the extreme sensitivity of the Government to any publicity at the moment'. Silence was duly kept but no answer ensued. The Chief Executive of the HEA was instructed in March 1989 to delay the start of the fieldwork for an estimated 2 months until the matter had been discussed in a higher Cabinet Committee. At the end of the same month, the HEA requested that its part of the work (subject to a separate contract) was put on ice until a decision was reached. Plans were now seriously disrupted as deadlines passed and fieldwork timetables were interrupted.

By June, concern was being raised elsewhere and the Chairman of the MRC's Committee on Epidemiological Studies of AIDS wrote to the Chief

Medical Officer in support of the study, expressing 'dismay' at the delay (N. E. Day, 5 June 1989). In July, the study's advisory group members wrote to the Minister (David Mellor, QC) requesting a meeting to discuss the study, while the All-Party Parliamentary Group on AIDS wrote supporting the study and urging early funding in the absence of scientific grounds for delay.

The researchers received no further information until the lead story in *The Sunday Times* on 10 September 1989. The front page news feature reported that the study had been personally vetoed by the then Prime Minister, Margaret Thatcher, on the grounds of its intrusiveness and its unacceptability to the British people. This was followed by widespread discussion in the press and other media. The All-Party Parliamentary Group wrote in protest to the Secretary of State (Kenneth Clarke, QC), reminding him that the decision 'flies in the face of the advice given by your Department and the Chief Scientist's office' and noting the high response rate achieved in the feasibility study (Lord Kilmarnock, 15 September 1989). A group of Scottish scientists followed suit by arguing that 'it is unprecedented for a post-war British Government to overturn the recommendation of a Research Council in this way' (3 October 1989). Sir Klaus Moser expressed concern at the Government's decision at the British Association for the Advancement of Science meeting in September, and was widely reported in the press (*New Scientist*, 23 September 1989), while these events were the subject of an editorial in *Nature* (Maddox, 1989).

The source of the decision as described in the press was never communicated directly to the researchers. In late September, the ESRC wrote to inform the applicants that it had received a letter from the Department of Health stating that 'in all the circumstances it is not appropriate for the Government to support it and, more generally, that it would not be right for the Government to sponsor the survey', and expressing regret that the ESRC would not be able to provide support. After enquiries had been made, the survey team learned that the Wellcome Trust would be willing to consider an application for funding of the study. The Trust undertook peer review of the proposal with unprecedented speed, and on 15 October 1989 announced a grant of £900 000 to be awarded to researchers at SCPR, St Mary's Hospital, Imperial College and UCMSM. Time had been lost, and much work on sampling and interviewer recruitment had to be repeated. However, the stage was set for the main study to begin. The first interview was completed in May 1990 and the last one filed in November 1991, bringing the final sample to 18 876.

In the following chapters, we describe the scientific details of the design and validation of the survey method before turning to a detailed account of the findings.

References

ACSF Investigators (1992) AIDS and sexual behaviour in France. *Nature*, **360**, 407.

Aldhous, P. (1992) French venture where US fear to tread. *Science*, **257**, 25.

Anderson, R.M., Medley, G.F., May, R.M. & Johnson, A.M. (1986) A preliminary study of the transmission dynamics of the human immunodeficiency virus (HIV), the causative agent of AIDS. *Journal of Maths, Applied Medicine & Biology*, **3**, 229–63.

Bone, M. (1978) *Family Planning Services: Changes and Effects*. HMSO, London.

Bone, M. (1986) *Population Trends: Trends in Single Women's Sexual Behaviour in Scotland*. HMSO, London.

British Market Research Bureau (1987) *AIDS Advertising Campaign, Report on Four Surveys during the First Year of Advertising, 1986–7*. British Market Research Bureau, London.

Carballo, M., Cleland, J., Carael, M. & Albrecht, G. (1989) A cross national survey of patterns of sexual behaviour. *Journal of Sex Research*, **26**, 287–99.

Chesser, E. (1956) *The Sexual, Marital and Family Relationships of the English Woman*. Hutchinson's Medical Press, London.

Cochran, W.G., Mostelier, F. & Tukey, J.W. (1953) Statistical problems of the Kinsey Report. *Journal of the American Statistical Association*, **48**, 673–716.

Coxon, A. (1988) The numbers game. In Aggleton, P. & Homans, H. (eds) *Social Aspects of AIDS*. Falmer Press, Lewes.

Dunnell, K. (1979) *Family Formation 1976*. HMSO, London.

Ellis, H. (1948) *The Psychology of Sex*. Heinemann, London.

England, L. (1950) A British sex survey. *The International Journal of Sexology*, **3**, 148–56.

Farrell, C. (1978) *My Mother Said . . . The Way Young People Learned about Sex and Birth Control*. Routledge & Kegan Paul, London.

Fay, R.E., Turner, C.F., Klassen, A.D. & Gagnon, J.H. (1989) Prevalence and patterns of same-gender sexual contact among men. *Science*, **243**, 338–48.

Ford, C.S. & Beach, F.A. (1952) *Patterns of Sexual Behaviour*. Eyre & Spottiswoode, London.

Freud, S. (1953) Introductory lectures on psychoanalysis. In Strachey, J. (ed.) *The Standard Edition of the Complete Psychological Works of Sigmund Freud*, vol. 16. Hogarth Press and the Institute of Psychoanalysis, London.

Gagnon, J.H. (1988) Sex research and sexual conduct in the era of AIDS. *Journal of AIDS*, **1**, 593–601.

Gorer, G. (1955) *Exploring English Character*. Cresset Press and Criterion Books, London.

Hethcote, H.W. & Yorke, J.A. (1984) Gonorrhoea: transmission dynamics and control. Lecture notes. *Biomathematics*, **56**, 1–105.

Johnson, A.M. (1988) Social and behavioural aspects of the HIV epidemic – a review. *Journal of the Royal Statistical Society Series A*, **151**, 99–114.

Johnson, A.M. (1992) Epidemiology of HIV infection in women. In Johnstone, F.D. (ed.) *Baillière's Clinical Obstetrics and Gynaecology*, 6th edn, pp. 13–31. Baillière Tindall, London.

Johnson, A.M., Wadsworth, J., Elliott, P. *et al.* (1989) A pilot study of sexual lifestyle in a random sample of the population of Great Britain. *AIDS*, **3**, 135–41.

Kinsey, A.C., Pomeroy, W.B. & Martin, C.E. (1948) *Sexual Behaviour in the Human Male*. W.B. Saunders, Philadelphia.

Kinsey, A.C., Pomeroy, W.B., Martin, C.E. & Gebhard, P.H. (1953) *Sexual Behaviour in the Human Female*. W.B. Saunders, Philadelphia.

Lanval, M. (1950) *An Inquiry into the Intimate Lives of Women*. Cadillac Publishing Company, New York.

Maddox, J. (1989) Sexual behaviour unsurveyed. *Nature*, **341**, 181.

Masters, W. & Johnson, V. (1966) *Human Sexual Response*. Churchill, London.

Masters, W. & Johnson, V. (1970) *Human Sexual Inadequacy*. Churchill, London.

McManus, T.J. & McEvoy, M. (1987) Some aspects of male homosexual behaviour in the United Kingdom. *British Journal of Sexual Medicine*, **14**, 110–20.

Melbye, M. & Biggar, R.J. (1992) Interactions between persons at risk for AIDS and the general population in Denmark. *American Journal of Epidemiology*, **135**, 593–602.

Office of Population Censuses and Surveys (1985) *General Household Survey*. OPCS, London.

Potts, M., Anderson, R. & Boily, M.-C. (1991) Slowing the spread of human immunodeficiency virus in developing countries. *Lancet*, **338**, 608–12.

Reinisch, J.M., Ziemba-Davis, M. & Sanders, S.A. (1990) Sexual behaviour and AIDS: lessons from art and sex research. In *AIDS and Sex: An Integrated Biomedical and Biobehavioural Approach*, pp. 37–80. Oxford University Press, Oxford.

Reiss, I.L. (1986) *Journey into Sexuality: An Exploratory Voyage*. Prentice Hall, New Jersey.

Report of a Working Group (Chairman: Sir David Cox) (1989) *Short Term Prediction of HIV Infection and AIDS in England and Wales*. HMSO, London.

Report of a Working Group (Chairman: Professor N. Day) (1990) AIDS in England and Wales to end 1993. Projections using data to end September 1989. *Communicable Diseases Report*, 1–12.

Schofield, M. (1965) *The Sexual Behaviour of Young People*. Longman, London.

Schofield, M. (1973) *The Sexual Behaviour of Young Adults*. Allen Lane, London.

Spencer, L., Faulkner, A. & Keegan, J. (1988) *Talking about Sex*. SCPR, London.

Sundet, J.M., Kvalem, I.L., Magnus, P. & Bakketeig, L.S. (1988) Prevalence of risk-prone behaviour in the general population of Norway. In Fleming, A.F., Carballo, M. & Fitzsimons, D.F. (eds) *The Global Impact of AIDS*. Alan R. Liss, London.

US Committee on AIDS Research and the Behavioral, Social and Statistical Sciences (1989) *Sexual Behaviour and Intravenous Drug Use*. National Academy Press, Washington.

Wadsworth, J. & Johnson, A.M. (1991) Measuring sexual behaviour. *Journal of the Royal Statistical Society Series A*, **154**, 367–70.

Weeks, J. (1981) *Sex, Politics and Society: The Regulation of Sexuality since 1800*. Longman, New York.

Weeks, J. (1985) *Sexuality and its Discontents*. Routledge & Kegan Paul, London.

Wellings, K., Field, J., Wadsworth, J., Johnson, A.M., Anderson, R.M. & Bradshaw, S.A. (1990) Sexual lifestyles under scrutiny. *Nature*, **348**, 276–8.

Winkelstein, W., Lyman, D.M., Padian, N. *et al.* (1987) Sexual practices and risk of infection by the human immunodeficiency virus. *Journal of American AIDS*, **257**, 321–5.

Wodak, A. & Moss, A. (1990) HIV infection and injecting drug users: from epidemiology to public health. *AIDS*, **4**, S105–S109.

Chapter 2
Designing the Survey

KAYE WELLINGS & JULIA FIELD

The National Survey of Sexual Attitudes and Lifestyles (NATSAL) was conceived and planned within the public health context of the AIDS epidemic, its aims, as already stated, being to assist in the prevention of further spread of HIV and in the planning and provision of health care services for those already affected. The study needed to reflect these aims and those involved in its design were ever mindful of the uses to which the data would be put.

Since this survey was originally expected to draw extensively on public funds, and since there was no certainty that these funds would be available on a regular basis, the research instrument was designed to provide data which would assist health care professionals working in many areas of sexual health: psychosexual counselling, the prevention of STD and family planning, for example. This was the policy driven objective, but although of the greatest practical urgency, it was not the only one guiding the content of the survey. In addition, the hope was that the survey would stimulate further social enquiry in this field, addressing questions raised by previous research and posing fresh ones by generating new hypotheses.

At the start of the survey, a number of decisions had to be taken on the measurement objectives, the mode of data collection and the size and nature of the sample. These deliberations were not made independently of each other. The method of data collection chosen, for example, influenced the sampling frame and the measurement objectives determined its composition and structure. Decisions about the method of data collection and the sampling frame had to be made at an early stage, before detailed questionnaire development and testing. The design process, the decisions taken and their rationale are described in this chapter.

The measurement objectives of the survey

The measurement objectives of the study were defined as follows.
1 To quantify components of sexual history, such as numbers of partners in particular time intervals and age at first sexual intercourse, in a representative sample of the British population.

2   To measure the prevalence and distribution of different patterns of sexual orientation.

3   To measure the frequency and extent of experience of particular sexual practices.

4   To measure attitudes towards sexual behaviour and knowledge of possible associated health risks, and to examine their relationship with behaviour.

5   To determine the demographic characteristics of those whose current sexual lifestyle puts them at greatest risk of HIV and other STDs.

6   To assess changes in sexual lifestyles through generational comparisons of sexual histories.

The research variables

The measurement objectives, in turn, generated a list of variables to incorporate in the questionnaire design.

1   Past sexual history:
   (a) age at first heterosexual and homosexual sexual experience, and circumstances;
   (b) age at first heterosexual intercourse; identity of partner; nature of relationship (for example, casual encounter, permanent one-to-one relationship);
   (c) timing of subsequent heterosexual experience.

2   Recent experience:
   (a) current relationship;
   (b) nature of relationship;
   (c) experience of marriage, cohabitation, divorce, separation.

3   Sexual orientation:
   (a) prevalence and distribution of different modes of sexual orientation;
   (b) extent to which orientations are discrete or continuous;
   (c) stability of sexual orientation over time;
   (d) attitude towards different orientation(s).

4   Sexual practices:
   (a) frequency of sex;
   (b) past and current experience of different sexual practices (non-penetrative sex, vaginal and anal intercourse, orogenital sex);
   (c) patterns of sexual practices.

5   Sexual partners:
   (a) numbers and gender of sexual partners in different time intervals;
   (b) duration of partnerships in the last 5 years;
   (c) experience of monogamy, serial monogamy, concurrent partners, in last 5 years;

(d) experience of paying for sex.

6 Sexual health:

(a) knowledge and awareness of risk of AIDS and HIV;

(b) experience of infertility, abortion, miscarriage, unplanned pregnancy;

(c) attendance at STD clinics;

(d) sources of advice on sexual health;

(e) experience of recreational drug use;

(f) HIV antibody testing.

7 Risk reduction behaviour:

(a) perceived degree of control over sexual health and life course;

(b) knowledge of, motivation towards and experience of safer-sex practices;

(c) use of contraceptives.

8 Psychosocial factors influencing sexual behaviour:

(a) extent and strength of social influences – parents, family, friends, school;

(b) persistence of these influences over time;

(c) attitudes towards aspects of sexual lifestyles, for example celibacy, monogamy, abortion, pre-marital and extra-marital sex, homosexuality.

9 Demographic variables for purposes of subgroup analysis of: gender, age, marital status, occupation, educational level, household size and composition, ethnic identity and area of residence.

Method of data collection

Decisions about the method of data collection centred on the nature, breadth and complexity of the information sought. The sensitive and personal nature of information about sexual behaviour meant that potential respondents would need to be convinced of the necessity for such enquiry before committing themselves to participation. A personal interview approach would allow interviewers to explain the rationale fully, to provide reassurance and to encourage contact with the research team where necessary. This would have been less easily achieved using a postal survey.

The amount of data to be collected also favoured a personal interview. Interviews of the duration planned (on average, just under 1 hour for a quarter of the sample, and 40–45 minutes for the remainder) may be acceptable for face-to-face interviews but are less so for postal or telephone surveys. The complexity of the data sought and the need for careful definition of terms and extensive filtering and routing instructions were also more suited to face-to-face interviewing. The restrictions on interview techniques, chiefly the impossibility of using show-cards, militated against a telephone survey. In addition, in a telephone survey the interviewer has little control over whether the interview is conducted in comfort or out of earshot of other household members.

Both postal (Sundet *et al.*, 1988) and telephone (RUHBC, 1989; ACSF Investigators, 1992) surveys on the subject of sexual behaviour have been carried out successfully in Britain and other countries. However, a high proportion of individuals are still without telephones in Britain, particularly young people. The absence of an efficient sampling method for telephone interviewing was a further drawback (Collins & Sykes, 1987; Foreman & Collins, 1991). An early postal pilot was attempted but achieved a very poor response. On balance, the use of personal interviews seemed best suited to the specific objectives and social context of this study.

Designing the questionnaire

Development work

Several stages of fieldwork took place during the course of the 2-year development and pilot phase of the research leading to the implementation of the main stage.

Qualitative research to guide questionnaire design

The first phase of fieldwork consisted of a series of 40 in-depth interviews, carried out by members of the research team and by SCPR's specialist interviewers, with men and women from a wide age range, all social classes and both urban and rural areas (Spencer *et al.*, 1988). A topic guide was used, but the interviews were unstructured and lasted over 1 hour. The main aim of these exploratory interviews was to discover the extent of sexual information that members of the public were willing to disclose, the source of any discomfort, the terminology preferred and understood, and the accuracy with which people were able to recall sexual experiences, such as numbers of partners, lengths of relationships and when they occurred. The results of this process formed the basis for designing the structured questionnaire.

Questionnaire piloting

Draft versions of the structured questionnaire were tested in a first round of small-scale pilot studies, using experienced interviewers. Following questionnaire amendment on the basis of this exercise, further similar pilot studies took place using both new and experienced interviewers. These pilot stages facilitated refinement of the questionnaire in readiness for the feasibility survey and provided valuable experience that was to guide other aspects of the study, such as introducing the survey on the doorstep, wording introductory letters and training interviewers.

Feasibility study

Given the nature of the investigation, a feasibility study was considered necessary to assess the acceptability of the survey, the extent to which it would produce valid and reliable results and the sample size needed to obtain accurate estimates of minority behaviour. This was a large-scale test of the instrument, the target being an achieved sample of around 1000 interviews from a stratified random sample of addresses selected from the sampling frame according to a design similar to the one intended for the main survey (see Chapter 3). Fieldwork took place between September and November 1988. The target response rate of 65% was achieved and experiments on question wording and order successfully resolved remaining design dilemmas. The results, reported elsewhere (Wellings *et al.*, 1990), formed the basis of the application for funding of the main study.

The format of the instrument

Decisions about the sequence and structure of the questionnaire were based on a number of considerations. In particular, there were concerns to minimize interviewer bias, to maximize clarity and to provide a sequence of questions which would lead to reliable and coherent responses.

A key aim was to facilitate the development of good rapport between respondent and interviewer. Direct questions of a personal nature that might be considered intrusive were avoided early in the schedule, before such a rapport had developed. The questionnaire was constructed so that relatively neutral questions led on to more intimate and sensitive ones. It opened with requests for information on general health, weight, height, smoking, drinking and health-related behaviour, and moved on to family background and other social influences and then gradually into memories of early sex education and first sexual experiences. The order of these questions also served as an *aide-mémoire* for the respondent, providing a contextual framework into which life events could be placed to help in ordering them and to aid recall.

The core questions on sexual lifestyle, covering age at first intercourse, numbers of heterosexual and homosexual partners, frequency of sex, experience of different practices and so on, occupied the central section of the interview.

Attitudinal questions, inviting views on, for example, sex before marriage, outside marriage and between people of the same gender, were placed towards the end of the questionnaire. This was done so that respondents could report their own behaviours before the point at which a moral judgement on behaviour was requested of them. The final part of the interview collected information on marital status, occupation, education and ethnic identity.

A decision had to be made about whether to use a face-to-face method of delivery, self-completion or both, and in what combination. In making the choice, the advantages of the face-to-face presentation of questions in terms of opportunities for providing clarification were obvious. On the other hand, a self-completion component containing the more sensitive questions would go some way towards reducing possible bias that might be introduced if some respondents were reluctant to disclose sensitive information except in complete privacy. The challenge lay in finding a mix that combined optimally the merits of each.

The decision was taken to include all questions relating to sexual partners and practices in a booklet to be completed by the respondent in the presence of, but out of the view of, the interviewer. Self-completion had also proved to be a successful approach in the previous pilot carried out by Gallup. This also contained questions on abortion, infertility, STD clinic attendance, HIV testing and drug use. The booklet was to be completed by the respondent and sealed in an envelope bearing only a number as a means of identification.

The face-to-face component of the questionnaire contained some personal questions of a sensitive nature, relating to first heterosexual experiences and to sexual orientation, since responses to these were needed in order to decide whether a booklet should be given at all. This strategy also provided an opportunity to compare responses in face-to-face interviews with those in self-completion. The booklet was not given to respondents with no sexual experience at all, or to those aged 16 or 17 who had not experienced heterosexual intercourse.

Responses to the more personal questions asked in the face-to-face part of the interview were elicited through the use of show-cards. For example (at question 31a), a female respondent reporting having felt sexually attracted 'more often to females, and at least once to a male' would select and report letter L from the choice on the card. This technique was introduced in advance of the first sex-related questions in order to properly familiarize the respondent with the technique. It served to protect respondents both from verbalizing sexually explicit terms and from being overheard by any other household members. (Wherever practicable, interviewers sought to secure privacy for the interview.)

Two versions of the questionnaire were developed, the longer version containing the full module of attitude questions already referred to, and more detailed questions on family background and influences, first intercourse and sex education than the shorter version. The long version was intended for a quarter of the sample (which would be a systematic, random subset, fully representative of the total selected) and the reduced module for three-quarters.

Wording the questions

The second stage in constructing the questionnaire was to decide on precise question format. This was developed from several sources, including a review of previous work and, most importantly, the qualitative research that had been carried out with the express purpose of guiding questionnaire design.

Choice of language: formal or informal?

An early decision was needed on whether there should be some flexibility in the questionnaire to allow respondents to use their own language. Much of the preparatory work, including the literature search, seemed to point naturally to the use of the respondent's own language in the wording of the questionnaire. Many researchers counsel matching the language of the interview with that of the respondent on the dual grounds that only thus will a rapport be forged with the interviewer, facilitating maximum possible disclosure, and only thus can precise understanding of the questions by the respondent be ensured. Kinsey, for example, cautions against the use of scientific terms, advising instead the use of the vernacular (Kinsey *et al.*, 1948).

Several recent surveys have successfully adopted this formula. Project Sigma (1989), for example, asked its sample of gay men for their meaning of a particular term before imposing its own definition, in order to determine precisely what was being measured: '*Suppose someone asked you "How many sexual partners have you had this month?" What must have happened sexually for a person to "count" as your sexual partner?*' Similarly, in a survey based on a mixed-race sample in the USA (AIMN, 1988), the interviewer handed the respondent a list of sex-related terms — for example, penis, anus, semen, masturbation, and so on — and asked: '*Before we start, can you please tell me what word you use in ordinary conversations to refer to each of the following sexual terms*'. Having translated the concept into the respondent's language, the interviewer then substituted the respondent's preferred term for each formal term contained within the instrument.

The arguments in favour of using the respondent's own terms are self-evident and do not need rehearsing. In the context of this survey, however, there were practical problems generated by the scale of the survey, the broad generality of the population to be sampled and the chosen questionnaire format. Tailoring language to each participant is somewhat less feasible in the case of a large-scale, heterogeneous, general population sample, where there is a wide diversity in terms of sexual orientation and practices, than it is with a purposive sample drawn from a relatively homogeneous group. Added to this was the problem of format; the inclusion of a self-completion component presented few possibilities for negotiating meanings of terminology. Of equal importance was the need to use terms which would have precise behavioural definitions.

Respondents' preferences for terminology

The qualitative phase of development work revealed a number of difficulties that needed to be resolved. The use of terms, their meaning and respondents' preferences for use were all explored in the course of this work. Interviewers were instructed to encourage and prompt respondents to provide an account of a particular experience, behaviour, practice or relationship and then to ask what term they would use to describe such a phenomenon (for example, 'What would you generally call the person you've just described?'). Alternatively, the interviewer picked up a term used by the respondent and asked what he or she was describing (for example, 'What would count as a sexual partner for you?'). The interviewer was able to move backwards and forwards between a concept and the term representing it to probe language preferences and the 'fit' between various standard terms and their use.

Sexual behaviour is rarely spoken about publicly and as a result the language used to describe it is impoverished and inappropriate. There was a wide diversity of language styles used to describe sexual behaviour, ranging from the biblical ('couple', 'copulate', 'fornicate') to the vernacular ('screw', 'fuck'); from the euphemistic ('doing it', 'having it') to the romantic ('making love'); and from the lay terms ('having sex', 'sexual intercourse') to the scientific ('coitus').

The terms used varied not only between respondents but also within the pattern of use at each interview. Respondents were seldom consistent in their style of language throughout the interview, often moving between different expressions. There was some evidence, too, that the use of terms changes with experience and through time. Use of terms varies with the nature of the relationship and with the life stage of the respondent.

Another difficulty that came to light as a result of the qualitative work was the possible discordance between words the interviewer felt comfortable using and those the respondent felt comfortable with. Some respondents expressed a clear preference for the vernacular; others used a more basic term themselves, but were less happy hearing it used by the interviewer. Whilst espousing the use of the vernacular, Kinsey acknowledged this difficulty and issued the following word of caution (Kinsey *et al.*, 1948): 'One must know and use the vernacular terms with a fine sense of their properties and their exact meanings in each group. Their awkward use may damage instead of building rapports'.

Conversely, there was some evidence of discomfort on the part of interviewers when frank language was used by respondents. The importance of remembering that research can be threatening to the *researcher* as well as to the respondent has also been noted elsewhere (Sieber & Stanley, 1988).

Our own experience showed that the use of respondents' own language would be unlikely to provide the required standardization. Instead, it had rather the reverse effect, demonstrating that the meaning of terms depended on the context in which they were used.

Towards the end of the qualitative, in-depth interviews, respondents were asked to state explicitly their preferences for terms and style of language. A general consensus emerged for the use of formal language, with the proviso that explanations should be provided where necessary. In deference to both respondents' and interviewers' expressed preferences, and because of the research team's concern for precise definitions, formal terms were used throughout the questionnaire, both in the face-to-face interview and the self-completion booklet.

The use of standard terms, and the provision of fixed definitions for them, perhaps lays the study open to the charge of narrow operationalism, and possibly also to the criticism that it neglected or disregarded respondents' own meanings. The justification for the decision to rely on standard terms for this survey lies in the study's purposes. One of the aims, as previously described, was to provide data that would help in predicting the future spread of HIV infection, which necessitated being absolutely clear what had taken place in practical and physiological terms. In this context, it is essential to measure, as precisely as possible, at what intervals, with what frequency and with whom specific sexual acts defined in concrete terms have taken place.

The problem of understanding

Having decided on standard terms, it was important to ensure that the meaning attached to each term used would also be standard, precise and sufficiently well understood to represent the same behaviour throughout the sample population (Cantril & Fried, 1944). Everyday English, as it is used in colloquial speech, is often ambiguous; for the purposes of the survey, definitions were needed that would be precise enough to measure accurately the range and consistency of sexual behaviour.

Terms and expressions needed to be as neutral as possible and to avoid causing offence or appear judgemental. At the same time, they needed to be easily understood, and it was not always easy to avoid resorting to technical terms. The qualitative research showed that there were few terms whose meaning was universally understood. The meaning of such terms as 'vaginal sex', 'oral sex', 'penetrative sex' and 'heterosexual' is taken for granted in much health education literature, but considerable misunderstanding remains.

In addition to a simple lack of understanding of many terms, the developmental work unearthed another difficulty, namely a tendency to attribute to unfamiliar terms meanings associated with unorthodox or bizarre sexual practices. By contrast, what was classified as 'normal' sex did not seem to need a distinguishing term to define it, and it was often described in euphemisms whose meanings were far from precise enough for research purposes.

Terms held different meanings for different people. This was clearly illustrated by the term 'sexual partner'. Examples from the qualitative work showed the concept to be variously defined according to the strength and durability of the relationship and the extent to which it was socially institutionalized. For most people, the term signified some kind of sexual activity between two people, but for some it excluded their spouse and for others it included a partner with whom sex had not taken place recently. The essential component of the definition in the context of this survey – the physical sexual experience – was neither necessary nor sufficient in the meanings respondents imputed to the concept. Yet it was crucial to the validity of the study that the indicators used measured only, and no more than, what we wanted them to measure.

As a result, it was necessary to define terms in concrete practical ways. For example, 'partners' were defined as 'people who have had sex together just once, or a few times, or as regular partners, or as married partners', and a heterosexual partner was defined as someone with whom the respondent had vaginal, oral or anal sexual intercourse. In the face-to-face section of the interview schedule, interviewers were provided with explanations to offer to respondents. Whenever possible, the language most commonly understood by respondents in the qualitative work was used to amplify questions, parenthesizing lay terms as alternatives for interviewers to use; for example: '. . . *at what age did you start menstruating (having periods)?*' (question 33b). The self-completion booklet was prefaced with a glossary of key terms, such as: 'Vaginal sexual intercourse: a man's penis entering a woman's vagina'. (The text of the glossary can be found in full in the Appendix 1.)

Pains were taken to avoid conveying to respondents that definitions of terms imposed any moral or 'correct' meaning on them. The glossary in the self-completion booklet was introduced as being 'just to make sure that everyone applies the same meaning to certain terms we use'.

It was not within the remit of this study to explore the importance or emotional salience that different forms of sexual expression and relationships have for individuals. Large-scale, quantitative surveys of this kind are not best suited to exploring the richness and complexity of sexual expression. Small-scale, in-depth qualitative studies are better suited to this task.

Question wording: the example of sexual practices

A starting point for quantitative estimates is to ensure that common definitions are attached to specific acts. As previously discussed, it was clear from the development work that, for heterosexual respondents, the term 'having sex' was generally equated with vaginal intercourse. It was necessary to state explicitly which activities were being referred to. Questions investigating the occurrence of any kind of sexual activity that could result in the exchange of bodily fluids were expanded for clarity. For example, 'When, if ever, was the last occasion you had sex with a woman? *This means vaginal intercourse, oral sex, anal sex?*' (booklet, question 1a, male version); and 'When, if ever, was the last occasion you had *vaginal sexual intercourse* with a woman?' (booklet, question 3a, male version).

Most of the problems of comprehension were ironed out at the early qualitative stages of investigation, or else at the pre-feasibility study piloting stages. However, one or two emerged during the course of the feasibility study, an example of which is described below.

One of the main strategies of health education interventions to encourage risk reduction has been to encourage people to adopt sexual practices that do not involve the exchange of bodily fluids. It was therefore of central interest to investigate how widespread such practices are; that is, forms of sexual expression which avoid vaginal intercourse and anal and oral sex. The intention was to assess the prevalence of mutual masturbation, although it was clear from the development work that the term 'masturbation' was unacceptable.

Question 3 in the booklet asks about heterosexual practices, questions 3a–d being about vaginal intercourse, oral sex and anal intercourse respectively. Question 3e originally asked: '*When, if ever, was the last occasion you had any other form of genital contact with a woman, that did not also involve vaginal intercourse, oral or anal sex?*' This was piloted in advance of the feasibility study with apparently no misunderstanding, but results from the feasibility study showed high proportions – 40% (157) of men, and 44% (225) of women – who claimed *never* to have had genital contact without intercourse. The conclusion from the data, that some four out of 10 respondents had limited their sexual experience to full sexual intercourse, was intuitively difficult to accept. It seemed more likely that this was the result of a large number of respondents misunderstanding the question, and again the qualitative work shed some light on this. In the knowledge that what sounded unfamiliar was often perceived as unorthodox and unacceptable, the expression 'genital contact without intercourse' could have been perceived as some kind of sexual aberration or bizarre practice. The question was revised and repiloted and a more easily understood, if rather convoluted, version was produced: '*When was the last occasion you had **genital contact with a woman NOT involving intercourse?*** (For example, stimulating sex organs by hand but not leading to vaginal, oral or anal intercourse.)' The addition of the words in parentheses resulted in much higher rates of reporting for this practice (see Chapter 6).

Reliability and validity

Attempts at obtaining quantitative data on sexual behaviour must rely on self-reports because the objective verification of such intimate acts is virtually impossible. Mechanisms for ensuring reliability (the potential of the research instrument to replicate the results, and the extent to which findings are generalizable to the population as a whole) and validity (whether the question measures what it is intended to measure) were therefore uppermost in our minds in question development. Two important aspects of reliability and validity are the twin problems of veracity and accuracy of recall.

It is widely assumed that people will be reluctant to tell the truth about aspects of their sexual experience. Yet we have no reason to believe that this is more problematic in studies of sexual practices than in other aspects of human behaviour. Potential problems relating to people's ability to recollect accurately and report their experience honestly beset investigation into many aspects of human behaviour. Topics on which people might be tempted to give less than honest replies include drinking and smoking behaviour, frequency of having a bath or shower, reasons for absences from work, negative views about racial minorities and earnings from all sources (Belson, 1966). Researchers display few reservations about investigating these areas of behaviour on the grounds of doubtful disclosure.

Difficulties encountered in this respect were no greater than anticipated, and if anything rather less so. Clearly, this is an area in which the interviewer effect could threaten validity of response. The greater the sensitivity about a topic, the stronger the temptation to modify the truth. A question may be considered sensitive for a number of reasons (Lee & Renzetti, 1990) – because it probes socially disapproved attitudes or behaviour, for example, or because it attempts to make public material which would normally be kept private. Kudos attaches to some, and opprobrium to other, sexual practices, as is the case for other activities, such as eating and drinking or earning money. Some activities which respondents were asked to reveal are not only socially disapproved but actually illegal (anal sex between a man and a woman in England and Wales, for example).

Encouraging reliable responses

A number of design features can be built into the methodology to try and guard against this effect (Smith & Hyman, 1950). One solution is to pose 'permissive' questions, those which, by their wording, imply acceptance of the behaviour in question. Some researchers on sexual behaviour (Kinsey *et al.*, 1948; Coxon *et al.*, 1988) advocate using leading questions of the type '*When did you last . . . ?*' or '*When was the first time you . . . ?*', thereby placing the onus of denial on the respondent. The use of such questions is generally criticized, on the grounds that they introduce bias in favour of *over-reporting* the behaviour in question. However, leading questions may on some occasions be used intentionally to counteract a tendency in the opposite direction, i.e. the tendency to *under-report* behaviour that is socially unacceptable or felt to be unorthodox (Kinsey *et al.*, 1948).

   The technique of using leading questions was used in a more moderate form in NATSAL; for example, questions of the type '*When did you first . . . ?*' included 'never' amongst the response options.

   A guarantee of confidentiality can also do much to ensure veracity of response (see also Chapter 3). Reassuring respondents of the confidentiality of the survey was of the greatest importance in relation to the self-completion booklet, which contained the more intimate and personal questions. Answers to these were not seen even by the interviewers, who gave respondents instructions to place the booklet in the envelope provided and to seal it, on completion. This was reinforced in the printed instructions on the front cover page of the booklet itself:

Confidentiality

The questions in this booklet are mostly very personal. Your answers will be treated in strict confidence; the interviewer does not need to see them.

*When you have finished, put the booklet in the envelope and seal it. Your
name will not be on the booklet or envelope.*

Memory error

The problem of accuracy of recall, in common with that of veracity, is not
exclusive to research into sexual behaviour. Social survey researchers
regularly rely on the memories of respondents for their data. Inevitably
this introduces questions about validity. The literature on memory research
is not extensive, but what studies there are point inescapably to the
fallibility of memory-dependent information.

The assumption is that memory decays progressively with time, so that
recent events are recalled more reliably than remote ones (Hunter, 1957).
Yet there are many instances where this effect is reversed. Older people
may remember events in their distant past in detail, forgetting what
happened yesterday. According to the literature on the subject we cannot
assume a direct relationship between the rate of forgetting a particular
event and the time lapsed since its occurrence. There may be a number of
intervening variables, such as the emotional significance of an experience,
its associations with other events and the motivation to retain the memory.

Certainly, events like first intercourse seem sufficiently salient emotionally to be recalled by most people without difficulty. In the feasibility
study the question was asked: *'How old were you when you first had
sexual intercourse with someone of the opposite sex or hasn't this happened?'* (question 19). Only 8/557 (1.5%) of women and 7/420 (1.7%)
of men failed to remember the age at which they first had sexual intercourse. (In the main study the proportion was even smaller; see Chapter
4.)

Memory error is more likely to occur in the context of recollections of
lifetime sexual partners and accounts of different sexual practices. Recall
will be easiest for those with fewest partners, and for those whose relationships have been socially regulated in some way, e.g. through
engagement or marriage, or a shared home. It is likely to be more
difficult for those with large numbers of partners. This is worrying because
the experience of these respondents may be of greater interest in terms of
identifying the characteristics of those at high risk.

Particularly in relation to the disclosure of sensitive information, it is
never easy to know whether inaccuracies are a product of a simple lapse
of memory, of unconscious repression or of deliberate concealment. Here
the boundary between the twin problems of veracity and recall becomes
blurred. People may not lie intentionally but may be unable to give
a truthful account because of the difficulty of retrieving censored information. It has been shown that errors in recall are not random but vary

with social expectations (Withey, 1954). Forgetting may be a process of active blocking rather than of passive decay. Kinsey reminds us that the effect of this can be to reverse any possible advantageous effects of recent recall on accuracy since recent events may be most subject to censorship.

The difficulties in interpreting respondents' reports of subjective data are increased when reporting is not about present events but about those recollected from the past. This may be because of a tendency to modify selectively recollection of past feelings according to the value system currently held. Asked simply whether the first *sexual experience* was with a man or a woman, a respondent might be more likely to give an answer that excludes past behaviour that is now considered unacceptable.

Aiding the process of recall

Efforts were made to explore by what means error caused by imperfections in recall might be reduced. Large-scale quantitative surveys have their limitations in eliciting data that are difficult to recall. Recall can be more a process of gradual reminiscence than of instant recollection. Probably the most successful techniques facilitating this are those involving a slow, careful process of retrieval more akin to the therapeutic method than to survey research. Good qualitative work can do much to uncover hidden experiences in the respondent's past, and our own experience in the early in-depth interviews was that respondents did a good deal of 'remembering' during the course of an interview. By contrast, the fully structured questionnaire in general allows only a 'one-shot' approach to response that does not permit reflection and revision. What comes to mind first may not always bear the closest correspondence with reality.

All the same, there are techniques that can be used in the design of a questionnaire to ease the process of recall. In so far as recall seems prone to something akin to the social desirability response, the problem may respond, to some extent, to the same kinds of methodological devices designed to deal with the problem of honesty. The order in which different time periods are set out in a question also influences recall. This was particularly important for questions requiring an estimate of numbers of sexual partners over different time periods – a lifetime, or in the last 5 years, 2 years, 1 year, 6 months or 3 months. In order to assess the effect of order in our questionnaire, two versions of the questionnaire were piloted. Version A set out the intervals with the shortest time period first and the longest last, and version B was in reverse order. In fact, version B proved the more satisfactory alternative. The proportion of respondents who were unable to give responses to this question was higher in version A compared with B for all intervals except the shortest.

Order effect

A further consideration was the order in which points on rating scales might best be listed to elicit the most reliable responses. There is some evidence, although not entirely conclusive (Bradburn & Mason, 1964; Quinn & Belson, 1969; Belson, 1981), that bias arises because of a tendency to endorse the first item on a scale rather than the last *and* to endorse the more 'favourable' response in a set of options. Since scaled items are often set out, for convenience, with favourable items first, social desirability bias and order effect can be additive. One way of attempting to reduce this effect is to reverse the scale; that is, to place the *least* acceptable response first. This was particularly important for questions on sexual orientation, which used a Kinsey-type scale (see Chapter 7) to probe highly sensitive information. The initial formulation for the feasibility survey was as follows.

I have felt *sexually attracted*:

- only to a person, or people, of the opposite sex;
- mostly to people of the opposite sex;
- about equally to people of the opposite sex and to people of the *same* sex as me;
- mostly to people of the same sex as me;
- only to a person, or people, of the same sex as me.

I have never felt sexually attracted to anyone at all.

I have had some *sexual contact or experience*:

- only with a person, or people, of the opposite sex;
- mostly with people of the opposite sex;
- about equally with people of the opposite sex and with people of the *same* sex as me;
- mostly with people of the same sex as me;
- only with a person, or people, of the same sex as me.

I have not had any sexual contact or experience with anyone at all.

It could not be determined without large-scale testing whether the scales would work better with the more widespread behaviour pattern (sex with people of the opposite sex) at the top of the scale, or in reverse order. There seemed to be sound arguments for both versions. Given the 'first-item' bias and, in this particular case, given the stigma attached to same-gender sex (making 'opposite sex' the favourable option), it would seem logical to assume that any order effect bias would be increased by putting the 'favourable' option of 'opposite sex' first on the scale. At the same time, this needed to be balanced against a consideration of the sense of the question. A key problem in formulating sexual orientation questions stems from the fact that the English language provides one word, 'sex', to describe both 'gender' and, for want of a better term, 'libidinous expression', which gives rise to considerable potential for misinterpretation. Putting 'opposite sex' first might serve to clarify the meaning of 'same sex' when it appeared further down the list.

The opportunity was taken, in the feasibility survey, to carry out split-run experiments to test for order effect. Version A had 'same sex' at the top, while version B had the scale in reverse order ('opposite sex' at the top). Roughly half the pilot sample received each version. At the same time, the order in which the two scales were presented was varied: half the sample were asked first about attraction and then about experience, while for the other half the order was reversed. Results could not only be examined in terms of differences in reporting between these four groups but also checked for concordance with responses about homosexual experience given in the self-completion booklet. Table 2.1 summarizes the results for both interview and booklet.

As these figures for men show, the results from version B ('opposite sex' first) showed greater consistency with data from the self-completion booklet. Concordance was 91.0% for version B and 80.3% for version A. Not unexpectedly, a larger proportion of men reported homosexual contact in the booklet than in the interview in version B, but the high proportion in version A (13.3%) reporting homosexual contact in the interview but not in the booklet gives some indication of the extent of misunderstanding from listing the responses in this order.

These results seemed to justify the conclusion that the source of possible error was more one of misunderstanding the terms used than of order effect. It was decided to abandon the terms 'same sex' and 'opposite sex' and opt for the terms 'female' and 'male' (for example: *I have felt sexually attracted . . . only to females, never to males*'). It was not desirable to use 'woman' and 'man' because of the risk of pre-adult

Table 2.1. Correspondence in reporting any male homosexual experience between the face-to-face interview and the self-completion booklet in the feasibility survey

| | Question wording | |
| | Version A (%) | Version B (%) |
Any homosexual experience		
Booklet only	6.4	6.9
Interview only	13.3	2.1
Booklet and interview	2.0	2.6
Neither	78.3	88.4
Base	203	189

experiences being discounted. It was also decided to order the scale to start with the most familiar orientation.

Single occurrence events vs habits

Events like first intercourse (which by definition can only occur once), marriage or births of children (which occur rarely) have advantages for recall. The literature on memory research confirms that incidence is easier to recall than frequency (Hornsby & Wilcox, 1989). Thus questions such as '*When was the first time you . . . lived with a partner/lived away from home?*', or dates of single-occurrence events (birth of babies, menarche, etc.), produce more valid results than regular occurrences (e.g. frequency of intercourse).

Knowledge of this effect is turned to methodological advantage simply by converting as many questions as possible into the type requiring incidence as the answer in preference to frequency. For example, if the measurement objective is to establish *average* frequencies of intercourse, a more reliable method might avoid questions of the type 'How often do you have sex?', substituting instead 'When did you last have sex?'

Research has showed that people tend to transfer *into* the period in question, events which actually took place *outside* it, at either end (Gray, 1955). This was particularly relevant, in relation to sexual partnerships and sexual practices, in deciding whether to ask about a fixed period of time, such as a 'typical week', or about a period ending on the day before the interview, such as the last 7 days. This made the case for taking the memory period up to the point immediately before the interview, so closing the door to one set of transfers.

Internal and external validity

The empirical investigation of sexual behaviour offers few opportunities for triangulating data, for reasons mentioned above. Recent attempts to address this problem include test–retest repeatability (Saltzman *et al.*, 1987), comparisons between retrospective reports and diary keeping (McLaws *et al.*, 1990), comparison of self-completion with face-to-face interviews (Klassen *et al.*, 1989) and validation against external data sets. A method of ascertaining validity in this survey was to examine logical tests of consistency in the questionnaire. These opportunities occurred naturally in the course of developing the structure for respondents to follow. For example, those reporting age at first sexual intercourse in the questionnaire should report at least one heterosexual partner in the booklet. In the questionnaire used in the feasibility survey, 101 consistency checks within and between interview and self-completion items were built into the research instrument and 62 of these revealed no inconsistencies. Where errors occurred in the remaining 39 checks, the majority pointed to inadvertent rather than deliberate errors, often related to question design or layout. This corresponds with the conclusion of Marquis *et al.* (1986) that while there are undoubtedly problems of unreliability in surveys on sensitive subjects, misreporting of personal information is often as much a function of question design as of unwillingness or inability to report.

The external validity of these data can be assessed by comparing responses with independent data sets. These checks were also carried out at the main stage of the survey and are described in Chapter 3.

Sampling

Sample size and type

The feasibility study (Wellings *et al.*, 1990) provided the necessary information about the acceptability of a study on sexual behaviour and the data allowed a more informed decision on the sample size needed. The need for reliable prevalence estimates of less common behaviours, such as paying for sex or injecting drugs, indicated that a general population sample, randomly selected from a reliable sampling frame, was required. Alternatives to simple random sampling were considered, such as designs that would improve sampling efficiency (for example, to oversample those with the highest-risk behaviour), but without prior data the appropriate strata on which to oversample were difficult to assess. On the basis of random sampling, adequate precision was required to estimate the prevalence of behaviours as rare as one in 100, even within subgroups of the sample that could be as small as 500. These considerations led to an estimate that a sample of around 20 000 achieved interviews was needed.

Population coverage

A key consideration concerned the lower and upper limits of the age range of the sample, since the ages at which people begin and end their sexual careers vary widely. A lower age range of 16 was agreed on the assumption (borne out by the feasibility study) that a sizeable proportion of young adults would already be sexually experienced, representing an important group for health education targeting. Many younger teenagers are also sexually active under the age of sexual consent, but this could have led to difficulties in obtaining parental permission to interview their children on this topic. Surveys designed specifically for this age group are probably more appropriate. The questionnaire was carefully designed to protect sexually inexperienced respondents from being asked questions which were not relevant to them.

A decision relating to an upper age limit was more difficult. Qualitative work had shown that older people found the subject more intrusive and were less willing than younger people to agree to be interviewed. This was borne out by the fact that the response rate even among the oldest age group (45–59) was slightly below that in other age groups (see Chapter 3).

The decision to impose a cut-off point of 59 years for inclusion in the survey was also guided by the survey's measurement objectives. Many of the topics about which the survey was to collect data are known not to affect older people greatly. Sexually transmitted infections are rarely found amongst older people, and problems of infertility and unwanted pregnancy no longer affect older women. Intrusion into this personal area of life was therefore less justified for older people, and excluding them allowed the concentration of resources on the groups of most urgent concern at the present time. We hope that future replication of the survey might extend the age range to cover all age groups.

Sampling frame

Using personal interview as the data collection method narrowed the choice of sampling frame to the electoral register (ER) and the postcode address file (PAF), each of which has advantages and disadvantages (Todd & Butcher, 1982; Lynn & Lievesley, 1992). The ER, a list of individuals eligible to vote in Britain, is available for use approximately 6 months after collection of the information. Because of the estimated 10% change in registrations each year due to deaths, new entrants and home movers (OPCS, 1987; Butcher, 1988), it quickly becomes outdated. This drawback can be largely overcome by treating the register as a list of addresses instead of a list of individuals, but the coverage of addresses is incomplete and the excluded elements are a seriously biased subset of the population. For example, young people, ethnic minorities and the highly mobile are disproportionately likely to live at addresses not on the ER (Todd & Butcher, 1982). Recently, the number of registered electors has fallen, possibly due to failure to register because of fears about the Community Charge.

The small users' PAF, a regularly updated computer-held file of largely residential addresses, is free from problems of failure to register or of mobility of residents (Butcher, 1988). Not only is the PAF's coverage of residential addresses superior to that of the ER, omissions are more likely to be random and not biased in any particular direction (Dodd, 1987), and so are unlikely to be directly related to any of the variables of interest to this study. The definition of a 'small user' is one created by the Post Office, with its particular need for delivering mail: the PAF includes businesses with small volumes of mail and could exclude a few private households or residential institutions receiving a high volume of mail. However, the major disadvantage of the PAF is that it contains no information about individuals resident at each address; that is, it does not list the names of residents or how many there are. Consequently, addresses can only be selected with equal probabilities. A sampling procedure that requires that only one person per household is interviewed means that those who live alone have a higher chance of selection than do individuals who live in larger households.

Both the PAF and the ER exclude the homeless, and the PAF also excludes some elements of the institutionalized population. However, less than 1% of the population is resident in institutions and the large majority are elderly people who would not have been eligible for this survey. The PAF was chosen for this survey mainly on the grounds of its superior coverage of private residential addresses. The biased coverage of the ER would have been particularly serious in this case because sexual behaviour is likely to be associated with the known correlates of coverage, such as age and mobility.

The objectives of the study, the qualitative research and the experience of previous researchers in the field guided the development of the final research instrument. Extensive pre-piloting, culminating in the feasibility study, established its robustness. The results of the feasibility study, through measures of response rate, sample representativeness and validity, demonstrated the general acceptability of the survey to the British population and the potential of the methods developed to achieve the research objectives. This gave the authors, the scientific referees and the funding agency the necessary confidence to proceed to the main stage of the survey.

Summary

All aspects of the design of the survey – the content of the questionnaire, the method of data collection and the sample size and frame – reflected the aims and objectives of the survey. Of particular concern was the need to ensure that the data would be valid and reliable and that the survey would be acceptable to the study population. The sensitive nature of the information to be gathered heightened the necessity to convince participants of the need for the survey, of the confidential nature of the enquiry and of the credentials of the investigators.

A prolonged period of careful development work – comprising qualitative research to guide the design and piloting of the questionnaire, followed by a feasibility survey to test the response rate, the represent-ativeness of the sample and the acceptability of the investigative techniques – enabled questions relating to the reliability and validity of the data to be resolved prior to the main stage of the survey.

The complexity of the data and the need for the careful definition of terms led to the choice of a personal interview rather than a telephone survey or postal questionnaire. The format of the personal interview, part face-to-face, part self-completion, combined both components in a way likely to achieve optimal results in terms of maximizing response rates and eliminating bias.

The questionnaire was fully structured and scheduled. The language used in the questionnaire – formal, neutral terminology – and the pro-vision of concrete, practical definitions reflected the wide variety of definitions and meanings attached to terms, a lack of understanding of some words and a dislike of others. It also reflected the stated preferences of interviewers and respondents.

A random probability sample of around 20 000 was required in order to investigate the distribution of behaviours within the population and to measure the prevalence of those which are relatively uncommon. The age range of 16–59 reflected the aim of the survey to provide information of value in the context of sexual health, covering broadly the reproductive age range, but was also prompted by evidence of some decline in response and recall amongst older respondents at the feasibility stage of the survey.

Although the selection of the procedures was guided by considerations related to the subject-matter, the actual procedures themselves were no different from those used in other surveys.

References

ACSF Investigators (1992) AIDS and sexual behaviour in France. *Nature*, **360**, 407–9.

AIMN (1988) AIDS in a multicultural neighborhood. Questionnaire. Bayview–Hunter's Point Foundation for Community Improvement, San Francisco.

Belson, W.A. (1981) *The Design and Understanding of Survey Questions*. Gower, London.

Belson, W.A. (1966) The effects of reversing the presentation order of verbal rating scales. *Journal of Advertising Research*, **6**(4), 30–7.

Bradburn, N.M. & Mason, W.M. (1964) The effect of question order on responses. *Journal of Marketing*, **1**(4), 57–61.

Butcher, R. (1988) The use of the Postcode Address File as a sampling frame. *The Statistician*, **37**, 15–24.

Cantril, H. & Fried, E. (1944) The meaning of questions. In Cantril, H. Gauging Public Opinion. Princeton University Press, Princeton.

Collins, M. & Sykes, W. (1987) The problems of non-coverage and unlisted numbers in telephone surveys in Britain. *Journal of the Royal Statistical Society (Series A)*, **150**(3), 241–53.

Coxen, A. (1988) Re numbers game. In Aggleton, P. & Homans, H. (eds) Social aspects of AIDS.

Dodd, T. (1987) A further investigation into the coverage of the Postcode Address File. *Survey Methodology Bulletin 21*. OPCS, London.

Foreman, J. & Collins, M. (1991) The viability of Random Digit Dialling in the UK. *Journal of the Market Research Society*, **33**(3), 218–27.

Gray, P.G. (1955) The memory factor in social surveys. *Journal of the American Statistical Association*, **50**, 270.

Hornsby, P.P. & Wilcox, A.J. (1989) Validity of questionnaire information on frequency of coitus. *American Journal of Epidemiology*, **130**(1).

Hunter, I.M.L. (1957) *Memory*. Pelican, London.

Kinsey, A.C., Pomeroy, W.B. & Martin, C.E. (1948) *Sexual Behavior in the Human Male*. W.B. Saunders, Philadelphia.

Klassen, A.D., Williams, C.J., Levitt, E.E., Rudkin-Mincot, H.G., Miller, H.G. & Gunjal, S. (1989) Trends in premarital sexual behaviour. In Turner, C.F., Miller, H.G. & Moses, C.E. (eds) *Sexual Behaviour and AIDS*. National Academy Press, Washington DC.

Lee, R.M. & Renzetti, C.M. (1990) The problems of researching sensitive topics. *American Behavioral Scientist*, **3**(5), 510–28.

Lynn, P. & Lievesley, D. (1992) *Drawing General Population Samples in Great Britain*. SCPR, London.

Marquis, K.H., Marquis, S. & Polich, M. (1986) Response bias and reliability in sensitive topic surveys. *Journal of the American Statistical Association*, **394**, 381–9.

McLaws, M.L., Oldenburg, B., Ross, M.W. & Cooper, D.A. (1990) Sexual behaviour in AIDS-related research: reliability and validity of recall and diary measures. *Journal of Sex Research*, **27**, 265–87.

Office of Population Censuses and Surveys (1987) *Central Postcode Directory Guide*. OPCS, Titchfield.

Project Sigma (1989) *Briefing Document: A Digest of Early Findings of Project Sigma*. Department of Social Sciences, South Bank Polytechnic, London.

Quinn, S. & Belson, W.A. (1969) The effects of reversing the presentation order of verbal rating scales in survey interviews. Survey Research Centre, London School of Economics and Political Science, London.

RUHBC (1989) CATI: LAH AIDS questionnaire by month. Research Unit in Health and Behavioral Change, University of Edinburgh, Edinburgh.

Saltzman, S.P., Stoddart, A.M., McCusker, J., Moon, M.W. & Mayer, K.H. (1987) *Public Health Reports*, **102**, 692–7.

Sieber, J.E. & Stanley, B. (1988) Ethical and professional dimensions of socially sensitive research. *American Psychologist*, **43**, 49–55.

Smith, H.L. & Hyman, H. (1950) The biasing effect of interview expectations on survey results. *Public Opinion Quarterly*, **14**(3).

Spencer, L., Faulkner, A. & Keegan, J. (1988) *Talking about Sex*. SCPR, London.

Sundet, J.M., Kvalem, I.L., Magnus, P. & Bakketeig, L.S. (1988) Prevalence of risk-prone sexual behaviour in the general population of Norway. Abstracts 4, Global Impact of AIDS Conference, London.

Todd, J. & Butcher, B. (1982) *Electoral Registration in 1981*. OPCS, London.

Wellings, K., Field, J., Wadsworth, J., Johnson, A.M., Anderson, R.M. & Bradshaw, S.A. (1990) Sexual lifestyles under scrutiny. *Nature*, **348**, 276–8.

Withey, S.B. (1954) Reliability of recall of income. *Public Opinion Quarterly*, **18**, 197–204.

Table 3.1. Outcome of sampling: alternative assumptions

	No assumptions about eligibility	Assumptions about eligibility	
		CASRO	NATSAL
Total addresses issued	50 010	50 010	50 010
Out-of-scope addresses	5 980	5 980	5 980
No eligible resident	14 228	14 228	14 228
Language problem/sick/away		562	
	14 228	14 790	14 228
No contact after 4+ calls	1 027	1 027	1 027
Estimated ineligible		369	226
Complete refusal of information	1 761	1 761	1 761
Estimated ineligible		632	387
Potentially eligible	29 802	28 239	29 189
Completed interviews	18 876	18 876	18 876
Response rate (%)	63.3	66.8	64.7

The method adopted by the Council of American Survey Research Organizations (CASRO) (McQueen, 1992) excludes those who are sick, away from home or unable to speak English and then uses the proportion of ineligible households observed in the sample to adjust the denominator. Using this method, 32.3% of addresses where no contact was made or all information refused can be estimated to be outside the eligible age range and excluded from the denominator, resulting in a response rate of 66.8% (Table 3.1). The observed proportion of ineligibles is likely to be an overestimate, since households whose members are older are easier to contact than households composed of younger people. The mean number of calls made by an interviewer before making contact with an ineligible household was 1.62, compared with 3.03 calls for eligible households (Table 3.2). In all, 22% of calls were made to addresses where all household members were aged 60 or above. It therefore seems likely that a lower proportion of non-contactable households would be ineligible than would be the case with contactable households. A more realistic estimate might be the proportion of calls made to obtain an ineligible household (22%). When 22% of non-contacts and complete refusals are excluded from the base as ineligible, the response rate is 64.7%.

While allowing that the variations in survey methods and in response definitions make exact comparisons difficult, the response rate of this study compares favourably with previous studies of sexual behaviour in

Table 3.2. Outcome by number of calls at address where eligibility of respondent was established

Outcome	Number of cases	Total number of calls	Mean number of calls
Ineligible			
All household members 60+ years	14 228	23 093	1.62
Eligible			
Refusals	7 517	24 714	3.29
Sick/away	562	1 441	2.56
Completed interviews	18 876	55 614	2.95
Total	26 955	81 769	3.03

$$\text{Proportion of calls to ineligible households} = \frac{23\,093}{23\,093 + 81\,769} = 22.0\%$$

Britain and with those in other countries. For the first time in 1988, and again in 1989, the General Social Survey in the USA (Smith, 1988) included personal questions on sexual behaviour. In 1989, the overall response rate was 77.6%, and 8.8% of the respondents refused to answer the sexual behaviour questions. Recent social surveys of a less sensitive nature do not appear to have achieved markedly higher response rates, suggesting that people are only slightly less willing to answer questions on sexual behaviour than to respond to any other survey. In 1989, the response rate in the General Household Survey (GHS) (OPCS, 1991) for complete household cooperation was 74.2% and for British Social Attitudes (Jowell *et al.*, 1990) it was 69%.

Gender of interviewer

Traditionally, interviewers have been women, but in recent years the proportion of male interviewers has been steadily increasing in the SCPR panel. Intuitively, there might seem to be good reasons to try to match the gender of the interviewer to the gender of the respondent, but in a study where the gender of the respondent is not known in advance of the attempt to make contact, this was not a practical possibility. Nevertheless, potential respondents were offered the choice of a male or a female interviewer if there appeared to be any hesitation about agreeing to give the interview. In the development stage of the study, respondents had been asked about their preference for the gender of the interviewer. The majority had no clear preference either way. Of those who expressed

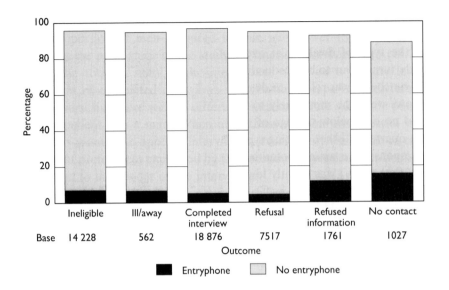

Fig. 3.2. Effect of entryphone on outcome at address.

there was information on age and gender for most selected individuals even if they did not then participate. Non-response was more common among men than among women (Table 3.5), the difference being mainly due to failure to make contact and proxy, rather than direct, refusals. The refusal rate increased with increasing age.

The importance to any study of a good response rate is undeniable and is used to judge the quality of survey estimates. The problem of measuring the presence of response bias and its effect on the particular variables that a survey has been designed to investigate is endemic to

Table 3.5. Gender and age group of selected respondents by outcome (%)

Outcome	Men	Women	Missing	16–24	25–34	35–44	45–59	Missing	All selected individuals
Sick/away	2.3	1.9	13.9	1.5	1.6	1.9	2.3	5.5	2.1
Refusal	31.8	24.3	76.4	20.9	21.6	23.7	29.9	80.5	27.7
Proxy	*5.6*	*2.5*	*13.9*	*3.6*	*2.8*	*3.2*	*3.6*	*14.3*	*4.0*
Parental	*0.3*	*0.2*	*0.0*	*1.5*	*0.01*	*0.02*	*0.0*	*0.2*	*0.3*
Personal	*21.8*	*19.4*	*51.5*	*12.6*	*16.0*	*18.1*	*24.1*	*55.5*	*20.6*
No contact	*4.1*	*2.2*	*5.9*	*3.2*	*2.8*	*2.4*	*2.2*	*10.5*	*3.1*
Completed interview	66.0	73.9	11.9	77.6	76.8	74.4	68.0	13.7	70.0
Base*	12 296	14 558	101	4 298	7 256	6 304	7 438	1 659	26 955

* All addresses except deadwood, ineligible, refusal of all information, no contact, lost in post or rejected as unusable; numbers, not percentages.

survey research but is largely ignored. Suspicion is readily voiced, how-ever, when the subject is as sensitive as sexual behaviour. We cannot know whether the non-responders are typical of the population with respect to sexual behaviour and several possible sources of bias exist. For example, this sample (like other PAF sample surveys) could not include homeless people. Homeless people form a very small minority of the whole population, but might possibly include a disproportionate number of prostitutes and those who inject drugs. On the other hand, the refusal rate increased with increasing age and older people were least likely to have practised high-risk behaviours or to have had multiple partners in the recent past.

Data preparation

Editing and coding

All completed questionnaires were subjected to a thorough clerical editing and coding stage before the data were keyed to computer. The edit inspection looked for missing information and inconsistencies. If the nature of an omission, error or inconsistency was such that correction was possible because the correct information was present (and clear) elsewhere in the questionnaire, then a correction was made. Other incon-sistencies were unchanged because it was neither possible nor appropriate to attempt to decide which piece of information was correct. The pre-sence of an inconsistency was coded at the end of the data record. A more detailed description of the inconsistency codes is given in a later section (p. 62). 'Don't know/can't remember' codes and 'Not answered' (information missing) codes were also introduced at this stage.

There were only two open-ended questions that needed subsequent coding from responses recorded verbatim. One was a question on under-standing of the phrase 'safer sex' (interview, question 43). A code frame of 44 items was developed from a listing of answers to 100 questionnaires. There was allowance for coding up to seven responses per respondent. The other question that required post-coding was the respondent's occu-pational details, from which socioeconomic group and social class class-ifications were derived (OPCS, 1980).

Once clerical editing and coding were complete and the data had been keyed to computer, a computer edit program was applied. This checked for missing data, for correct routing and for correct code ranges for each variable. For numerical fields, such as weight, height and numbers of partners, upper and lower limits were set and records that fell outside those limits failed the edit initially. All edit failures were referred back to the questionnaire and appropriate action was taken to amend the record

behaviour. Therefore the self-completion booklet was not given to those who, in questions 19 and 31 in the face-to-face interview, reported no sexual experience at all with either males or females (see Chapter 2). As an extra precaution against intrusiveness, respondents aged 16 or 17 were not given the booklet if they had never had heterosexual intercourse after the age of 13, even if they had had some heterosexual experience. In all, 3.8% of men and 3.4% of women were not given the self-completion booklet but some assumptions could be made about their sexual experience and partnerships and these are not considered as item non-response.

Item non-response can arise in any survey for a variety of reasons. There may be misunderstanding of a question or of routing instructions on a questionnaire. Inability to remember the information requested or objections to particular questions may be other causes of item non-response. Item non-response can be minimized with good questionnaire design and interviewing technique, but for self-completion questionnaires researchers must rely on careful and unambiguous question wording and layout and sensitive treatment of topics that could cause offence. Thus, by selecting the methodology of self-completion, the researchers accepted a trade-off between a possible increase in item non-response and a probable improvement in the reporting of socially censured behaviour.

In the face-to-face interview, the level of item non-response was low and did not reach 2% even for questions as sensitive as age at first heterosexual intercourse. However, despite a careful introduction to the self-completion booklet, 3.7% of men and 4.0% of women failed to complete it. Once a respondent had agreed to complete a booklet, the level of item non-response within it was low, below 5% for most of the questions. Similar reluctance to answer questions on sexual behaviour was found in the US General Social Survey (Smith, 1988), where 6.1% of those agreeing to answer questions on important social topics refused to answer questions on sexual behaviour.

Respondents found dates to be the most difficult information to recall. Parts of the booklet asked for details such as the month and year of the first and the most recent sexual intercourse with the three most recent partners in the last 5 years. Information on these dates was missing in up to 8% of the cases, which may reflect the difficulty that the respondents had in recalling the information with sufficient accuracy. Ten per cent of men who reported having paid for sex did not respond to the question on the number of partners that they had paid. This deficit could reflect an unwillingness to disclose the information (despite having disclosed that they had paid for sex at all) or a difficulty in remembering the number. Taking this evidence with that of the inconsistency coding, it seems more likely that item non-response was associated with difficulty of recall rather than with an unwillingness to disclose sensitive information.

Demographic representativeness of the sample

Clearly, good comparative data are not available for the variables at the core of this study (that is, population-based estimates of sexual behaviour), but the demographic characteristics of the achieved sample can be compared with other sources. It is not always obvious how to select the most appropriate data for comparison. Since completion of census forms is a legal requirement for households, census data should be the most complete and reliable, but in the most recent census (1991), there is some doubt about the completeness of coverage (OPCS, 1993). All surveys, including those sponsored by the Government, are subject to potential response bias.

Distribution of men and women

Comparing the achieved sample with 1991 census figures (OPCS, 1993), we would expect 49.7% of the sample to be men, but (after weighting the data) the proportion is 44.4%. A deficit is present in all age groups, a finding that is common to many other surveys, particularly sex surveys (Sundet *et al.*, 1988; Catania *et al.*, 1992; Spira *et al.*, 1993). This appears to be due to greater difficulty in contacting selected male respondents and to proxy refusals rather than to higher rates of direct refusal.

Age distribution

When the age distribution of the achieved sample is compared with the 1991 census figures (OPCS, 1993), only small differences are apparent (Fig. 3.4). The most marked under-representation was among older respondents (men aged 50–59 and women aged 55–59), which was balanced by over-representation of younger age groups.

Distribution of ethnic groups

A comparison is made with the Labour Force Survey (LFS) (OPCS, 1990) of the distribution among different ethnic groups, although the age bands are not identical (Table 3.6). The LFS presents figures for men and women combined, but the upper limit of the oldest age group is retirement age; that is, 64 for men and 59 for women. Comparisons must be treated with caution, but there is no evidence that people from ethnic minorities are under-represented (unless they are under-represented in both surveys). The proportion who self-identify as black is higher than in the LFS, and the proportions of all other non-white groups are similar to the LFS estimates.

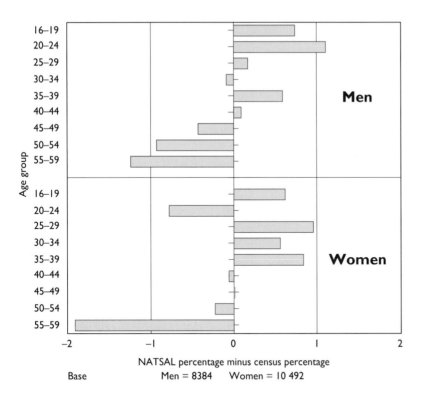

Fig. 3.4. Age distribution of survey sample compared with data from the 1991 census. [Source: interview, question 1a]

Table 3.6. Distribution of ethnic origin compared with the LFS (%) [Source: classification question 17]

	NATSAL			LFS*		
	16–29	30–44	45–59	16–29	30–44	45–65
White	93.2	93.8	95.6	93.3	94.5	95.8
Black†	2.4	1.8	1.8	1.6	1.0	1.2
Indian	1.5	1.7	0.9	1.7	1.6	1.2
Pakistani	0.7	0.5	0.3	0.8	0.7	0.5
Bangladeshi	0.3	0.1	0.1	0.2	0.1	0.1
Chinese	0.3	0.2	0.1	0.3	0.4	0.2
Other‡	1.2	1.5	0.8	1.1	0.9	0.4
Not answered	0.3	0.4	0.4	1.0	0.7	0.8
Base	6 903	7 020	4 953	12 068	11 354	10 318

* LFS (1990) figures reported for men aged 45–64 and women aged 45–59.
† LFS groups West Indian, Guyanese, African.
‡ LFS groups Arab, Mixed, Other; NATSAL groups Other, Asian, Other.

Table 3.7. Distribution of marital status compared with GHS (1990) (%)
[Source: classification question 1]

	NATSAL		GHS	
	Men	Women	Men	Women
Single	30.2	21.4	28.0	21.5
Cohabiting	7.2	8.0	6.3	6.4
First marriage	48.9	51.7	53.8	55.5
Later marriage	8.4	8.9	6.9	7.2
Separated	1.4	2.6	1.2	2.0
Divorced	3.4	5.6	2.9	5.1
Widowed	0.6	1.9	0.7	2.3
Weighted base	8 378	10 483	6 516	7 101
Missing	6	9		

Distribution of marital status

The distribution of the sample according to marital status shows some minor differences when compared with the GHS (1991) (Table 3.7). The differences are not confined to any particular age group. They may be due in part to the question format, which was designed with the analysis of sexual behaviour in mind, not simply the description of civil status. The categories were listed in the following order – married (and living with spouse), cohabiting with a partner of the opposite sex, cohabiting with a partner of the same sex, widowed, divorced, separated or single – and the interviewer was instructed to read the list only as far as necessary to elicit a response. Whether or not those who were married had been married before was discovered at a later question. This ordering lays greater emphasis on living arrangements than on civil status, so the data may not be strictly comparable with the GHS.

Distribution of socioeconomic groups

To compare socioeconomic groups with an external data source, the GHS is taken (Table 3.8) and a collapsed version of the 17-category OPCS classification is used. Excluded from the bases are full-time students, the armed forces and people who had never worked or could not be classified. Even so, the comparison is not exact for two reasons: the GHS figures for men cover the age group 16–64, and the present survey did not obtain occupation details for anyone who had not worked in the

Table 3.8. Distribution of socioeconomic group compared with GHS figures (%)
[Source: classification questions 7–10]

	NATSAL		GHS	
	Men	Women	Men*	Women
Professional	7.1	1.9	8.0	1.0
Employers and managers	20.5	10.1	20.0	9.0
Intermediate non-manual	8.9	17.0	10.0	19.0
Junior non-manual	10.2	35.2	7.0	33.0
Skilled manual and own account non-professional	35.0	6.7	37.0	8.0
Semi-skilled manual and personal services	14.6	23.4	14.0	23.0
Unskilled manual	3.6	5.6	3.0	6.0
Base	7 790	8 908	6 673	6 392

* Men aged 16–64.

previous 10 years. Despite the need for caution in pressing the comparison, the socioeconomic profiles obtained by the two surveys are quite close. The biggest difference occurred in the junior non-manual category – this survey had 3.2% more men and 2.2% more women in this group than did the GHS – but this was balanced by deficits in the categories immediately higher and lower.

Other external checks on validity

In addition to the comparisons of demographic characteristics, comparisons are made below between other items covered in the survey and the nearest equivalent data from external sources.

Height, weight and body mass index

One check on the validity of self-reported data concerned height, weight and body mass index (BMI). Respondents answered questions about their height and weight in whatever units they chose. For comparison, data from the Health and Lifestyle Survey (Cox, 1987) were used, in which qualified nurses weighed and measured a random sample of British respondents using standardized scales. Despite this difference in method of obtaining the measures, the results are reassuringly close (Table 3.9). Men reported a 2 cm excess and women a 1 cm excess in mean height compared with the Health and Lifestyle data. Small discrepancies (1.8 kg

Table 3.9. Comparison of reported and measured height, weight and BMI
[Source: interview, question 6]

	Men			Women		
	NATSAL (reported)		Health and Lifestyle (measured)	NATSAL (reported)		Health and Lifestyle (measured)
Height (m)						
Mean	1.77		1.75	1.63		1.62
SD*	0.073		0.075	0.069		0.065
Base†	7 975		2 493	9 996		3 122
Missing	33			48		
Weight (kg)						
Mean	77.1	77.1‡	75.3	63.1	62.7‡	62.7
SD	12.02	11.89‡	12.31	11.61	11.45‡	11.73
Base†	7 948	5 990‡	2 493	9 898	7 671‡	3 024
Missing	57			158		
BMI						
Mean	24.6		24.7	23.8		24.0
SD	3.47		3.73	4.43		4.32
Base†	7 922		2 493	9 870		3 024
Missing	84			189		

* Standard deviation.
† All respondents aged 18–59.
‡ Statistics restricted to respondents 'sure' of their weight.

for men and 0.4 kg for women) were also seen in mean weight, but when the analysis was restricted to those respondents who were sure of their weight, there was no difference in mean weight for women between self-reported and measured data. Comparisons of BMI (the ratio of weight in kilograms to the square of height in metres) were close, with mean discrepancies of 0.1 for men and 0.2 for women. The data show no major discrepancies and very little evidence of exaggeration of fashionable characteristics such as increased height for men or reduced BMI for women.

Therapeutic abortions

Female respondents were asked, in the self-completion booklet, about previous experience of termination of pregnancy. This is a relatively

Table 3.10. Abortions in the last year
[Source: booklet, question 14]

Age group	Rates per 1000 women aged 16–44		95% confidence interval	Base*	Missing
	Great Britain†	NATSAL			
16–19	25.2	23.5	14.5–35.0	953	25
20–24	27.1	21.4	14.1–31.5	1 208	56
25–29	18.1	14.5	8.9–22.0	1 460	76
30–34	12.0	8.9	4.8–16.2	1 292	71
35–39	7.5	6.1	2.3–12.0	1 199	77
40–44	2.7	4.0	1.3–9.5	1 225	76
Total	15.3	12.7	10.2–15.5	7 338	381

* All women respondents aged 16–44.
† OPCS (1991); Scottish Health Service (1991).

sensitive question and the reported rates can be compared with national data since therapeutic abortion is statutorily notifiable. Abortion rates calculated from the study data for women show a close approximation to national figures (OPCS, 1991; Botting, 1991; Scottish Health Service, 1991) (Table 3.10). There is a strong age trend, and for each 5-year age band the 95% confidence interval is consistent with the combined official notifications for England, Wales and Scotland.

There is the possibility that the national figures are inflated because a very small number of women have two abortions within a year and women from abroad may give addresses in Great Britain, thus reducing the validity of a direct comparison with data from this study. However, the relative completeness of reporting of therapeutic abortions contrasts markedly with studies carried out in the 1970s. Dunnell (1979) found that fewer than half the expected number of abortions were reported in her 1976 study of family formation in Britain, and a similar discrepancy was reported by Tietze & Dawson (1973) in New York.

Internal consistency of the data

A further measure of data validity is that of internal consistency between responses to different questions in the questionnaire. The questionnaire was designed in such a way that there were many opportunities for checking internal consistency. For example, respondents were asked to give information about homosexual experience during the face-to-face interview, using show-cards, and again in more detail in the self-completion booklet. This device deliberately provided more than one opportunity for disclosure. Thus an inconsistency could arise if a respondent felt more confident in reporting homosexual behaviour in the self-completion booklet than in the face-to-face interview. Such inconsistency may simply reflect the respondent's level of confidence in the anonymity of the method.

Inconsistency can also arise from memory error. For example, a respondent may have reported two sexual partners in the last 5 years, but when completing the detailed information on the three most recent partners may have discovered that, on reflection, three partners fell into the last 5 years.

In all, 185 inconsistency checks were carried out on each questionnaire. Of men, 78.6% had no inconsistencies, 19.2% had one or two and the remainder had between three and eight; of women, 82.4% had no inconsistencies, 16.2% had one or two and the remainder had between three and seven. Overall, the majority of the inconsistency codes had none or very few cases recorded against them; only 28 revealed 50 cases or more, half of which had 100 cases or more. The single most frequently occurring inconsistency (503 cases) was the reporting of one sexual partner ever in the interview and two or more partners in the self-completion booklet. Within the self-completion booklet, 230 respondents reported homosexual experience that was not recorded in the face-to-face interview. Also, within the data obtained in the booklet there were some inconsistencies between the recency of the last sexual intercourse and the recency of particular sexual practices.

These findings indicate that, in general, respondents were more willing to reveal socially censured behaviour in the self-completion booklet than in the face-to-face interview, confirming that the decision to use this method for the most sensitive questions had been appropriate.

Statistical considerations

Sampling errors

As with most personal interview surveys, a simple random sample of addresses was not a viable possibility for practical and economic reasons. A systematic multistage sample design was chosen as a good approximation, and this resulted in clusters of addresses within local authority wards. However, the standard statistical techniques used throughout the analysis of the data assume that the sample was obtained from a simple random sample of the parent population. The effect of the departure from simple random sampling in terms of precision can be estimated from the ratio of the true variance (incorporating the clustered design of the sample) to the variance calculated under the assumption of simple random sampling (Groves, 1989). The design factor (DEFT) is defined as the square root of this ratio. The values of DEFT can be used simply as multipliers to adjust the values of the individual standard errors obtained under the assumption of simple random sampling to give an estimate of the true standard error allowing for the design effect of the sampling procedure. This leads to an assessment of the loss of precision inherent in the sample design for individual variables.

Complex standard errors and DEFT values have been calculated (using the software CLUSTERS; Verna & Pearce, 1986) for a selection of demographic and sexual behaviour variables. A DEFT value of 1 implies that the clustered sample has the same precision as a simple random sample of the same size. Departures from 1 show the increasing effect of the sample design. Occasionally DEFT can take a value less than 1, which seems to be anomalous. However, the variance estimates are themselves subject to sampling variation. It is theoretically possible for a clustered sample to yield greater precision than a simple random sample, but DEFT values less than 1 are unlikely to occur.

For the demographic variables (Appendix 3, Table A3.3), the values of DEFT range from 1.034 (for men looking after the home full-time) to 1.955 (for Asian women). This range of values compares favourably with those obtained by other surveys (Heath *et al.*, 1985). Those few values of DEFT greater than 1.5 are for variables to do with race and religion. This is due to the geographically clustered distribution of people from particular ethnic groups; religious affiliation is closely associated with ethnic group. Sexual behaviour variables are shown in the same format in Appendix Table A3.4 and show DEFT values ranging from 1.064 (for women with three or four heterosexual partners) to 1.349 (for women who used no contraception at their first heterosexual intercourse). These values span a narrower range of values than the demographic variables.

Statistical presentation of the data

All results are presented separately for men and women and they are derived from weighted data. The weights are not integers, but the bases have been rounded to the nearest integer and there may be small rounding errors in the bases. Similarly, percentages may sometimes add to slightly more or slightly less than 100, due to rounding.

Respondents have been assigned to a social class using the same procedure as the 1981 census, with three main exceptions. First, where respondents are economically active, either their current or previous occupation has been used to allocate a social class, but, unlike the census, only if this occupation was within the last 10 years. Secondly, a person on a Government scheme is classified with respect to their previous job, if they have had one. Finally, if a person is unemployed but waiting to take up a job, then the future job is used for classification. If respondents are married or living with a partner, then their partner's occupation is classified in the same way. In the majority of analyses, 'household social class' has been used. This is represented by the respondent's or partner's social class, whichever is the higher. For the remainder, social class is allocated on the basis of the respondent's occupation. The use of a household social class does have several advantages, but there remains the problem of young people who have never worked and therefore cannot be classified.

Key variables are tabulated for a standard selection of demographic characteristics in Tables in Appendix 3, where missing values are listed explicitly (but not included in the calculation of percentages). More detailed analyses within each chapter have been carried out after excluding missing values. Throughout the handling of the data, no assumptions were made about any missing items, with a few key exceptions, intrinsic to the questionnaire. From the structure of the questionnaire (Appendix 1) it is clear that a number of skips were made in order to avoid redundant questions. This structure has been incorporated into the assumptions that can be made about questions that were skipped. For example, 3.8% of men and 3.4% of women reported in the face-to-face interview that they had never had heterosexual intercourse (question 19a) and no homosexual experience (question 31b), so they were not asked to complete the booklet. The assumption was then made that they had had no homosexual or heterosexual partners, and the self-completion questions were interpreted accordingly.

No formal hypotheses have been tested on the bivariate analyses but a range of multivariate techniques had been used for data reduction and formal hypothesis testing. Broad attitudinal variables have been constructed by combining the responses to particular questions on attitudes to sexual behaviour using principal components. Events that may not have taken place yet, such as age at first sex, have been analysed using survival analysis. Logistic regression has been used to explore the relationships between dichotomous response variables and a variety of explanatory variables. The results have been presented as odds ratios (with 95% confidence intervals) adjusted for all other factors in the model. An odds ratio of 1 implies equivalence of risk; therefore, where the 95% confidence interval includes 1, the results are consistent with there being no excess (or reduced) risk.

Summary

This survey of 18876 individuals was carried out over the period May 1990 to November 1991, using a systematic probability sample drawn from the PAF. The achieved sample was broadly representative of the population of Great Britain aged 16–59. The response rate was in line with many sample surveys on various aspects of social behaviour as well as those on sexual behaviour. When compared with other official and sample survey sources, frequency distributions over a number of variables, including demographic information, are similar. In common with most other sample surveys, however, the possibility of bias cannot be ruled out completely. Internal consistency between different data items is high, particularly since the information sought was complex, sensitive and, in some cases, distant in time.

References

Botting, B. (1991) Trends in abortion. *Population Trends*, **64**, 19–29.
Catania, J.A., Coates, T.J., Stall, R. *et al.* (1992) Prevalence of risk related factors and condom use in the United States. *Science*, **258**, 1001–6.
Cox, B. (1987) Body measurements (heights, weights, girth, etc.). Chapter 4. In Cox, B.D., Blaxter, M., Buckle, A.L.S. *et al.* Health and Lifestyle Survey. Health Promotion Research Trust, London.
Dunnell, K. (1979) *Family Formation 1976*. HMSO, London.
Farrell, C. (1978) *My Mother Said . . . The Way Young People Learned about Sex and Birth Control*. Routledge & Kegan Paul, London.
Fay, R.E., Turner, C.F., Klassen, A.D. & Gagnon, J.H. (1989) Prevalence and patterns of same gender sexual contact among men. *Science*, **243**, 338–48.
General Social Survey (1988) Number of sex partners and potential risk of sexual exposure to Human Immunodeficiency Virus. *Morbidity and Mortality Weekly*, **37**, 565–8.
Gorer, G. (1971) *Sex and Marriage in England Today*. Nelson, London.
Groves, R. (1989) *Survey Errors and Survey Costs*. Wiley, New York.
Heath, A.F., Jowell, R.M. & Curtice, J.K. (1985) *How Britain Votes*. Pergamon Press, Oxford.
Johnson, A.M., Wadsworth, J., Wellings, K., Bradshaw, S.A. & Field, J. (1992) Sexual lifestyles and HIV risk. *Nature*, **360**, 410–12.
Jowell, R., Witherspoon, S. & Brook, L. (1990) *British Social Attitudes: The Seventh Report*. Gower, London.
Kish, L. (1949) A procedure for objective respondent selection within the household. *Journal of the American Statistical Association*, **44**, 380–7.
Kraft, P., Rise, J. & Gronnesby, J. (1989) Prediction of sexual behaviour in a group of young Norwegian adults. *NIPH Annals*, **12**(2), 27–44.
McQueen, D.V., Robertson, B.J. & Nisbel, L. (1991) *Data Update: AIDS-Related Behaviour Knowledge and Attitudes, Provisional Dates*. No. 27. RUHBC. University of Edinburgh, Edinburgh.
Melbye, M. & Biggar, R.J. (1992) Interactions between persons at risk for AIDS and the general population of Denmark. *American Journal of Epidemiology*, **135**, 593–602.
Office of Population Censuses and Surveys (1980) *Classification of Occupations*. HMSO, London.

Office of Population Censuses and Surveys (1990) *Labour Force Survey, 1989*. HMSO, London.

Office of Population Censuses and Surveys (1991) *Abortion Statistics. Legal Abortions Carried out under the 1967 Abortion Act in England and Wales, 1990*. HMSO, London.

Office of Population Censuses and Surveys (1991) *General Household Survey, 1989*. HMSO, London.

Office of Population Censuses and Surveys (1993) *1991 Census. Age, Sex and Marital Status*. HMSO, London.

Platek, R. & Gray, G.B. (1986) On the definitions of response bias. *Survey Methodology*, **12**, 12–27.

Ross, M. (1988) Prevalence of classes of risk behaviour for HIV infection in a randomly selected Australian population. *Journal of Sex Research*, **25**, 441–50.

Schofield, M. (1968) *The Sexual Behaviour of Young People*. Longman, London.

Schofield, M. (1973) *The Sexual Behaviour of Young Adults*. Allen Lane, London.

Scottish Health Service (1991) Scottish Health Statistics. ISD Publications, Edinburgh.

Smith, T. (1988) A methodological review of the sexual behaviour questions on the 1988 and 1989 GSS. *National Opinion Research Centre University of Chicago GSS Methodological Report 65*.

Spencer, L., Faulkner, A. & Keegan, J. (1988) *Talking about Sex*. Social and Community Planning Research, London.

Spira, A., Bajos, N. & ACSF Investigators (1993) *Les comportements sexuels en France*. La documentation Française, Paris.

Sundet, J., Kvalem, I., Magnus, P. & Bakketeig, L. (1988) Prevalence of risk-prone sexual behaviour in the general population of Norway. In Fleming, A.F., Carbaliv, M. & Fitzsimons, D.F. (eds) *The Global Impact of AIDS*, pp. 53–60. Alan R. Liss, London.

Tietze, C. & Dawson, D.A. (1973) *Induced Abortion: A Fact Book. Reports on Population/Family Planning, 14*. The Population Council, New York.

Van Zessen, G. & Sandfort, T. (1991) *Seksualiteit in Nederland*. Swets & Zeitlinger.

Verna, V. & Pearce, N. (1986) CLUSTERS (a package program for the computation of sampling errors for clustered samples, version 3). *International Statistics Institute, ISIRC Technical Report: 131*.

Wellings, K., Field, J., Wadsworth, J. *et al.* (1990) Sexual lifestyles under scrutiny. *Nature*, **348**, 276–8.

Chapter 4
First Intercourse between Men and Women

KAYE WELLINGS & SALLY BRADSHAW

There seems little doubt that first sexual intercourse remains an event of immense social and personal significance. The status of virginity, which is still of great cultural and legal importance, is technically defined in terms of experience of sexual intercourse. The apparent ease with which individuals are able to recall the first occasion on which coitus took place (fewer than 1% of respondents were unable to do so) also testifies to the fact that it is a memorable event. In addition, the event has major health implications, since it marks initiation into the sexual act, which, unprotected, carries a risk of adverse outcomes, such as unplanned pregnancy and sexually transmitted infection. The importance of collecting robust data on early sexual experience to guide the provision of services and the design of educational and preventive strategies is particularly important in Britain, where levels of teenage pregnancy are higher than in other countries in Europe (Jones *et al.*, 1985).

In relation to early sexual experience, the occurrence of first intercourse – its timing, the circumstances that surround it and its consequences – is therefore of central interest in the context of this study. At the same time, this one event alone is likely to be an unreliable indicator of the onset of sexual activity generally. Sexual behaviour involves a variety of practices which do not necessarily culminate in intercourse. Sexual practices that may be seen as preliminary to intercourse for many older adults may, for younger people, be an end in themselves. As a result, data were collected on age at first sexual experience as well as age at first sexual intercourse. This chapter describes only first heterosexual experiences. The timing of homosexual experiences is discussed in Chapter 7.

Questions asked

Two questions were asked in the face-to-face section of the questionnaire eliciting reports of early sexual behaviour. Respondents were handed show-cards on which were printed the questions: '*How old were you when you first had sexual intercourse with someone of the opposite sex or hasn't this happened?*', and '*How old were you when you first had any type of experience of a sexual kind – for example, kissing, cuddling, petting – with someone of the opposite sex (or hasn't this happened either)?'* In addition, respondents were asked the age of their partner at the time, whether it was also their first time, and whether contraception was used. Additional questions probing the nature of the relationship, the circumstances surrounding the event and feelings about its occurrence were asked only of those receiving the longer version of the questionnaire (see Chapter 2). This accounts for the major differences in bases throughout the present chapter.

It was not one of the aims of this survey to explore the extent and circumstances of sexual intercourse that occurred in childhood, and the research instrument used would have been inadequate and inappropriate to the task. Consequently, although respondents were initially asked when they had had sexual intercourse for the first time *ever*, they were asked to confine subsequent accounts to their first experience of intercourse *after* the age of 13 (1.2% of men and 0.4% of women reported experiencing sexual intercourse before the age of 13). All the following analysis in this chapter refers to intercourse that took place after the age of 13.

Age at first intercourse

By current age

Since first intercourse occurs only once in a lifetime, analysis of the data from successive birth cohorts in the sample allows secular trends to be described with some confidence. Experience of the event cannot change throughout a person's lifetime, though reflections on and attitudes towards the reporting of it can. The existing literature on the subject already provided evidence of major changes in age of first sexual intercourse during recent decades (e.g. Schofield, 1965; Farrell, 1978; Dunnell, 1979). Three trends were identified: a progressive reduction over the years in the age at which first intercourse occurs; an increase in the proportion of young women who have had sexual intercourse before the age of sexual consent; and a convergence in the behaviour of men and women.

The decline in the age at which first intercourse occurs

As Table 4.1 and Fig. 4.1 clearly show, one of the most striking trends to emerge from these data is the strong relationship between current age and age at first intercourse. Age at first intercourse decreases with the current age of the respondent, becoming successively lower in the more recent birth cohorts.

Analysis by 5-year age groups (Table 4.1) shows clearly the pattern

made to assess the degree of correspondence between women's recollections in this survey and those collected contemporaneously in others. In 1964, 14% of the boys and 5% of the girls in Schofield's sample of young people aged 15–19 reported having had sexual intercourse by the age of 16. In the corresponding sample aged 41–45 at the time of interview in this survey, 14% of men and 4% of women had had sexual intercourse by the age of 16. Similarly, 31% of the boys and 12% of the girls in Farrell's sample of young people aged 15–19 in 1974 reported having had intercourse by the age of 16, compared with 21% of men and 9% of women in the corresponding age group (those aged 31–35) in our sample. (Farrell notes a possible tendency for boys to exaggerate their sexual experience at the time of reporting.)

The dramatic decrease in age at first intercourse over recent years is equally marked for age at first sexual experience (Table 4.2); the median age has dropped from 16 to 14 for women and from 15 to 13 for men through successive age cohorts from 45–59 to 16–24. The data indicate that sexual experience in the broader sense tends to precede sexual intercourse by some time. While only 2.7% of women and 9.3% of men of all ages had experienced sexual intercourse before the age of 15, 33.8% and 55.8% respectively reported having had some sexual experience before this age. Not surprisingly, as Table 4.3 shows, the age at which first sexual experience occurs tends to be strongly associated with the age at first intercourse. For men whose first sexual experience

Table 4.2. Age at first experience and first intercourse by age group and gender [Source: interview, questions 19a,b]

	Median age				Median time lag between (1) and (2)	Base
	First experience (1)	Base	First intercourse (2)	Base		
Men						
16–24	13	1 462	17	1 475	3	1 397
25–34	14	2 336	17	2 340	3	2 299
35–44	14	2 105	18	2 111	3	2 070
45–59	15	2 046	19	2 054	4	2 000
Women						
16–24	14	1 842	17	1 867	2	1 795
25–34	15	3 223	18	3 236	2	3 192
35–44	15	2 558	18	2 569	3	2 537
45–59	16	2 916	20	2 937	4	2 822

Table 4.3. Quartiles for age at first intercourse by age at first experience
[Source: interview, question 19b]

Age of first intercourse	Median			Base
	1st	2nd	3rd	
Men				
<13	15	16	18	1 982
13–15	16	17	18	3 571
16–17	18	19	21	1 452
18–19	19	21	24	461
20–24	22	24	26	229
25+	26	28	30	83
Women				
<13	15	17	18	818
13–15	16	17	19	4 599
16–17	17	19	21	3 373
18–19	19	20	22	1 103
20–24	21	22	24	432
25+	26	28	33	88

occurred before the age of 13, the median age at first intercourse was 16, compared with a median of 19 for those for whom it occurred between 16 and 17.

The interval between first experience and first intercourse seems to be diminishing over time, more markedly for women than men (Table 4.2). The median time lapse between the two events for women in the age group 45–59 was 4 years or more, 2 years longer than for women aged 16–24, and for men, 4 years for those in the oldest age group, and 3 for those in the youngest.

First intercourse before the age of 16

Alongside a decline in the median age of first intercourse can be seen a parallel increase in the proportion of young people experiencing sexual intercourse before the age of 16 (Fig. 4.1 & Table 4.4) (16 is the age for a woman before which a man is acting unlawfully if he has sexual intercourse with her — see p. 230).

A sizeable minority of young people are now sexually active before 16 (Table 4.4). Of women aged 16–19, 18.7% had experienced sexual intercourse before the age of 16 compared with fewer than 1% of those aged over 55–59; for men the equivalent proportions are higher — 27.6% of men in the youngest age group compared with 5.8% of men aged 55–59

Gender differences in age at first experience

There is a widespread belief that men differ from women in sexual behaviour, that they have a higher sex drive and a lower tolerance of sexual
abstinence, and that they are more easily sexually aroused (Bancroft,
1989). However, a shift towards greater convergence between the sexes is
documented in recent literature on the subject, particularly that from the
USA. Several studies in the past two decades have shown a decline in
differences in attitudes and behaviour between men and women, towards
a single standard for both (Christiansen & Gregg, 1970; Robinson &
Jedlicka, 1982; Orr *et al.*, 1989).

This trend seems to be broadly confirmed in this survey, although the
convergence between men and women is more apparent in the data for
first intercourse than in those for first sexual experience (Table 4.2). First
intercourse still takes place later for women than for men, but the gap
between the sexes has been closing in recent birth cohorts. For those over
the age of 25 at the time of interview, the median age for men is 1 year
earlier than it is for women, whilst for those under the age of 25 the
median is the same for both sexes (Table 4.1). The gap between men and
women also narrows with respect to the proportions reporting first intercourse under the age of 16 (Table 4.4). Compared with women, the
proportion of men who are sexually active before 16 is higher in all age
groups, but the ratio of men to women who experienced intercourse
before the age of 16 has narrowed from 7:1 in the oldest age group
(55–59), to 1.5:1 in the youngest (16–19).

The data for first intercourse for successive birth cohorts, then, show a
consistent pattern of decreasing age at first occurrence, together with an
increase in the proportions with experience before the age of 16, and
some convergence in the behaviour of men and women over time. These
trends are likely to reflect a combination of maturational effects and
social influences on sexual behaviour. Although it is not possible from
these data to attempt any conclusive explanation of these trends, some
attempt can be made to assess the interplay between biological and
cultural factors.

Biological effects

A trend towards earlier physical maturity, together with a progressive
relaxation in social mores governing sexual intercourse, could result in
the effects of biological and cultural influences being additive. An attempt
was made to separate biological–maturational from social–historical effects. Although there is no single reliable marker of sexual maturation in
men, menarche offers a useful indicator in women. If biological readiness

Table 4.5. Quartiles for age at first sexual experience by age at menarche

| Age at menarche | Median | | | Base |
	1st	2nd	3rd	
10 or younger	14	15	16	394
11–12	14	15	16	3 615
13–14	14	15	17	4 615
15 or older	15	16	17	1 564

Table 4.6. Quartiles for age at first sexual intercourse by age at menarche
[Source: interview, question 33b; booklet, question 21]

| Age at menarche | Median | | | Base |
	1st	2nd	3rd	
10 or younger	16	18	20	397
11–12	16	18	20	3 637
13–14	17	18	20	4 638
15 or older	17	19	21	1 579

played a major role, then some correlation between age at first inter-course and age of menarche, together with a decline in the age of menarche in recent decades, could be expected. In contrast to some US studies, which have shown little association between age at menarche and onset of sexual activity except amongst black teenagers (Kantner & Zelnick, 1972; Udry *et al.*, 1986), these data show a significant correlation between the two events (Tables 4.5 & 4.6). Median age at first sexual experience and first sexual intercourse for women who first menstruate at 15 or older is 1 year later than for those who do so under the age of 15.

Over the past century, age at menarche has declined in most developed countries. In 1900, the average age was probably around 14, and it has decreased steadily since (Tanner, 1962), levelling off in recent generations. These data show a small but significant fall in the mean age of menarche (Table 4.7) between the oldest age group (45–59) and women under 45.* Nineteen per cent of women aged 45–59 began

* Analysis of variance showed a significant difference at the 1% level between the mean age at menarche for the age group 45–49 and the three younger age groups. Half a year was added to the reported age at menarche when the means were calculated to take account of the fact that menarche reported at age 13, for example, could have occurred at any time between the ages of 13 and 14.

Table 4.7. Mean age at menarche by age group
[Source: interview, question 33b; booklet, question 21]

Age at interview	Mean age at menarche	95% confidence interval	Base
16–24	13.40	13.33–13.47	2 172
25–34	13.42	13.37–13.47	2 810
35–44	13.41	13.35–13.47	2 481
45–59	13.54	13.48–13.60	2 606

Table 4.8. Age at menarche by age group
[Source: interview, question 33b; booklet, question 21]

	Age at interview				
Age at menarche	16–24 (%)	25–34 (%)	35–44 (%)	45–59 (%)	All ages (%)
10 or younger	2.8	3.5	4.2	3.9	3.6
11–12	37.0	35.2	36.2	34.5	35.7
13–14	47.7	46.8	44.7	42.8	45.4
15 or older	12.6	14.5	14.9	18.8	15.3
Base	2 172	2 810	2 481	2 606	10 069

menstruating after their 15th birthday, compared with 12.6% of those aged 16–24. However, the percentage of women in this older age group who reported menstruating before the age of 11 was also greater than for the youngest age group (Table 4.8 & Fig. 4.4).

The data do not, however, show a marked fall in the age of menstruation, and certainly not on a scale sufficient to explain the scale of the changes in age at first intercourse. Despite the relationship between biological readiness and age at occurrence, the decline in the age at menstruation with successive age groups is not large enough to account for much of the decline in age at first intercourse in recent decades.†

† Combining the effect of current age and age at menarche in a life-table analysis shows that both are significant, but the log rank χ^2 statistics (1213 and 64) show that the effect of current age is stronger. In a stepwise analysis, current age entered the model first ($\chi^2 = 1213$), followed by age at menarche ($\chi^2 = 56$), indicating a strong association between current age and age at first intercourse and, in addition, a weaker association between age at menarche and age at first intercourse.

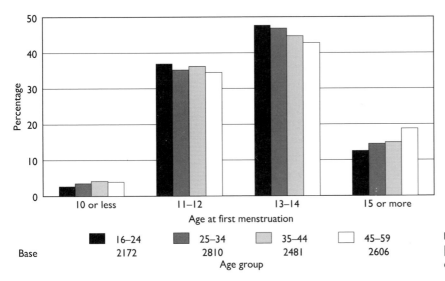

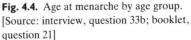

Fig. 4.4. Age at menarche by age group. [Source: interview, question 33b; booklet, question 21]

Cultural influences

Given the importance of social factors in determining the start of sexual experience, the historical backcloth against which these changes have taken place is of interest here. Amongst other things, the past three decades have seen marked changes in the employment status of women, a series of legal reforms in the 1960s liberalizing sexual behaviour (the Abortion Law Reform Act in 1967, for example), the advent of effective contraception and the extension of family planning services. Of these, the factor that is often held to be of paramount importance in explaining trends in first sexual intercourse is the availability of reliable birth control, in particular oral contraception. A number of empirical studies carried out in the 1970s found no association between pill use and sexual activity (Black & Sykes, 1971; Settlage *et al.*, 1973; Akpom *et al.*, 1976; Garris *et al.*, 1976; Reichelt, 1978). A more recent survey of Scottish women favours factors other than oral contraception as an explanation for the fall in age at first intercourse (Bone, 1986), and these survey data seem to support those conclusions. As Table 4.1 shows, age at first intercourse has declined progressively through each age group, but not uniformly so. As noted above, the fall is most marked for the older age groups. Median age at first intercourse is 2 years higher, at 21 years, for women aged 55–59 than it is for those 10 years younger. Thus the steepest decline occurred during the 1950s. Median age of first intercourse fell as much during this one decade as it was to do over the next 30 years. This irregular pattern is also apparent in the data for men.

A common assumption is that the advent of reliable birth control

methods (in the form of oral contraception) preceded and probably facilitated a lowering of age at first intercourse, by removing one of the
most powerful deterrents – the fear of unwanted pregnancy – from the
sexual act (Ayd, 1969). Yet although the pill was prescribed as early as
1961, it was not available in practice for unmarried women until 1972,
and it was not available regardless of ability to pay until 1975, so that the
women in the sample whose experience contributed to the most dramatic
fall in age at first intercourse would have been largely unaffected by these
events. This is not to say that efficient and accessible contraception has
not been influential in the lowering of age at first intercourse, but we
must look to other factors to explain the steep decline during the 1950s. It
seems as likely that legal and technological advance has occurred in
response to changing mores, as the reverse.

These data provide no evidence of a sexual revolution co-terminous
with the decade of the 1960s.

The influence of social class and education

Appendix Table A4.1 and Table 4.9 indicate marked variation with social
class, particularly for men. The median age at first intercourse for men of
all ages in social class I is 19, 3 years later than for men in social class V,
and for women in social class I it is 20, 2 years later than for women in
social class V. This relationship is not easily interpreted since social class is
measured at the time of interview, following a varying interval since first
intercourse. In the case of older respondents, the occupation recorded,
on which their social classification is based, is their current one, and may
be different from occupation at the time of first intercourse. Younger
respondents still in full-time education will be categorized as students, so
that their social class status will be as yet undetermined.

Findings of previous studies are equivocal on the relationship between
social class and age at first intercourse. Kinsey's data (Kinsey *et al.*, 1948,
1953) indicate striking social class differences: working class adolescents
experienced sexual intercourse at an earlier age than those from the
middle classes. However, more recent US studies have noted a lessening
of social class influences over time (Kantner & Zelnick, 1972; Fisher &
Byrne, 1981). Surveys of young German workers and students carried out
at the same time similarly indicate the disappearance of social class
differences in age at onset of sexual experience (Schmidt & Sigusch, 1971,
1972).

In Britain, however, social class differences seem to have persisted
later than in the USA and elsewhere in Europe. Studies in the 1970s
found age at first intercourse to be earlier amongst young people from
working class backgrounds than amongst those from middle class back-

Table 4.9. Median age at first intercourse by social class within age group
[Source: interview, question 19a]

Age group:	16–24								25–34							
Social class:	I	II	III NM	III M	IV	V	Other	Base	I	II	III NM	III M	IV	V	Other	Base
Men	18	17	17	16	16	16	18	1 472	18	17	17	16	16	16	18	2 337
Women	18	17	17	17	16	16	17	1 863	19	18	18	17	17	17	17	3 230

Age group:	35–44								45–59							
Social class:	I	II	III NM	III M	IV	V	Other	Base	I	II	III NM	III M	IV	V	Other	Base
Men	19	18	18	17	18	17	16	2 108	21	19	19	18	18	17	18	2 047
Women	19	19	18	18	18	18	18	2 565	22	20	20	19	20	20	20	2 933

grounds (Farrell, 1978; Dunnell, 1979), as have more recent studies (Forman & Chilvers, 1989; West *et al.*, 1993). Certainly, stratification of these data by age group (Table 4.9) shows no clear evidence of any lessening of social class effect through successive age cohorts, except perhaps for the oldest age group of men aged 45–59 at interview, amongst whom the social class effect was more marked than for men aged under 45.

There is evidence here that the trend towards diminishing differences between men and women in age at first intercourse identified above (p. 70), in common with many other behavioural trends, may have begun earlier among those in upper social class groups. For those aged 45–59, the median age at first intercourse for women in all social class groups is higher than it is for men, but the difference is greater the lower the social class. The gender difference is 3 years in social class V and 1 year in social classes I–III. By contrast, median age at first intercourse is the same for both men and women in the 16–24 age range, regardless of social class (with the exception of social class III manual). We see here another indication of a trend hinted at elsewhere in this book, of a general convergence between men and women with respect to sexual behaviour in specific subgroups of the population.

The relationship between age at first intercourse and social class is of interest in the context of cervical cancer. Epidemiological studies have suggested the importance of early sexual experience with multiple partners in the aetiology of this disease, the incidence of which is higher amongst women in lower social class groups (Boyd & Doll, 1964; Wynder, 1969). Recent studies exploring this relationship have found that although working class women experienced sexual intercourse earlier, social class had no obvious impact upon numbers of sexual partners (if anything, working class women accumulated fewer sexual partners than those in higher social classes), suggesting that early age at first intercourse, rather than multiple partners, may be a more useful focus in explaining the higher incidence of cervical cancer amongst working class women (Harris *et al.*, 1980; Brown *et al.*, 1984; Mant *et al.*, 1988). The data from this survey on the relationship between social class and both age at first intercourse and numbers of sexual partners (see Chapter 5) add further support to these conclusions.

US data show that age at first sexual intercourse also increases with educational level (e.g. Klassen *et al.*, 1981). The interaction between age at first intercourse, education, social class and current age of respondent is complex. Social class and education are clearly interrelated, and both are related to current age, as people acquire qualifications and move through social grades during their lifetime. At the same time, educational level also decreases with increasing age, with the secular trend towards spending longer in full-time education. It is assumed that educational level will influence age at first intercourse. However, in many cases young people will experience first intercourse before completing their education, and it might equally be the case that the age at which the event occurs might itself wield an effect on the level of educational achievement.

The differential according to educational level (represented by highest qualification achieved) is apparent for all ages and both sexes (Table 4.10). Median age at first intercourse increases with educational level, and the effect is particularly marked for graduates. The major difference between graduates and non-graduates is also manifest in the analysis of intercourse before the age of 16. Compared with their graduate peers, non-graduate men are more than three times as likely to have sex before their 16th birthday, and non-graduate women more than one and a half times as likely. Only one in four male graduates had experienced sexual intercourse before the age of 18, compared with more than half non-graduates.

Multivariate analysis was used to assess the strength of the relationship between first intercourse before 16 and current age, social class and educational level. Although education and social class are related, they each have an independent effect on age at first intercourse once the effects of current age have been accounted for, that of education being stronger than that of social class. This analysis confirmed the association between education to at least O level standard and a reduced likelihood

Table 4.10. Median age at first intercourse by education within age group
[Source: interview, question 19a]

Age group:	16–24						25–34					
Education:	Degree	A level	O level/CSE	Other	None	Base	Degree	A level	O level/CSE	Other	None	Base
Men	18	17	16	17	16	1 471	18	17	17	17	16	2 334
Women	18	17	17	17	16	1 862	19	18	17	18	17	3 228

Age group:	35–44						45–59					
Education:	Degree	A level	O level/CSE	Other	None	Base	Degree	A level	O level/CSE	Other	None	Base
Men	19	18	17	17	17	2 104	21	19	19	18	18	2 041
Women	20	19	18	18	18	2 566	21	21	20	20	20	2 931

of intercourse before 16. The relationship between social class and age at first intercourse is likely to be more tenuous, since social class measures current rather than contemporary socioeconomic status.

The influence of ethnic group

The relationship between racial origin and age at first intercourse is similarly complex. Ethnic influences appear to have an important effect on adolescent sexual behaviour through cultural or contextual mechanisms (Furstenberg *et al.*, 1987), but they may also operate through structural factors influencing family income and marital status. Table 4.11 shows the relationship between race and religion and first intercourse before 16. As can be seen, those of Pakistani, Bangladeshi and Indian origin are much less likely to report sexual intercourse having occurred before the age of 16 than are those from other ethnic groups, and this is especially marked for women, little more than 1% of whom report first intercourse before this age. Black men and women are more likely to report sexual intercourse before the age of 16, though the excess for women is more marginal. US data have also shown that black Americans begin sexual experience earlier than white Americans (Klassen *et al.*, 1981; Hofferth, 1988).

Not surprisingly, median age at first intercourse is higher for Asian groups and lower for blacks, compared with whites (Appendix 3, Table

Table 4.11. Proportion of respondents reporting first sexual intercourse before 16 by ethnic group and religion
[Source: interview, question 19a]

	Men		Women	
	(%)	Base	(%)	Base
Ethnic group				
White	18.9	7749	8.0	9760
Black	26.3	157	9.6	218
Pakistani, Bangladeshi, Indian	10.7	186	1.1	189
Other	14.0	120	5.0	139
All ethnic groups	18.8	8212	7.9	10307
Religion				
Church of England	13.4	2039	5.1	3403
Roman Catholic	19.5	731	5.1	1171
Other Christian	14.6	882	5.7	1538
Non-Christian	10.8	342	4.6	383
None	22.7	4240	12.3	3834
All religious groups	18.8	8234	7.8	10329

A4.1). What is of interest is that gender differences are more pronounced for minority ethnic groups. Whilst the median age at first intercourse for those who are white is 18 for both men and women, for those who are black it is 17 for men and 18 for women, and for Asians it is 20 for men and 21 for women.

The relationship between religion and early intercourse is also explored in Table 4.11. Those reporting no religious affiliation were more likely to experience intercourse before the age of 16, and the differences are more marked for women than men. Respondents belonging to the Church of England or other Christian Churches (excluding the Roman Catholic Church) were less likely to experience sexual intercourse before the age of 16, and those from non-Christian religions even less likely to do so. More surprisingly perhaps, given the position of the Roman Catholic Church on sexual behaviour, those reporting Roman Catholic affiliation are no less likely than those reporting other affiliations to report intercourse before the age of 16, and if anything slightly more so. It is possible that the effects of religious beliefs and sexual behaviour are reciprocal. Sexual behaviour may reflect the influence of religion, but the converse might also be true, as religious beliefs which do not support a preferred pattern of behaviour may be allowed to lapse. These bivariate relationships are likely to be confounded by other effects, and particularly

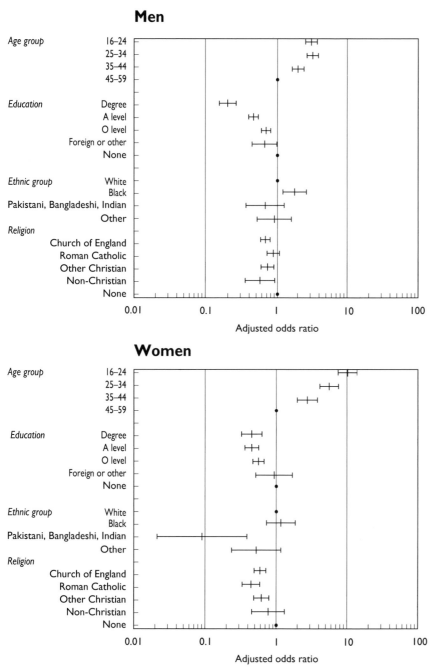

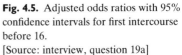

Fig. 4.5. Adjusted odds ratios with 95% confidence intervals for first intercourse before 16.
[Source: interview, question 19a]

that of age, since temporal trends in religious affiliation have changed over time, along with falling age at first intercourse.

A logistic regression model was used to look at the relationship between current age, religion, race and educational qualifications and the likelihood of first intercourse occurring before the age of 16. The adjusted odds ratios and their 95% confidence intervals are shown in Fig. 4.5. Social class was not included in this analysis because of its close association with educational qualifications, and because of the possibly greater relevance of education to early intercourse. For both men and women, age remained the most important factor; increasing age at interview was associated with decreasing likelihood of reporting first sexual intercourse before the age of 16. For both men and women, intercourse before the age of 16 was less likely to have occurred if the respondent was educated at least to O level or if any religious affiliation was acknowledged (except Roman Catholic for men and non-Christian for women). First sexual intercourse before 16 was less likely for women of Pakistani, Indian or Bangladeshi racial origin (the confidence intervals are wide due to the relatively small numbers in this category) and more likely for men who were black.

Regional differences

It should be noted that information on regions is related to the current residence of respondents, and in a mobile population it cannot be assumed that this is where first intercourse occurred. This might partly account for the absence of clear regional differences in the data. According to popular stereotypes, it might be expected that first intercourse would take place earlier on average in the 'permissive' South than in the 'puritanical' North. Our data show no sign of this (Appendix 3, Table A4.1). Median age for women in East Anglia and Scotland is 1 year later than for those in other areas, but there is no clear pattern for men. Nor in these data does there seem to be the clear rural–urban divide found in other data, where age at first intercourse is earlier in cities compared with the country (Klassen *et al.*, 1981; Ford & Bowie, 1989).

Contraception at first intercourse

The risks of unplanned pregnancy amongst the young make the question of contraception at first intercourse an important focus in the context of sexual health. Contraceptive use at first intercourse varies both with current age and with age at which the event occurred. Since there is also a relationship between current age and age at first intercourse, there is clearly the potential for some confounding of these effects.

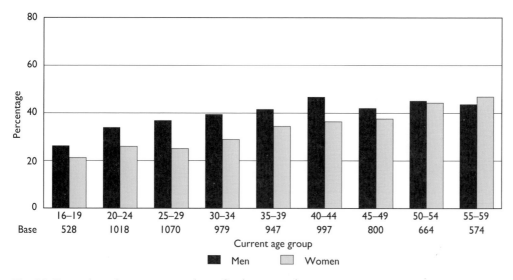

Fig. 4.6. Proportion using no contraception at first intercourse by current age.
[Source: interview, question 23]

As Fig. 4.6 shows, men are more likely than women, and older
respondents more likely than younger ones, to report not having used
contraception at first intercourse. Non-use of contraception at first intercourse has declined steadily over recent decades, and was reported by
fewer than a quarter of women and fewer than a third of men aged
16–24. Failure to use contraception does not necessarily signify risk of
unplanned pregnancy; a proportion of respondents – higher in older age
groups (see p. 95) – were married at first intercourse and may have
intended to become pregnant. (Failure to recall of contraceptive practice
at first intercourse is low for all respondents and only marginally higher
for the older respondents.)

The likelihood of no contraception being used also varies with age at
first intercourse (Fig. 4.7). Where intercourse occurs before 16, nearly
half of young women and more than half of young men report no method
used either by themselves or by their partner. This proportion falls
sharply to 32% of women and 36% of men aged 16 and over at first
intercourse. This might reflect a lack of confidence to seek contraceptive
supplies or advice or, alternatively, the sporadic nature of sexual activity
in this age group. It emphasizes the particular vulnerability of this group
to unplanned pregnancy.

With regard to specific methods, the evidence is that the condom is
the most commonly used method of contraception at first intercourse, and
that its use has been increasing over recent years. Condoms are more

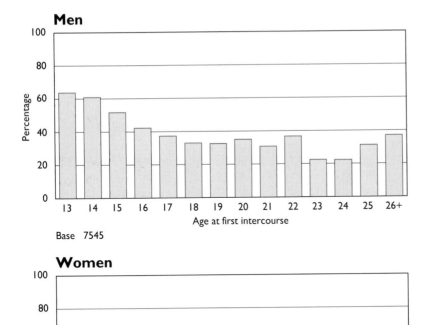

Men

Base 7545

Women

Base 9553

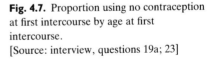

Fig. 4.7. Proportion using no contraception at first intercourse by age at first intercourse.
[Source: interview, questions 19a; 23]

commonly used by young people aged 16–24 than by those in any other age group. Half of all women and nearly as many young men in this age group report condom use at first intercourse, compared with little more than a third for other age groups. Figure 4.8 shows a recent sharp increase in the prevalence of condom use at first intercourse. The rise began in the mid 1980s; throughout the two decades before this, condom use remained remarkably stable despite fluctuations in the popularity of the pill in the wake of reports of possible adverse side effects (Royal College of General Practitioners, 1977; Vessey *et al.*, 1977; Pike *et al.*, 1983). This supports the view that the revival of the method in the 1980s was largely attributable to AIDS public education, suggesting considerable success in motivating public response.

The use of 'other method' (predominantly oral contraception) is

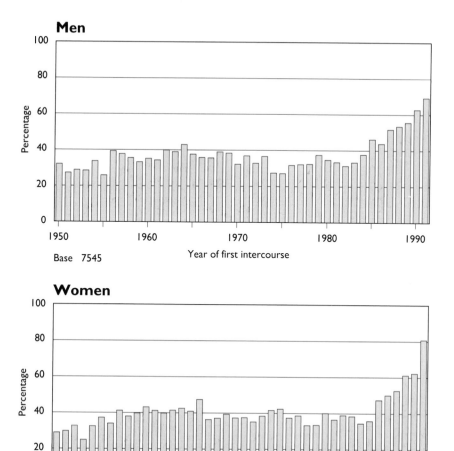

Men

Women

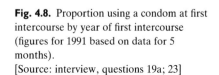

Fig. 4.8. Proportion using a condom at first intercourse by year of first intercourse (figures for 1991 based on data for 5 months).
[Source: interview, questions 19a; 23]

highest among women now aged 25 to 34, 28% of whom used this method of contraception at first intercourse. The proportion falls to 20% of 16- to 24-year-olds, possibly because of reports of adverse side effects of oral contraceptive use amongst young nulliparous women (Pike *et al.*, 1983) (Fig. 4.9). Reports of the use of 'other method' increase with age at which first intercourse occurs. The necessity for professional consultation for a medical prescription could be a deterrent to younger women (Fig. 4.10).

Experience of first intercourse

Relatively little is known about the context in which first sexual intercourse occurs: the stimulus to the event, influences on decision-making,

Men

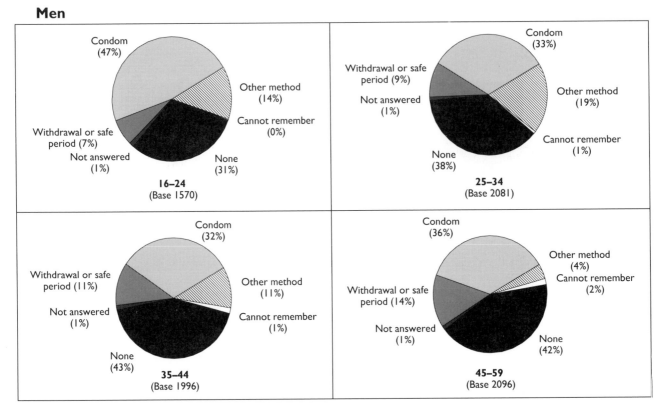

Fig. 4.9. Contraceptive use at first intercourse by current age.
[Source: interview, question 23]

the nature of the relationship with the first partner and the feelings provoked by the experience. The circumstances in which first intercourse occurs vary widely and this study cannot provide more than superficial insights into this important event. Some of the contextual data from the survey are discussed below, together with their implications for the age at which first intercourse occurs and whether contraception is used.

Age of partner

All respondents were asked the age of the person with whom they first had sexual intercourse and whether or not it was the first time for them. Only 2% of men and fewer than 1% of women reported never having known how old their first partner was, whilst 13% of women and 14% of men had no knowledge of whether or not they were also virgins. The younger men were at first intercourse, the less likely they were to have known whether or not their partners were also virgins, whilst for women

Women

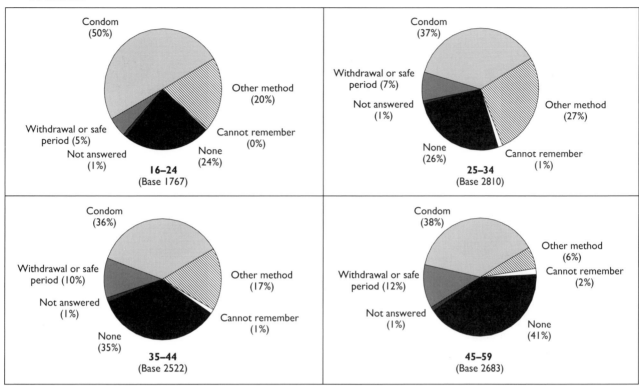

Fig. 4.9. *Continued*

the reverse was true. Similar findings have been reported by Zelnick &
Shah (1983).

Men's partners at first intercourse tend to be roughly the same age as
themselves (Fig. 4.11 & Table 4.12). This holds even for those who
reported early intercourse; nearly two-thirds of men aged under 16 at first
intercourse had partners who were also under 16. (The possibility that
men believed their partners to be older than they actually were cannot be
ruled out, particularly where the woman was under 16.) Where men's
partners were of discordant age, whether they were older or younger
varied with the age at which first intercourse occurred. The older the man
was at first intercourse the more likely it was to have taken place with a
partner younger than himself, and vice versa. However, there is no
evidence of widespread initiation of young men into sex by older women.

For women, the pattern is different. An older partner at first intercourse is the norm. Of women aged 13–17 at first intercourse, 75% had
partners older than themselves, and 75% of those aged 18–24 at first

Men

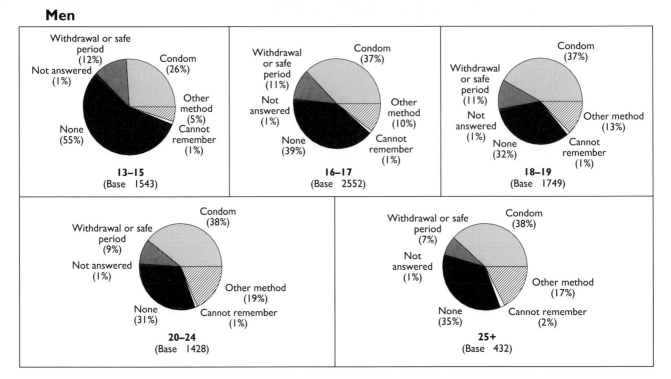

13–15
(Base 1543)

- Withdrawal or safe period (12%)
- Not answered (1%)
- None (55%)
- Condom (26%)
- Other method (5%)
- Cannot remember (1%)

16–17
(Base 2552)

- Condom (37%)
- Withdrawal or safe period (11%)
- Not answered (1%)
- Other method (10%)
- None (39%)
- Cannot remember (1%)

18–19
(Base 1749)

- Condom (37%)
- Withdrawal or safe period (11%)
- Not answered (1%)
- Other method (13%)
- None (32%)
- Cannot remember (1%)

20–24
(Base 1428)

- Condom (38%)
- Withdrawal or safe period (9%)
- Not answered (1%)
- Other method (19%)
- None (31%)
- Cannot remember (1%)

25+
(Base 432)

- Condom (38%)
- Withdrawal or safe period (7%)
- Not answered (1%)
- Other method (17%)
- None (35%)
- Cannot remember (2%)

Women

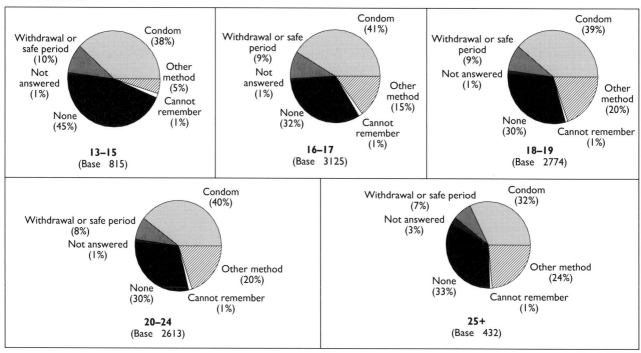

13–15
(Base 815)

- Condom (38%)
- Withdrawal or safe period (10%)
- Not answered (1%)
- Other method (5%)
- Cannot remember (1%)
- None (45%)

16–17
(Base 3125)

- Condom (41%)
- Withdrawal or safe period (9%)
- Not answered (1%)
- Other method (15%)
- Cannot remember (1%)
- None (32%)

18–19
(Base 2774)

- Condom (39%)
- Withdrawal or safe period (9%)
- Not answered (1%)
- Other method (20%)
- Cannot remember (1%)
- None (30%)

20–24
(Base 2613)

- Condom (40%)
- Withdrawal or safe period (8%)
- Not answered (1%)
- Other method (20%)
- Cannot remember (1%)
- None (30%)

25+
(Base 432)

- Condom (32%)
- Withdrawal or safe period (7%)
- Not answered (3%)
- Other method (24%)
- Cannot remember (1%)
- None (33%)

Fig. 4.10. Contraceptive use at first intercourse by age at first intercourse.
[Source: interview, questions 19; 23]

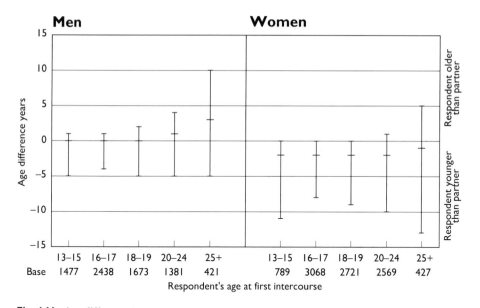

Fig. 4.11. Age difference between respondent and partner age at first intercourse. (Difference = median difference with 95th and 5th centiles in years between age of respondent and partner at first intercourse.)
[Source: interview, questions 19a; 21a]

Table 4.12. Quartiles of age difference in years between partner and respondent at first intercourse
[Source: interview, questions 19a; 21a]

Age at first intercourse	Median			Base
	1st	2nd	3rd	
Men				
13–15	−2	0	0	1 477
16–17	0	0	0	2 438
18–19	0	0	1	1 673
20–24	0	1	2	1 381
25+	0	3	6	421
Women				
13–15	−4	−2	−1	789
16–17	−4	−2	−1	3 068
18–19	−4	−2	0	2 721
20–24	−4	−2	0	2 569
25+	−5	−1	1	427

Table 4.13. Context of first intercourse by age at occurrence [Source: interview, questions 19a, 24, 25, 26b, 28]

	Age <16		Total	
	Men (%)	Women (%)	Men (%)	Women (%)
Nature of relationship				
Prostitute (men only)	1.2	—	1.6	—
Met for first time	4.6	3.3	4.4	0.8
Met recently	15.8	8.7	13.1	3.8
Known but not steady	42.0	28.6	28.6	16.5
Steady	35.5	57.9	42.9	51.4
Cohabiting	0.4	0.0	0.4	0.8
Engaged	0.6	1.3	3.0	10.5
Married	0.0	0.0	6.1	15.9
Rape (women only)	—	0.3	—	0.3
Base	391	217	1 909	2 405
*Planning**				
Spur of the moment	44.2	38.0	31.1	25.6
Expected soon	28.9	37.9	39.1	43.4
Expected then	10.5	9.2	10.9	12.1
Planned then	2.7	2.0	3.8	3.5
Planned in advance	13.7	12.9	14.5	15.5
Base	392	216	1 784	2 002
Feelings				
Too soon	24.4	58.5	12.3	25.5
Waited too long	1.8	1.6	7.1	3.1
About right	73.8	39.9	80.6	71.4
Base	381	214	1 864	2 344
*Main factor**				
Curiosity	40.5	23.2	27.1	14.1
Carried away	11.0	11.2	10.0	8.6
Peer group	13.9	9.4	8.4	4.4
Natural course	15.9	8.8	26.0	24.3
Drunk	3.6	6.7	4.0	2.7
To lose virginity	9.0	1.2	7.1	1.1
In love	6.2	39.5	17.3	44.9
Base	387	195	1 748	1 924

* Excludes those married at first intercourse.

Table 4.14. Context of first intercourse by age group of respondent
[Source: interview, questions 19a, 24, 25, 26b, 28]

Age group:	16–24		25–34		35–44		45–59	
	Men (%)	Women (%)	Men (%)	Women (%)	Men (%)	Women (%)	Men (%)	Women (%)
Nature of relationship								
Prostitute	0.0	—	0.9	—	1.7	—	3.4	—
Met for first time	4.3	1.9	5.5	0.7	3.6	1.1	4.4	0.2
Met recently	17.0	6.9	14.0	5.1	11.5	3.0	10.5	1.2
Known but not steady	29.5	23.3	28.3	18.6	31.6	14.2	25.1	12.1
Steady	48.3	62.5	46.8	61.7	40.5	51.1	36.7	33.8
Cohabiting	0.4	1.7	0.3	0.9	1.0	0.8	0.0	0.1
Engaged	0.6	2.8	1.6	7.8	3.6	15.5	5.7	13.6
Married	0.0	0.8	2.6	5.3	6.7	13.8	14.2	38.5
Rape	—	0.1	—	0.0	—	0.5	—	0.5
Base	393	428	520	698	518	614	477	665
*Planning**								
Spur of the moment	27.1	24.0	30.7	20.8	29.9	26.4	37.1	33.8
Expected soon	40.4	40.2	38.3	42.1	44.3	46.1	34.9	45.2
Expected then	12.2	12.9	10.6	13.2	8.1	11.5	13.6	10.2
Planned then	5.0	5.3	2.8	3.0	3.6	3.3	4.2	2.8
Planned in advance	15.3	17.5	17.6	20.9	14.2	12.7	10.3	8.0
Base	393	424	507	656	481	520	403	401
Feelings								
Too soon	15.6	36.9	10.1	29.4	12.5	24.3	11.7	15.3
Waited too long	3.1	0.8	6.7	1.6	9.2	3.8	8.8	5.5
About right	81.3	62.4	83.1	69.0	78.3	71.9	79.6	79.3
Base	388	413	508	689	507	601	451	641
*Main factor**								
Curiosity	30.7	23.6	32.5	15.1	23.7	8.4	20.8	9.5
Carried away	4.5	6.3	8.2	6.6	12.6	8.3	14.6	14.5
Peer group	7.2	4.1	7.2	6.3	8.8	3.8	10.5	2.5
Natural course	23.1	23.2	25.0	26.9	29.7	25.7	25.6	19.8
Drunk	6.6	5.2	3.8	2.0	2.3	2.8	3.9	1.1
Lose virginity	11.2	0.2	8.8	1.6	6.3	1.1	2.2	1.0
In love	16.7	37.5	14.4	41.5	16.7	49.9	22.4	51.6
Base	387	409	492	632	474	488	395	396

Note: Excludes respondents unable to recall, uncertain or with no opinion.
* Excludes those married at first intercourse.

Table 4.15. Proportion using no contraception at first intercourse by nature of the relationship
[Source: interview, questions 23; 24, 25, 26b, 28]

| | Using no contraception | | | |
| | Men | | Women | |
	(%)	Base	(%)	Base
Nature of relationship				
Prostitute	75.4	30	—	—
Just met for the first time	46.8	85	67.6	19*
Met recently	40.0	244	47.7	90
Known but not steady	49.1	540	43.6	394
Steady relationship	29.8	809	30.1	1 218
Living together (but not married or engaged)	—	8†	30.6	20
Engaged to be married	37.5	54	32.4	248
Married	29.1	115	38.5	377
Other	—	8†	65.5	15*
Planning‡				
Spur of the moment	54.4	551	56.5	510
Expected soon	34.3	693	32.5	854
Expected then	35.2	194	23.0	241
Planned then	32.8	68	19.3	67
Planned in advance	24.9	258	13.4	307
Feelings				
Too soon	50.0	226	47.6	594
Waited too long	33.7	128	34.4	70
About right	36.6	1 483	29.5	1 654
Main factor				
Curiosity	43.9	468	34.8	269
Carried away	50.2	174	46.3	161
Peer group	52.6	146	45.2	83
Natural course	26.2	449	25.5	466
Drunk	63.2	69	64.2	51
To lose virginity	40.4	120	31.2	20
In love	30.1	300	31.4	851

Note: Excludes respondents unable to recall, uncertain or with no opinion.
* Note small base.
† Base <10.
‡ Excludes those married at first intercourse.

start a family. More than two-thirds of women whose partner at first intercourse was someone they had met for the first time used no contraception; neither did nearly half of those for whom it was someone they had met recently, and fewer than a third of those in a steady relationship. The increased likelihood of lack of contraceptive protection with a non-steady partner may be a cause for concern, as this is the group most likely to suffer and least likely to welcome an unplanned pregnancy.

Factors associated with first intercourse

Respondents receiving the long questionnaire were asked to choose from a selection of response options relating to the circumstances surrounding first intercourse. The selection of these was guided partly by the early development work for the survey, and partly by the desire to achieve some comparability with Schofield's (1965) survey of young people, in which this question was also asked. Respondents were asked to mention any of several factors they considered to apply to themselves, and then to try to identify the single main factor obtaining at the time. Show-cards providing pre-coded responses contained the following statements.

- I was curious about what it would be like.
- I got carried away by my feelings.
- Most people in my age group seemed to be doing it.
- It seemed like a natural 'follow on' in the relationship.
- I was a bit drunk at the time.
- I wanted to lose my virginity.
- I was in love.
- Other particular factor (*specify*).
- None of these applied.

The question assumes both awareness and accurate recall of contributory and motivating factors at the time. Both assumptions are questionable, and we need to accept that many of the responses may well be rationalizations after the event. It is also possible that a response bias is operating here too, since some options – e.g. being drunk – are less socially acceptable than others.

Factors most commonly associated with first intercourse were curiosity (cited by 55% of men and 42% of women), and that it seemed a natural progression in the relationship (cited by 45% of men and 50% of women). There were, however, marked gender differences in the choice of factors. Whilst curiosity was the factor most commonly selected by men, for women it was 'being in love'. Fifty-eight per cent of women reported this as an associated factor, compared with only 30% of men. These findings are similar to those in other studies (Reiss, 1967; Kraft *et al.*, 1989).

Looking at the *main* factor associated with first intercourse (Fig.

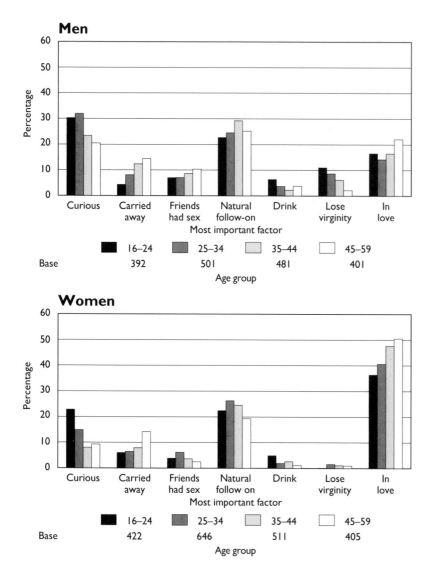

Fig. 4.13. Most important factor associated with first intercourse by current age. [Source: interview, question 26b]

4.13), there is little evidence of any return to an age of romanticism, certainly among women. The proportion of women who mention being in love as the main precipitating factor continues a slow decline through all age groups, from more than half the sample of 45–59 year olds (51.6%) to little more than a third (37.5%) of women aged 16–24. Men gave this as the main factor in first intercourse far less commonly than women, and the proportion doing so, after falling from 22.4% of 45–59 year olds to 14.4% of 25–34 year olds, rises slightly to 16.7% of 16–24 year olds.

Social pressure, particularly from peers, has been cited as a reason for young people having intercourse for the first time (Delameter & MacCorquodale, 1979). The two measures of this variable in the questionnaire relate to the responses, 'Most people in my age group seemed to be doing it' and, 'I wanted to lose my virginity'. Whilst it is not a key factor for either sex, men seem more susceptible to the 'herding instinct' than women − 8.4% of men and 4.4% of women mention the prevailing peer group norm as the most important factor (although this is an option respondents might have been least aware of at the time). There seems also to be more motivation for men to lose their virginity, and this increases with younger birth cohorts. For men aged 16–24 at interview, more than one in 10 gave this as the most important factor associated with first intercourse, compared with only one in 50 of those aged 45–59.

The use of alcohol is often associated with first intercourse, but there is little evidence of it being a major precipitating factor in these data. Younger respondents are more likely than older ones to report having been a 'bit drunk' at first intercourse, yet only 5.2% of women and 6.6% of men in the youngest age group of 16–24 report that being slightly drunk was the main factor associated with their loss of virginity, and 14% of men and 10% of women cite it as a contributory factor (Table 4.14). This factor is more likely to be cited by women for whom intercourse occurred before 16 (Table 4.13).

First intercourse seems to have been characterized by more planning and less spontaneity in recent years. Younger women in the sample were less likely than older women to report first intercourse having been mainly associated with being 'carried away by their feelings' (Table 4.14). This is consistent with the findings of recent US studies that have shown that many adolescents see their first experience of sexual intercourse as a conscious personal choice (Coles & Stokes, 1985; Bigler, 1989).

Contraception at first intercourse was far more likely to be used by either partner if intercourse was planned than if it was unplanned. Whilst more than half of women (56.5%) who reported that intercourse had occurred 'on the spur of the moment' reported no contraceptive use by themselves or their partner, only 14.5% of those who had planned the event (either by the respondent at the time or together with a partner in advance) did so.

Feelings about first intercourse

The majority of respondents recall their first intercourse as an event that both they and their partner agreed to, although there are some discrepancies between the perceptions of men and women. Men were more likely to report having been the more willing partner at first inter-course than women (8% vs 2%), and more likely to claim that both they and their partner were equally willing (85% vs 74%). Women were more likely to report having been persuaded than men (16% vs 1.5%). This may be influenced by women's expectations about the social appropri-ateness of compliance. Again, retrospective data need to be interpreted cautiously. In indicating what they felt about first intercourse, respon-dents may have unconsciously justified that long-ago decision by choosing responses that reflect their present-day morality. Reported incidence of coercion at first intercourse is rare, but it is more common for women than for men (1.7% vs 0.2%) (the phrasing here was 'would you say . . . that you were forced' (see Appendix 1, p. 400).

Most people, more than two-thirds of women and more than three-quarters of men, judged their first intercourse to have been well timed (Table 4.13). There are marked gender differences among those who did not: 25.5% of women reported feeling that the event took place too soon, compared with 12.3% of men, and 7.1% of men said that they waited too long, compared with 3.1% of women. Predictably, these views relate strongly to age at first intercourse. More than half (58.5%) of the women for whom first intercourse occurred under the age of 16 judged this to have been too soon, but less than a quarter of men (24.4%) did so. The

Table 4.16. Feelings about first intercourse by age at first intercourse [Source: interview, questions 19a; 28]

	Age at first intercourse				
	13–15 (%)	16–17 (%)	18–19 (%)	20–24 (%)	25+ (%)
Men					
Too soon	23.7	13.0	6.1	5.8	4.9
Waited too long	1.8	3.1	10.7	13.1	16.0
About right	71.5	81.2	81.2	79.4	76.9
No opinion	3.1	2.7	2.0	1.6	2.2
Base	394	656	409	338	110
Women					
Too soon	57.1	37.1	18.4	8.6	3.9
Waited too long	1.6	0.6	2.3	6.9	6.0
About right	39.0	60.0	77.3	82.0	87.3
No opinion	2.4	2.4	2.1	2.6	2.8
Base	219	775	700	614	88

Table 4.17. Quartiles for age at first intercourse by feelings about first intercourse
[Source: interview, questions 19a; 28]

	Median			
	1st	2nd	3rd	Base
Men				
Too soon	15	16	17	209
Waited too long	18	19	22	133
About right	16	17	19	1431
Don't know/no opinion	15	17	18	47
Women				
Too soon	16	16	18	600
Waited too long	19	20	22	82
About right	17	19	21	1672
Don't know/no opinion	17	18	20	59

median age at first intercourse for men for whom it was 'about right' was
17, for those for whom it was 'too soon', 16, and for those who felt they
had waited too long, 19. For women, the comparable figures are 19, 16
and 20 (Tables 4.16, 4.17).

Multivariate analysis

The combined effects of factors surrounding first intercourse, and the
effects of current age and education on the likelihood of first intercourse
before age 16 and contraceptive use, were explored using logistic regression. The likelihood under the age of 16 (Fig. 4.14) was strongly related
to current age, as expected, but for both men and women the effects of
education were attenuated by factors surrounding the experience of first
intercourse. Intercourse under the age of 16 was more likely to take place
with a new partner than a steady one and to be motivated by curiosity
rather than being in love. Alcohol played a minor role for women but
not for men.

When contraceptive use at first sexual intercourse was considered
using similar variables (Fig. 4.15), both age and education remained
highly significant, with the youngest respondents and those with educational qualifications at least to O level standard being more likely to use
contraception than older or less educated respondents. Alcohol was
strongly associated with failure to use contraception, an effect that has
been documented elsewhere (Wight, 1993). Sex under the age of 16 and

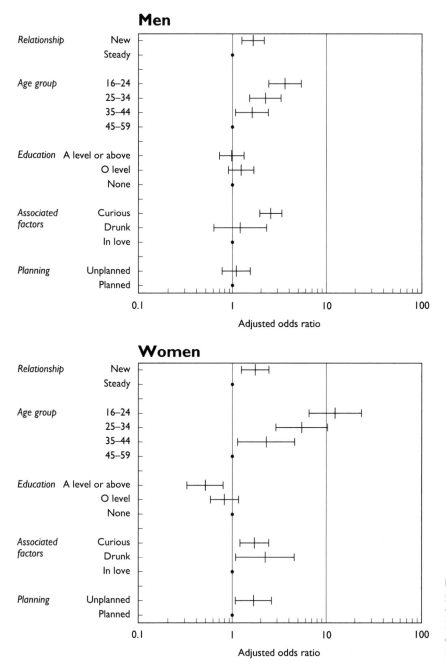

Men

Women

Fig. 4.14. Adjusted odds ratios for first intercourse before age 16 (excludes those who have never had sexual intercourse). Response options were grouped into categories for this model.
[Source: interview, question 19a]

lack of planning are also associated with no contraceptive use, again an effect noted elsewhere (Zelnick & Shah, 1983). In this context, the apparent trend towards greater planning noted above has positive implications for contraceptive use.

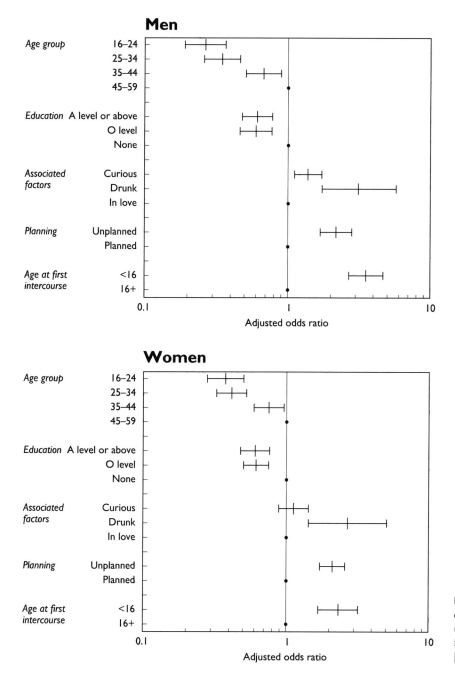

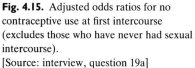

Fig. 4.15. Adjusted odds ratios for no contraceptive use at first intercourse (excludes those who have never had sexual intercourse).
[Source: interview, question 19a]

The comparison of these models is interesting. Whether or not first intercourse happens before age 16 is strongly associated with current age and weakly associated with the circumstances at the time. However, although the use of contraception on the first occasion is also associated with current age, it is strongly associated with factors surrounding the event itself. It is particularly striking that while those aged 16–24 are most likely to have intercourse under age 16, this is also the age group least likely to have intercourse without contraception.

Summary

The data for first heterosexual intercourse show a pattern of decreasing age at occurrence, together with an increase in the proportions reporting experience before the age of 16 and some convergence in the behaviour of men and women over time.

Perhaps the most notable of these trends is the sharp fall in the age at which first intercourse occurs. In the past four decades, the median age at first heterosexual intercourse has fallen from 21 to 17 for women and from 20 to 17 for men, while the proportion reporting its occurrence before the age of 16 has increased from fewer than 1% of women aged 55 and over to nearly one in five of those in their teens.

This change seems to have coincided with a period in which the traditional constraints on early sexual expression – social disapproval of sex before marriage, negative attitudes towards teenage sexuality and a fear of pregnancy – have been gradually lifted. The reduction of the interval between first sexual experience and first intercourse seems compatible with this interpretation of the change, whilst the evidence of increasing convergence between the behaviour of men and women suggests that these constraints may formerly have been greater for women than men.

These changes need to be seen in the context of liberalizing legal reforms, a relaxation of sexual attitudes and advances in medical technology. There is no evidence that any one factor is paramount in terms of explanatory importance.

Early intercourse is still associated with lower social class and lower educational level, but these effects seem to be weakening. The general impression is one of increasing homogeneity with respect to gender, occupational and education level and other sociodemographic variables.

Younger respondents are more likely to report early intercourse but more likely to report contraceptive use than are those who are older. The earlier first intercourse occurs, the less likely it is to be protected by contraceptive use, yet there is no evidence that a fall in the age of first intercourse has been accompanied by increased risk-taking in this respect. Young people today are more likely to be using contraception (most commonly the condom) at their first experience of sexual intercourse than were those of the previous generation.

The event of first heterosexual intercourse is associated with more planning and less spontaneity than was formerly the case, and contraceptive use tends to be associated with the former. The trend towards greater planning has positive implications for contraceptive use.

The majority of people have their first experience of sexual intercourse in an established relationship. Young women seem to be initiated by an older male partner, whilst men's first partners tend to be age peers. It is uncommon, and increasingly so, for first sexual intercourse to take place within marriage, and very rare for men's first sexual intercourse to be with a prostitute.

References

Akpom, C.A., Akpom, K.L. & Davis, M. (1976) Prior sexual behaviour of teenagers attending rap sessions for the first time. *Family Planning Perspectives*, **8**, 203–206.

Bigler, M.O. (1989) Surveys of American adolescents have found that the average age of first intercourse ranges from 16–16.9 years. *Siecus*, Oct./Nov., 6–9.

Black, S. & Sykes, M. (1971) Promiscuity and oral contraception: the relationship examined. *Social Science and Medicine*, **5**, 637–43.

Bone, M. (1986) Trends in single women's sexual behaviour in Scotland. *Population Trends*, **43**, 7–14.

Boyd, J.T. & Doll, R. (1964) A study of the aetiology of carcinoma of the cervix uteri. *British Journal of Cancer*, **18**, 419–34.

Brown, S., Vessey, M. & Harris, R. (1984) Social class, sexual habits and cancer of the cervix. *Community Medicine*, **6**, 281–6.

Christiansen, H.R. & Gregg, C.F. (1970) Changing sex norms in America and Scandinavia. *Journal of Marriage and the Family*, **32**, 616–27.

Christopher, F.S. & Cate, R.M. (1985) Anticipated influences on sexual decision making for first intercourse. *Family Relations*, **34**, 265–70.

Coles, R. & Stokes, G. (1985) *Sex and the American Teenager*. Harper & Row, New York.

De Buono, B.A., Zinner, S., Daamen, M. & McCormack, W.M. (1990) Sexual behaviour of college women in 1975, 1986 and 1989. *New England Journal of Medicine*, **322**(12), 821–5.

Delameter, J. & MacCorquodale, P. (1979) *Premarital Sexuality*. University of Wisconsin Press, Madison.

Dunnell, K. (1979) *Family Formation 1976*. HMSO, London.

Farrell, C. (1978) *My Mother Said ... The Way Young People Learned about Sex and Birth Control*. Routledge & Kegan Paul, London.

Faulkenberry, J.R., Vincent, M., James, A. & Johnson, W. (1987) Coital behaviors, attitudes and knowledge of students who experience early coitus. *Adolescence*, **22**, 321–32.

Fisher, W. & Byrne, D. (1981) Social background, attitudes and sexual attraction. In Cook, M. (ed.) *The Bases of Human Attraction*. Academic, London.

Ford, N. (1993) The sexual and contraceptive lifestyles of young people: parts I and II. *British Journal of Family Planning*, **18**, 52–5; 119–122.

Ford, N. & Bowie, C. (1989) Urban–rural variations in the level of heterosexual activity of young people. *Area*, **21**(3), 237–48.

Forman, D. & Chilvers, C. (1989) Sexual behaviour of young and middle aged men in England and Wales. *British Medical Journal*, **298**, 1137–41.

Garris, L., Steckler, A. & McIntyre, J.R. (1976) The relationship between oral contraceptives and adolescent sexual behaviour. *Journal of Sex Research*, **12**(2), 135–46.

Harris, R.W.C., Brinton, L.A., Cowdell, R.H. *et al.* (1980) Characteristics of women with dysplasia or carcinoma *in situ* of the cervix uteri. *British Journal of Cancer*, **42**, 359–69.

Hofferth, S.L. (1988) Trends in adolescent sexual activity, contraception and pregnancy in the United States. In Bancroft, J. & Reinisch, J. (eds) *Adolescence and Puberty*, Third Kinsey Symposium. Oxford University Press, New York.

Jones, E.F., Forrest, J.D., Goldman, N. *et al.* (1985) Teenage pregnancies in developed countries: determinants and policy implications. *Family Planning Perspectives*, **17**, 53–63.

Kantner, J.F. & Zelnick, M. (1972) Sexual experience of young unmarried women in the United States. *Family Planning Perspectives*, **4**, 9–18.

Kinsey, A.C., Pomeroy, W.B. & Martin, C.E. (1948) *Sexual Behavior in the Human Male*. W.B. Saunders, Philadelphia.

Kinsey, A.C., Pomeroy, W.B., Martin, C.E. & Gebhard, P.H. (1953) *Sexual Behavior in the Human Female*. W.B. Saunders, Philadelphia.

Klassen, A.D., Williams, C.J. & Levitt, E.E. (1981) *Sex and Morality in the US*. Wesleyan University Press, Middletown.

Kraft, P., Rise, J. & Gronnesby, J.K. (1989) Prediction of sexual behaviour in a group of Norwegian adults. *NIPH Annals*, **12**(2), 27–44.

Mant, D., Vessey, M. & Loudon, N. (1988) Social class differences in sexual behaviour and cervical cancer. *Community Medicine*, **10**(1), 52–6.

McCabe, M.P. & Collins, J.K. (1983) The sexual and affectional attitudes and experiences of Australian adolescents during dating: the effects of age, church attendance, type of school and socio-economic class. *Archives of Sexual Behaviour*, **12**, 525–40.

Orr, D.P., Wilbrandt, M.L., Brack, C.J., Raunch, S.P. & Ingersoll, G.M. (1989) Reported sexual behaviours and self-esteem among young adolescents. *American Journal of Diseases of Children*, **143**, 86–90.

Pike, M.C., Henderson, D.E., Krailo, M.D. *et al.* (1983) Breast cancer in young women and use of oral contraceptives. possible modifying effect of formulation and age of use. *Lancet*, **2**, 926–30.

RCGP Royal College of General Practitioners' Oral Contraceptive Study (1977) Mortality among oral contraceptive users. *Lancet*, **2**, 727–31.

Reichelt, P.A. (1978) Changes in sexual behaviour among unmarried women utilising oral contraception. *Journal of Population*, **1**(1), 57–68.

Reiss, I.L. (1967) *The Social Context of Premarital Sexual Permissiveness*. Rinehart & Winston, New York.

Robinson, I.E. & Jedlicka, D. (1982) Changes in sexual attitudes and behaviour of college students from 1965 to 1980: a research note. *Journal of Marriage and the Family*, **44**, 237–40.

Schmidt, G. & Sigusch, V. (1971) Patterns of sexual behaviour in West German workers and students. *Journal of Sex Research*, **7**, 89–106.

Schmidt, G. & Sigusch, V. (1972) Changes in sexual behaviour among young males and females between 1960 and 1970. *Archives of Sexual Behaviour*, **2**, 27–45.

Schofield, M. (1965) *The Sexual Behaviour of Young People*. Longman, London.

Schofield, M. (1973) *The Sexual Behaviour of Young Adults: A Follow-up Study to the Sexual Behaviour of Young People*. Allen Lane, London.

Settlage, D.S.F., Baroff, S. & Cooper, D. (1973) Sexual experience of younger teenage girls seeking contraceptive assistance for the first time. *Family Planning Perspectives*, **5**, 223–6.

Tanner, J.M. (1962) *Growth at Adolescence*, 2nd edition. Blackwell, Oxford.

Udry, J.R., Talbert, L.M. & Morris, N.M. (1986) Bio-social foundations for adolescent female sexuality. *Demography*, **23**, 217–27.

Vessey, M.P., McPherson, K. & Johnson, B. (1977) Mortality among women participating in the Oxford FPA Contraceptive Study. *Lancet*, **2**, 731–3.

West, P., Wight, D. & MacIntyre, S. (1993) Heterosexual behaviour of 18 year olds in the Glasgow area. *Journal of Adolescence* (in press).

Wight, D. (1993) Constraints or cognition? Young men and safer heterosexual sex. In Aggleton, P., Davies, P. & Hart, G. (eds) *AIDS: The Second Decade*. Falmer Press, Basingstone.

Wynder, E.L. (1969) Epidemiology of carcinoma *in situ* of the cervix. *Obstetric and Gynecological Survey*, **24**, 697–711.

Zelnick, M. & Kantner, J.F. (1980) Sexual activity, contraceptive use and pregnancy among metropolitan-area teenagers: 1971–79. *Family Planning Perspectives*, **12**, 230–7.

Zelnick, M. & Shah, F.K. (1983) First intercourse among young Americans. *Family Planning Perspectives*, **15**, 64–70.

Chapter 5
Heterosexual Partnerships

ANNE JOHNSON & JANE WADSWORTH

Patterns of sexual partnership may vary markedly. At any point in time, variation may occur between individuals, between social groups and between societies. For each individual, the nature and stability of sexual partnerships may vary through the lifecourse. Within a society, sexual lifestyle may alter through historical time (Weeks, 1981).

Previous work for this study, and that carried out by other observers in the late 20th century, provides evidence of the striking variability in the numbers of sexual partners reported by individuals over a given time period. While many people report one or a few partners, a small proportion report many partners (Centers for Disease Control, 1988; Johnson *et al.*, 1989, 1992; ACSF Investigators, 1992). In this chapter, the variability in numbers of heterosexual partners in different time intervals is described, and some of the possible influences on variation are discussed. Patterns of homosexual partnership are described in Chapter 7.

As in the description of other aspects of sexual behaviour, such as sexual practices (see Chapter 6), it is logical to assume that a number of factors may influence the formation of sexual partnerships. These include, for example, age and marital status. Those embarking on their sexual careers may be passing through a sexually experimental phase and experience a number of partner changes before establishing a longer-term and more committed relationship. Later in life, separation, divorce or widowhood may lead to the loss of a stable partnership and a return either to the formation of new partnerships or to a period of sexual abstinence. The lifecourse may thus substantially influence patterns of relationships. This influence must be distinguished from changes in sexual behaviour in historical time (or birth cohort effects), whereby cultural norms and behaviour are influenced by the changing social climate or legislative, medical, demographic or other factors (Weeks, 1981). It is perhaps worth emphasizing again, with a future historian's eye, that the study has been undertaken at the end of a period of at least 30 years during which there has been a rapid change in sexual mores, the availability of reliable contraception, effective treatment for most of the traditional STDs, a growth in international travel, the relaxation of legal constraints on male homosexuality, abortion and divorce and a more open attitude to sexual expression (see Chapter 1) (Dunnell, 1979). In addition to studying current behaviour patterns, we have therefore also examined the data for evidence of temporal trends, in so far as this is possible from retrospective information.

An understanding of patterns of partnerships is of interest to many different disciplines. From the anthropological point of view, comparisons between societies may allow conclusions to be drawn about the relative influences of nature and nurture on human sexual behaviour. From the sociological viewpoint, patterns of sexual partnership and family formation are a key component of social relations in contemporary Britain, while trends in sexual behaviour are an important aspect of the social history of the 20th century. For the educationalist, an understanding of the extent of sexual experience and of age at sexual debut (see Chapter 4) can inform sex education policy. For the epidemiologist, measurement of the frequency of partner change can improve understanding of the relationship between demographic characteristics and sexual behaviour, as well as the dynamics of STD transmission. Patterns of partner change are a key concern in the latter context since the risk of acquiring a sexually transmitted infection, including HIV, increases with the number of sexual partners with whom an individual has unprotected intercourse (May & Anderson, 1987; Holmes & Aral, 1991). In addition, the spread of STD is influenced by the extent to which those with many partners mix with those with few partners, an area that is more difficult to study from survey data (Hethcote & Yorke, 1984; Potts et al., 1991). Some limited aspects of sexual mixing have been analysed in this study, including patterns of age mixing and the extent to which men pay for sexual contact with women.

Methodological aspects

Question format

This chapter draws largely on the questions about the number and type of heterosexual partnerships, all of which were asked in the self-completion booklet. Question 7 asked about the number of opposite-sex partners in a series of different time intervals. Questions 10–12 asked for details of the three most recent partnerships in the last 5 years from those with more than one partner in that time. In addition, men were asked whether they had ever paid money for sex with a woman (Question 13), and about the number of women paid.

Qualitative research for this survey, as well as that of others (Spencer et al., 1988; Hunt et al., 1991), indicates that the definition of a sexual partner may vary considerably between individuals. Some may include as partners only those with whom penetrative vaginal intercourse took place, while others may include relationships that did not involve penetrative sex or involved only orogenital contact. The pilot work raised the suspicion that a small minority of respondents failed to include their spouse when assessing numbers of sexual partners. For these reasons, specific instructions were given to respondents in the question about the number of partners: 'Please include everyone you have ever had sex with, whether it was just once, a few times, a regular partner or your husband (wife)'. Heterosexual partners were defined as partners of the opposite sex with whom the respondent had had vaginal, oral or anal sexual intercourse.

Item non-response and coding assumptions

Questions on numbers of sexual partners were asked of all but a small minority of respondents who did not complete the booklet; 4.1% of women and 3.8% of men declined to complete the booklet and gave insufficient information in the face-to-face interview for any assumptions to be made about the numbers of heterosexual partners. For those who answered in the face-to-face interview that they had never had sexual intercourse and were not eligible to complete the booklet, the number of partners was assumed to be zero in the calculation of population estimates. (For further details, see Chapter 3, p. 55.)

Item non-response varied according to each question and was greatest for self-completion questions 10–12, which required further information for those with multiple partnerships in the last 5 years, a level of detail that it was difficult for some people to supply. For numbers of partners the non-response was in general below 5%.

Measurement precision

Questions about numbers of heterosexual partners were asked with respect to five different time periods: 1 month, 1 year, 2 years, 5 years and lifetime. It is important to collect data over several different time periods in order to capture the variability in sexual behaviour to assess patterns of partner change, as well as to identify possible secular trends. These are difficult to measure if data are restricted to relatively short time periods such as 1 year. However, the longer the time interval, the greater the problems of recall error. This is particularly true for 'lifetime' partners (so far). This summary statistic is complex since it is influenced by the number of years of sexual experience of the respondent, which is highly variable. It includes respondents who are embarking on their sexual careers, and who may form many new partnerships in the future, as well as those whose sexual careers are complete. It is also potentially the most inaccurate measure, especially for those in the older age groups, since they have a long period to recall and in which to acquire partners, and are likely to be those for whom the most active period is the most distant. However, the number of lifetime partners provides perhaps the most useful way of examining cohort effects in the data since, amongst the older age groups, this gave the only measurement of sexual behaviour many years ago.

These problems of measurement error must be borne in mind in the analysis and use of the data. For example, summary statistics, such as the mean of the distribution, frequently used in mathematical models, may be unstable over longer time intervals. For many analyses, it is more appropriate to use categories of behaviour in order to discern patterns of activity rather than using those that assume continuous distributions. This arises both as a result of possible measurement error and from the extreme positive skewness of the distribution, which is not amenable to simple normalizing transformation.

Results

Number of heterosexual partners in different time intervals

Table 5.1 shows the numbers of partners reported in the last year, in the last 5 years and ever (so far), stratified by age group and gender. One of the striking features of these data is the marked variability between individuals in the number of partners reported, and the extreme skewness of the distribution. For example, over the last 5 years, 65.2% of men and 76.5% of women reported no, or one, sexual partner. At the other end of the scale, 1% of men reported more than 22 partners and 1% of women reported more than eight partners. When the maxima are considered, it becomes evident that within this top 1% of the distribution are those with very active lifestyles. The maximum reported number of lifetime partners exceeded 4500 for men and 1000 for women. The corresponding 5-year estimate was 500 for men and 100 for women, and in the last year, 200 for men and 25 for women. There was a marked digit preference for multiples of 10, indicating the considerable difficulties that arise in accurately recording large numbers of partners, and the inherent inaccuracies that are likely to arise in reporting by these respondents, particularly if there is any bias resulting from rounding up or down.

Correspondingly, the mean and variance are strongly influenced by those reporting a very large number of partners. For example, for men the mean number of reported partners ever is 9.9, with a variance of 6575. The median for the same distribution is 4. Such extreme skewness may be unduly influenced by memory error, particularly among people with long and varied sexual careers, making the mean an unstable and potentially unreliable summary statistic. The shape of the distribution implies decreasing precision as time intervals increase and the period of recall lengthens, while the greatest inaccuracy is likely to occur amongst those with the largest number of partners. This high degree of variability has been commented upon previously and is a finding common to studies in many other populations (Centers for Disease Control, 1988; Anderson & Johnson, 1990; Wadsworth & Johnson, 1991; ACSF, 1992; Johnson *et al.*, 1992).

Table 5.1 also draws attention to the contribution of respondents in the top 1% of the distribution to the total number of reported partners. For example, 1% of men reported 16% of the partners in the last 5 years. For women, the equivalent figure is 12%. Recent attention has been drawn to the potential importance of those with particularly high numbers of partners (sometimes called 'core groups') in the maintenance of transmission of sexually transmitted organisms in a population (Holmes & Aral, 1991), and the influence of mixing between those with many partners and those with few in transmission dynamics (Hethcote & Yorke, 1984). The extreme skewness of the distribution lends support to the existence of such a high-activity group, and an understanding of the characteristics of those with very large numbers of partners is of great importance to STD epidemiologists. Nevertheless, such minorities in the population are not static, and the individuals in the upper centiles of the distribution may vary over time in response to the influences of marriage, parenthood, divorce, ageing, sexual fashion and the availability of partners.

Respondent's current age and heterosexual partnerships

Table 5.1 and Fig. 5.1 demonstrate marked variability in the distribution of the number of partners by age group. These effects are most marked over recent time periods (1–5 years). Men and women in the 16–24 age group are consistently those reporting the greatest numbers of sexual partners, despite being the group with the highest proportion of respondents who have not yet experienced heterosexual intercourse (20.7% of women and 20.4% of men). Amongst those aged 16–24, 11.2% of men and 2.5% of women reported 10 or more partners in the last 5 years. This higher number of partners per unit time is reflected in statistics for STD clinics, which indicate that the highest incidence of reported STD occurs in those aged 20–24 (PHLS, 1992).

The age differences in reported numbers of partners may be influenced by two factors. First, the youngest age groups are starting on their sexual careers, and may explore a series of relationships before (in the future) adopting a long-term relationship with a monogamous lifestyle. Second,

Table 5.1. Distribution of numbers of heterosexual partners in various time intervals by gender and age group
[Source: booklet, questions 7a,b,d]

	Men					Women				
	16–24	25–34	35–44	45–59	All	16–24	25–34	35–44	45–59	All
Lifetime										
0	20.4%	3.1%	1.9%	1.5%	6.6%	20.7%	2.1%	0.7%	1.5%	5.7%
1	16.3%	15.0%	20.5%	30.5%	20.6%	27.0%	30.8%	40.7%	57.7%	39.3%
2	9.8%	9.2%	10.7%	12.6%	10.6%	14.7%	18.3%	17.7%	16.6%	16.9%
3–4	19.4%	18.2%	17.1%	18.9%	18.4%	18.8%	22.5%	18.5%	12.9%	18.2%
5–9	17.9%	23.1%	20.9%	15.8%	19.4%	14.1%	16.7%	13.9%	7.4%	13.0%
10+	16.2%	31.4%	28.9%	20.8%	24.4%	4.6%	9.7%	8.5%	3.8%	6.8%
99th centile	45	86	75	100	75	18	25	28	20	25
Percentage of partners reported by 100th centile	11.4%	16.1%	21.4%	55.6%	30.3%	12.7%	18.3%	12.3%	19.6%	15.4%
Median	3	5	5	3	4	2	3	2	1	2
Mean	5.3	10.3	10.2	13.6	9.9	2.8	4.3	3.7	2.6	3.4
Variance	98.1	720.5	2838.5	22093	6575.1	25.9	315.0	42.2	196.7	165.3
Last 5 years										
0	20.6%	4.6%	4.5%	5.7%	8.7%	20.8%	3.1%	3.3%	11.3%	9.1%
1	20.1%	51.7%	72.6%	80.6%	56.5%	33.1%	67.6%	82.4%	81.9%	67.4%
2	11.8%	12.4%	9.4%	6.4%	10.0%	16.3%	14.3%	9.0%	4.9%	11.0%
3–4	20.2%	15.9%	7.5%	4.7%	12.0%	16.9%	10.3%	4.3%	1.7%	8.1%
5–9	16.1%	9.6%	4.2%	1.9%	7.9%	10.5%	3.8%	0.9%	0.2%	3.6%
10+	11.2%	5.8%	1.7%	0.7%	4.8%	2.5%	0.8%	0.2%	0.04%	0.8%
99th centile	35	25	12	6	22	15	8	5	3	8
Percentage of partners reported by 100th centile	11.4%	17.3%	11.5%	13.3%	16.0%	12.2%	10.7%	6.0%	7.1%	11.9%
Median	2	1	1	1	1	1	1	1	1	1
Mean	4.2	3.1	1.7	1.3	2.6	2.3	1.7	1.2	1.0	1.5
Variance	61.6	74.6	5.1	3.9	37.2	18.4	3.3	0.8	0.3	4.8
Last year										
0	26.9%	8.6%	6.8%	10.8%	13.1%	23.9%	6.7%	7.4%	19.3%	13.9%
1	46.2%	76.8%	84.1%	83.8%	73.0%	60.5%	86.8%	88.4%	78.9%	79.4%
2	14.3%	8.6%	6.1%	4.2%	8.2%	10.0%	4.9%	3.3%	1.6%	4.8%
3–4	9.1%	4.1%	2.1%	1.1%	4.1%	4.5%	1.3%	0.8%	0.2%	1.6%
5+	3.5%	1.9%	0.8%	0.1%	1.5%	1.0%	0.3%	0.1%	0	0.4%
99th centile	10	5	4	3	6	7	3	2	2	3
Percentage of partners reported by 100th centile	11.3%	14.0%	9.5%	4.6%	11.9%	8.3%	6.4%	10.1%	4.7%	8.1%
Median	1	1	1	1	1	1	1	1	1	1
Mean	1.4	1.2	1.1	1.0	1.2	1.0	1.0	1.0	0.8	1.0
Variance	5.2	8.9	1.1	0.3	4.0	1.8	0.3	0.2	0.2	0.5
Base	1984	2167	2051	2182	8384	2246	2899	2576	2771	10492
Missing	45	65	77	150	337	49	101	94	188	432

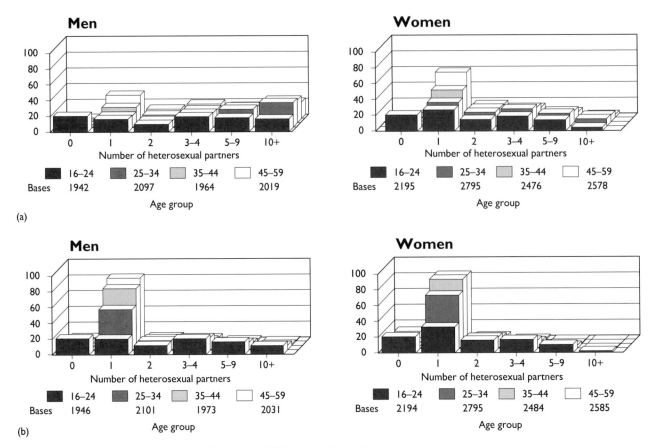

Fig. 5.1. Number of heterosexual partners (a) ever and (b) in the last 5 years by age group. [Source: booklet, question 7a,b]

age differences may reflect genuine generational changes in sexual behaviour influenced by the many different social and legislative issues previously discussed.

An examination of generational changes is more difficult from the data set, since there are differential problems of recall according to the length of time that an individual has been sexually active. For older people, it may be more difficult to remember what happened 30 years ago than for the youngest age group to reflect over only a 5-year period. Since the questions asked related to fixed time periods, rather than precise calendar years, it is not possible to reconstruct the precise sexual histories of older respondents when they were in their teens and twenties. Nevertheless, some evidence of temporal changes in sexual behaviour is available from the data on lifetime numbers of partners. Not surprisingly, the youngest age group (16–24) report fewer lifetime partners than those aged 25–44 because they have had less time to acquire many partners. For women and men, both the median number of partners (3 and 5 respectively), and the proportion reporting more than 10 partners (9.7% and 31.4% respectively), peak in the 25–34 age group, with a marked decline to 3.8% of women and 20.8% of men reporting more than 10 partners in the 45–59 age group (Table 5.1). Despite having a longer

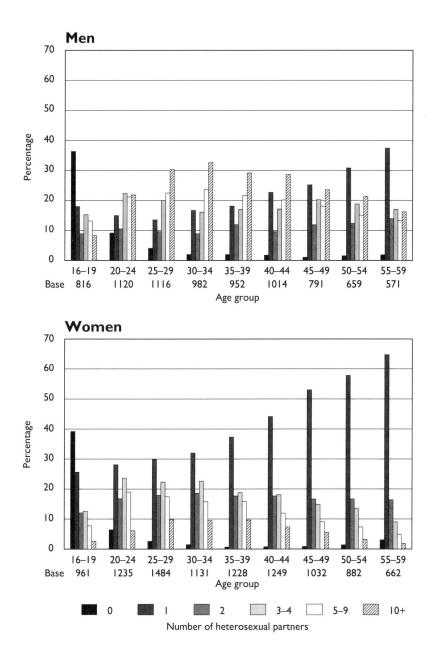

Fig. 5.2. Number of heterosexual partners ever by 5 year age groups.
[Source: booklet, question 7a]

1990; Smith, 1992; Wadsworth *et al.*, 1993). The differences become increasingly marked for increasing time periods. This may in part be a result of the greater variability in the distribution of number of partners with increasing time intervals, but may also reflect the greater difficulties of recall over time. In addition, those with very large numbers of partners have a large effect on summary statistics such as the mean. Consistency between genders would not necessarily be expected when 'lifetime' partners are considered because these involve widely differing time periods for different individuals.

It is unlikely that these explanations can account for all the differences observed, and we conclude that a number of social factors may influence reporting in contemporary Britain. British society still condones the behaviour of a man with many partners. This is illustrated by the language used to describe him ('stud', 'a bit of a lad'). On the other hand, a woman with many partners may be called a 'slag' or a 'tart', or other pejorative terms, for which no equivalent exists for the male. This double standard remains prevalent in the language, despite the apparent changes in attitudes towards female sexuality promoted by the women's movement, and the liberalization of attitudes towards sex outside marriage.

As Weeks (1981) has argued, relaxation in sexual mores as expressed in attitudes may not have changed to the extent sometimes implied in the terms sexual 'permissiveness' and 'revolution' (see Chapter 8). Social influences may still lead to reporting bias, characterized by exaggeration of the number of partners by men and under-reporting by women, whether this is deliberate, due to memory error, or unconsciously self-censoring.

Smith (1991) has considered the factors that may influence reporting in greater detail than is discussed here, and emphasizes the need for further empirical research in this area. Possible approaches include: the exploration of gender differences in mechanisms of recalling numbers of sexual partners; the use of calendar techniques to reconstruct detailed sexual histories; and qualitative methods to explore possible variation in definitions of a sexual partner. For example, men might be more likely to include as 'partners' those with whom they have had sexual contact not including intercourse, and women might discount them. In this survey in contrast to many others, a careful behavioural definition of a sexual partner was given. This may in part account for the smaller gender differences in reporting in the British data than in other surveys (Smith, 1992).

The influence of marital status

In a society that supports monogamy both socially and legally within marriage, but in which sex amongst the unmarried has become increasingly

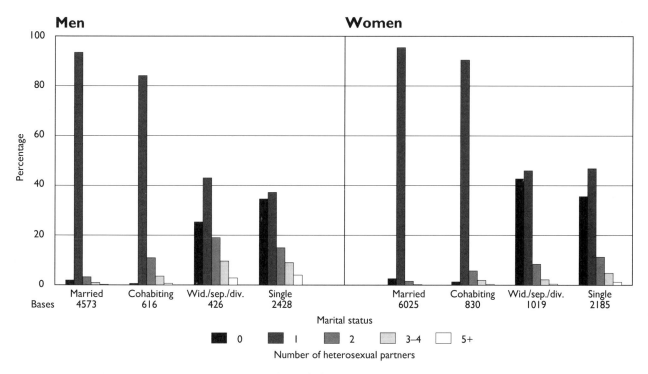

Fig. 5.4. Number of heterosexual partners in the last year by marital status.
[Source: booklet, question 7d]

accepted as the cultural norm (see Chapter 8), numbers of sexual partnerships might be expected to vary quite markedly by marital status. Figure 5.4 shows the overall distribution of numbers of heterosexual partners in the last year by marital status: 4.5% of men and 1.9% of women who are married reported more than one heterosexual partner in the last year (Table 5.2), and a tiny fraction (1.2% of married men and 0.2% of married women) reported *more than* two partners in the last year. Respondents who were neither married nor cohabiting were, not surprisingly, much more likely to have had no partner in the last year. At the same time, they were also much more likely to report multiple partners in the last year. Amongst single people, more than a quarter of men (28.1%) and close to a fifth of women (17.5%) reported two or more partners in the last year, while 13.1% of men and 6.1% of women reported more than two partners, a pattern that contrasts strikingly with that of married individuals. Those cohabiting occupy an intermediate position when compared with the married and single. Amongst these, 15.3% of men and 8.2% of women reported two or more partners in the last year.

These bivariate analyses may be confounded by the effects of age,

Table 5.3. Proportion reporting two or more heterosexual partners in the last year by marital status and social class
[Source: booklet, question 7d]

	I, II		III NM		III M		IV, V, other	
	(%)	Base	(%)	Base	(%)	Base	(%)	Base
Men								
Married	6.1	1989	3.6	1005	3.3	1053	2.2	526
Cohabiting	16.5	263	13.5	152	14.9	102	14.7	80
Single	26.7	453	32.0	319	34.2	600	24.1	1072
Widowed, separated, divorced	34.0	104	49.4	37	31.7	161	23.9	122
Women								
Married	2.1	2680	2.4	1209	1.3	1367	1.4	768
Cohabiting	8.0	263	12.6	206	4.7	190	6.5	130
Single	17.2	361	20.1	652	14.2	113	16.3	1066
Widowed, separated, divorced	13.2	193	11.8	231	10.4	61	10.2	532

behaviour has been limited, and in some cases conflicting. Dunnell (1979), in her 1976 study, found some evidence that women aged 16–24 in manual classes experienced both earlier first intercourse and earlier first pregnancy, basing social class classification either on the husband's occupation (for married women) or on the father's occupation (for single women). Class differences in experience of sex before marriage amongst women aged 20–49 were small, with no obvious social class trend. In her study of 16–19 year olds in 1974, Farrell (1978) found some evidence of earlier sexual experience amongst working class boys. Gorer (1971), in his 1969 study of English men and women, reported increased pre-marital intercourse, earlier intercourse and a weak trend towards increasing numbers of partners in manual social classes. However, these analyses did not attempt to control for age or marital status. Chesser's earlier study of women in 1954 (Chesser, 1956) suggests a similar class relationship for age at first intercourse and pre-marital sexual intercourse. Studies of cervical cancer (Brown *et al.*, 1984) have found that the risk of this condition is higher in those in manual social classes. This has been considered as possible evidence of different patterns of sexual behaviour between socioeconomic groups. Mant *et al.* (1988) found that women of lower social class attending family planning clinics reported an earlier age of first sexual intercourse, but fewer partners than women of higher social class.

Table 5.4. Proportion reporting two or more heterosexual partners in the last year by age and social class
[Source: booklet question 7d]

	I, II		III NM		III M		IV, V, other	
	(%)	Base	(%)	Base	(%)	Base	(%)	Base
Men								
16–24	24.4	249	28.8	313	34.0	461	23.4	914
25–34	13.6	783	11.7	437	14.4	540	20.9	341
35–44	10.1	932	5.3	365	11.4	422	6.8	254
45–59	7.3	845	4.1	398	4.9	494	2.8	291
All ages	11.5	2810	11.7	1513	16.0	1916	17.3	1800
Women								
16–24	11.4	279	19.7	649	7.5	242	16.0	1023
25–34	6.0	1071	7.2	595	3.7	564	9.6	567
35–44	4.1	1143	6.1	525	1.8	425	4.4	386
45–59	2.2	1033	1.9	529	0.5	501	2.4	518
All ages	4.7	3526	9.3	2297	2.8	1732	9.9	2496

The examination of the relationship between social class and heterosexual partnerships in the survey data has proved complex. No simple trend in behaviour in relation to social class is seen. Unstratified analysis of the relationship between social class and sexual partners (see Appendix 3, Tables A5.1A to 5.4B) suggests a weak trend of increasing numbers of sexual partners with lower social class. However, stratification of the data by marital status and age gives a more complex picture (Tables 5.3 & 5.4) of the likelihood of reporting two or more heterosexual partners in the last year. For those who are currently, or have ever been, married, and for cohabitees, there is a trend towards a greater likelihood of reporting multiple partners in the last year with higher social class. This effect is most marked for married men in social classes I and II (6.1% reported two or more partners in the last year compared with only 2.2% of men in social classes IV and V). However, for single men and women the class relationships are less clear, with men in social class III manual and non-manual and women in III non-manual being the most likely to report multiple partnerships.

Table 5.4 shows the same variable (two or more heterosexual partners in the last year) stratified by age group and social class. Men over 45 in social classes I and II were more likely to report multiple partners in the

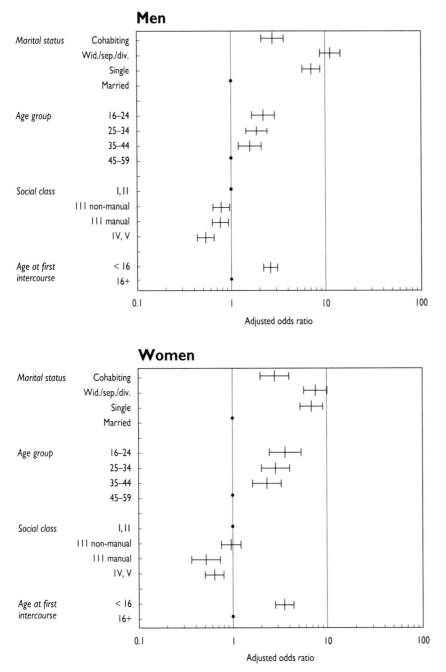

Men

Women

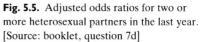

Fig. 5.5. Adjusted odds ratios for two or more heterosexual partners in the last year. [Source: booklet, question 7d]

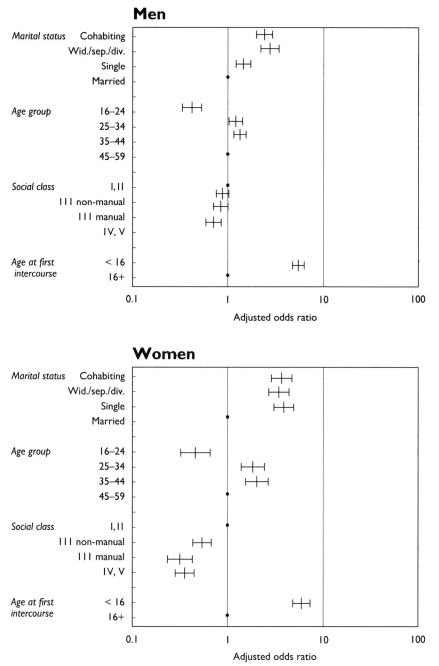

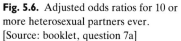

Fig. 5.6. Adjusted odds ratios for 10 or more heterosexual partners ever. [Source: booklet, question 7a]

married respondents, but there was less difference between the marital status categories than there was in models for the shorter time intervals, while the effects of social class and first sexual intercourse under the age of 16 remained similar.

By examining the effects of these demographic and behavioural factors simultaneously, it is possible to characterize those who report more partners in a given time interval. The effects of age were attenuated by the inclusion of other factors in the models. Whilst the youngest respondents were the most likely to report more partners in recent time intervals, partner change does not cease in the teens and twenties. The differences in these multivariate models between recent behaviour and lifetime behaviour reflect the influences of both birth cohort and life stages. Attenuation of the effects of age is particularly related to the effects of marital status, confirming the bivariate analysis where those outside married relationships (including, to a lesser extent, those cohabiting) are much more likely to be forming multiple partnerships at any stage in the lifecourse.

The pattern of sexual relationships: monogamy, serial monogamy and concurrent relationships

Simple counts of numbers of partners give some indication of the variability in the number of partnerships formed by individuals. They give less indication of the overall pattern of relationships and, in particular, whether they are serially monogamous (one beginning after another has finished) or whether partnerships are concurrent (where a new relationship begins during the course of an existing one.

Data of this nature, besides having intrinsic interest for the understanding of human sexual relationships, also have implications for the dynamics of STD transmission. If a sexually acquired infection is introduced into a new relationship with an individual who has other concurrent relationships, a larger number of people will be placed at risk of infection than in a situation of serially monogamous relationships that involve only one effective partnership. This holds true, provided that there is no further partner change during the infectious period of the organism and before it is treated.

Questions 10–12 in the booklet attempted to gather data on partnership patterns for all respondents who reported two or more partners in the last 5 years. Questions were limited to the most recent three sexual partners, but respondents were requested to give considerable detail on the type and duration of partnerships, and the age and gender of each partner.

Not surprisingly, this proved to be one of the most difficult questions for respondents to complete, and 9.7% of men and 7.3% of women with two or more partners in the last 5 years did not give all details about their three most recent partners. Difficulty arose particularly in the completion of dates of starting and ending the relationship. Since data were limited to the last three partnerships, information is not complete for the total number of partnerships reported in that period. Since respondents were asked to complete questions only about the three *most recent* partners, these should represent the partnerships recalled most easily for those with more than three. Non-response was highest for the youngest responders who also had the highest numbers of partners, due largely to the absence of complete dates by which to classify partnerships. These difficulties emphasize the problems of collecting such data over longer time periods, and were the basis of the research team's decision not to attempt to collect detailed data over the entire lifecourse.

Figure 5.7 shows the distribution of partnership timing in the last 5 years by age group. This includes both homosexual and heterosexual partnerships. Multiple partnership in the last 5 years was reported by 68% of the sexually active 16 to 24-year-old men and half the women, but the prevalence of monogamy increased rapidly with age to nearly 90% of men and 95% of women aged 45–59. Amongst those with multiple partnerships, serial relationships dominate the pattern for 16–24 year olds. For the entire sample, 15.1% of men and 7.6% of women reported concurrent relationships over the last 5 years. With increasing age, concurrent relationships become the dominant pattern amongst those

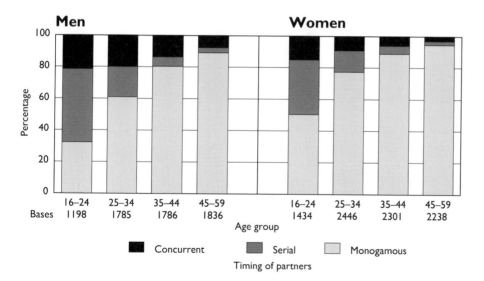

Fig. 5.7. Age group by timing of partners in the last 5 years (excludes all those with no sexual partner in the last 5 years).
[Source: booklet, questions 7b; 10–12]

with multiple partnerships, although the overall proportion who are monogamous increases. For example, in men aged 35–44, 13.8% reported concurrent partnerships and only 6.3% serial partnerships. This changing pattern over the lifecourse is presumably a reflection of the length and level of commitment to a particular relationship. As the proportion of individuals in married relationships increases with age, so additional relationships become increasingly likely to occur at the same time as, and outside, a long-term relationship.

Examining the data by marital status (Fig. 5.8) indicates that married people are far more likely to be monogamous than any other marital status group. Where multiple relationships occur, not surprisingly these are most likely to be concurrent. The influence of living with a partner as a measure of commitment to a relationship is unclear, since those who are cohabiting show patterns that are more like those who are single, divorced or separated than to those who are married (Fig. 5.8). Only 43.1% of cohabiting men and 59.9% of cohabiting women reported monogamy over the last 5 years, with 24.3% of men and 12.7% of women reporting concurrent partnerships. This relationship is likely to be attenuated by the influence of age (cohabitees being younger) and the likelihood that cohabiting relationships may be of shorter duration than 5 years. Nevertheless, it is striking that cohabitation does not appear to exert any strong influence on monogamy. This accords with the data in Table 5.2 and Fig. 5.5, which indicate that those cohabiting are more

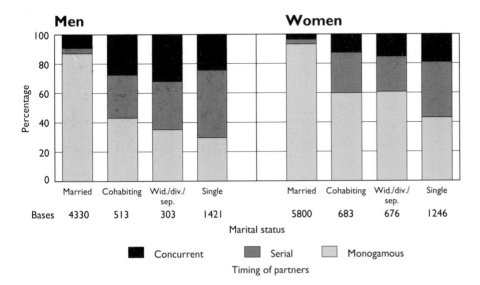

Fig. 5.8. Marital status by timing of partners in the last 5 years (excludes all those with no sexual partner in the last 5 years).
[Source: booklet, questions 7b; 10–12]

likely to report multiple partnerships independent of age, social class and age at first intercourse.

Age difference between partners

The age difference between partners is an important component of sexual behaviour. It also has implications for STD transmission, since, for example, men tend to have younger female partners. Women may be put at risk of STD at an earlier age by mixing with more experienced older partners at sexual initiation. This pattern is seen in the HIV epidemic in Africa, where women tend to become infected at an earlier age than men (Quinn *et al.*, 1986). The age difference between respondents and their first partner was discussed in Chapter 4 (p. 91).

Here, the age difference between respondents who have been sexually active in the last year and their most recent sexual partner (booklet, question 1d) is examined, as this gives the most contemporary estimate of age mixing between partners. The age difference is reported in Fig. 5.9 as the difference between the age of the respondent and the age of their most recent partner. The median is always greater than zero for men and has a negative value for women, indicating, not unexpectedly, that men

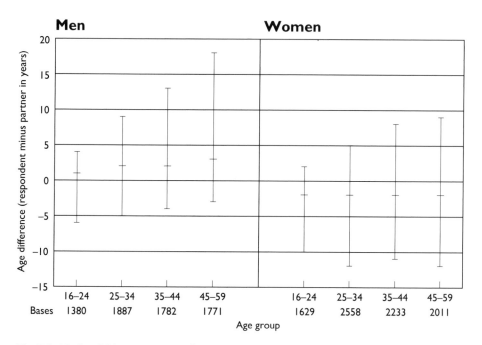

Fig. 5.9. Median (95th and 5th centiles) of age difference between heterosexual partners (excludes those whose most recent sexual partnership was more than a year ago). [Source: interview, question 1b; booklet, question 1d]

Table 5.6. Proportion of respondents with two or more heterosexual partners in the last year by age group and age of most recent partner
[Source: booklet, questions 1d; 7d]

Partner	16–24 (%)	Base	25–34 (%)	Base	35–44 (%)	Base	45–59 (%)	Base	All ages (%)	Base
Men										
6+ years older	53.8	63	25.9	84	13.1	50	3.7	26	28.3	233
3–5 years older	51.8	117	15.2	107	17.3	91	3.9	62	25.2	376
Within 2 years	35.2	962	12.6	955	6.9	815	3.7	688	15.8	3 420
3–5 years younger	33.9	217	15.2	496	4.8	396	3.1	453	11.7	1 562
6+ years younger	32.8	17*	24.1	244	17.3	428	11.9	541	16.5	1 230
Women										
6+ years older	23.8	305	7.5	465	4.6	393	2.2	313	9.0	1 476
3–5 years older	20.3	432	6.4	582	4.5	496	1.3	487	7.7	1 997
Within 2 years	19.0	839	5.5	1 253	2.5	1 052	1.6	965	6.6	4 110
3–5 years younger	26.2	48	12.1	166	13.8	116	5.0	102	12.4	432
6+ years younger	—	5†	17.5	90	10.8	174	8.4	141	11.5	410

* Note small base.
† Base <10.

tend to have younger women partners. For men there was an increase in the median age difference from 1 year in the youngest age group to 3 years in those aged 45 or more. For women the median age difference is 2 years for all age groups. Variation in the mean differences by age is shown in Appendix 3, Table A5.5. The gender difference in age mixing patterns presumably reflects the tendency for men to select increasingly younger female partners as they grow older, possibly through divorce and remarriage. Nevertheless, heterosexual partnership with an individual within 2 years of the age of the respondent is the most frequent combination throughout the lifecourse (Table 5.6).

Table 5.6 reports on the relationship between the age difference between partners and the likelihood of reporting two or more partners in the last year. For men the pattern is not straightforward. There is a tendency for men with older female partners to be more likely to report multiple partnerships in the last year, but the relationship varies with age. The relationship is strongest for the youngest men (16–24). For those aged 25–44, multiple partnerships were most frequently reported by those with female partners at both extremes of the age difference spectrum. For men over 45, those with partners 6 years or more younger than themselves were most likely to report two or more partners in the last year. The relationship appears to invert with increasing age. From these data it is not possible to conclude whether this is an age cohort or an ageing effect. However, one explanation might be that younger men with older female partners are more sexually adventurous and may be forming relationships with more sexually experienced women. Conversely, the oldest men with the youngest partners may be those who have recently experienced marital breakdown and adopted new relationships with younger women. The inverse pattern is seen for women, and the probability of reporting two or more partners in the last year is highest amongst women with the youngest male partners. This is consistent across all age groups with the exception of women aged 16–24, where no clear trend emerges.

Thus, patterns of age mixing and sexual behaviour appear to vary with gender and over the lifecourse. As women become older, they are more likely than men to be without a sexual partner (19.3% of women and 10.8% of men aged 45–59 reported no sexual partners in the last year; Table 5.1), while men become increasingly likely to form relationships with younger women partners.

Male experience of commercial sex

The extent to which men pay money for sex with women is poorly understood. Data in this area are sparse, but are relevant not only to an understanding of the spectrum of sexual expression but also to the potential spread of HIV and other STDs. The role of prostitute–client contacts in the spread of STD has through the centuries been a repeated subject for social and moral debate, but seldom the subject of rigorous scientific enquiry before the advent of AIDS (Pankhurst, 1913; Weeks, 1981; Brandt, 1987; Davenport-Hines, 1990). There is some evidence that prostitute–client contacts may have had a significant role in the transmission of gonorrhoea and syphilis in the late 19th and early 20th century, particularly in relation to the use of prostitutes by troops during wartime (Adler, 1980).

The role of prostitutes in STD transmission has been reviewed elsewhere (Darrow, 1983). Prostitutes remain at high risk of STD (Ward *et al.*, 1993) but in the late 20th century the overall contribution of commercial contacts to the burden of STDs is poorly understood. Prostitutes in urban centres in Africa were amongst the first to suffer a high prevalence of HIV infection, as were their clients (Piot *et al.*, 1987). In societies where there is a high prevalence of both untreated STD and unprotected intercourse with prostitutes, commercial sex may have a significant role in HIV transmission. Research in the USA and Europe suggests that transmission of HIV through sexual intercourse between female prostitutes and their clients has thus far been limited. Infection amongst prostitutes has been predominantly associated with injecting drug use and contact with non-paying partners. This may in part be attributed to the high levels of condom use with commercial partners as well as to the low prevalence of HIV amongst clients (Centers for Disease Control, 1987; Day *et al.*, 1988; Padian, 1988). The prevalence and characteristics of commercial sex are poorly understood, due primarily to the clandestine and frequently illegal nature of much activity associated with the sex industry and to the formidable methodological problems of estimating population size realistically.

If little is known about the nature of sex workers, even less is known about their clients. In particular, there are few estimates of the proportion of men who have experience of paying for sex or the frequency with which such contacts take place. This is a subject which few sexual behaviour studies have addressed. Time trend data are virtually non-existent because so much of the research in the last few decades has focused on women.

Amongst Kinsey's white, college-educated men, about 30% had had contact with a prostitute at least once, but only 4% had extensive experience (Gebhard & Johnson, 1979). More recent data based on probability samples are not available, although some questions on the subject were asked in the US volunteer sample surveys of the 1960s and 1970s. In his data, Kinsey found some evidence of a temporal decline in the use of prostitutes. Men born before 1900 in his sample reported greater frequency of sex with prostitutes than those born later (Kinsey *et al.*, 1948). A few studies have been carried out amongst clients of prostitutes in recent years, but these suffer from all the problems of volunteer samples and are unable to provide a denominator from which to estimate the prevalence of this behaviour amongst adult males.

Recently published surveys and those still in progress are beginning to provide data from probability sample surveys (ACSF Investigators, 1992; Johnson *et al.*, 1992). This survey included one question (question 13) in the self-completion booklet which asked men only whether they had ever paid money for sex with a woman, when was the most recent occasion, and how many women the respondent had paid. As with homosexual partnerships, paying for sex remains a stigmatized behaviour in contemporary British society, and the prevalence estimates derived should probably be regarded as minima. Women were not asked a similar question, since even such a large sample was inadequate to measure prevalence, which was likely to be exceedingly low. The extreme sensitivity of the enquiry at the time the survey was planned made us reluctant to include a question that might cause undue offence but yield little useful data.

Table 5.7 shows the proportion of men reporting paying for sex with a woman in various time intervals by age, marital status and social class;

Table 5.7. Proportion of men who have paid a woman for sex, by demographic characteristics
[Source: booklet, question 13]

	In the last 5 years (%)	Ever (%)	Ever Base
Age			
16–24	1.7	2.1	1 925
25–34	2.6	6.3	2 086
35–44	2.0	8.5	1 942
45–59	1.0	10.3	1 988
Marital status			
Married	1.0	7.2	4 498
Cohabiting	3.9	9.4	588
Widowed, separated, divorced	4.2	14.2	424
Single	2.3	4.1	2 431
Social class			
I	2.4	7.2	554
II	2.6	9.5	2 226
III NM	1.3	5.9	1 499
III M	1.4	6.0	1 888
IV	1.9	5.7	852
V	1.3	4.5	217
Other	1.2	4.1	698
Works away from home			
Yes	2.4	9.2	2 151
No	1.6	5.9	5 746
Homosexual partner ever			
Yes	7.0	16.3	312
No	1.6	6.4	7 626
All men	1.8	6.8	7 941

6.8% of men reported that they had paid for sex with a woman at some time, and 1.8% had done so within the last 5 years. There is a fivefold increase in the proportions who had ever paid for sex between the youngest and the oldest age groups (2.1% vs 10.3%). In contrast, recent experience (in the last 5 years) was most common amongst men aged 25–44. This indicates that for the older age group, paying for sex was for the majority a past rather than a recent experience. It is difficult to assess whether the decline in lifetime experience of prostitution with younger age is due to a cohort effect or simply due to the fact that younger people have fewer years of sexual experience. Given that recent experience is greatest in those aged 25–44 but 'lifetime' experience less prevalent, this may suggest that there has been a genuine decline in the prevalence of experience of commercial sex amongst men. This would be consistent with Kinsey's earlier findings and also with the increasing availability of non-commercial partners suggested by the rising proportion of women with 10 or more partners in their lifetime (Fig. 5.2).

Single men are the least likely ever to have paid money for sex (4.1%), although in the last 5 years married men are the least likely to have done so. Widowed, separated and divorced men are the most likely to have paid for sex ever or in the last 5 years (4.2%), a finding that is consistent with the relatively high frequency of partner change in this group discussed earlier. There is no clear social class gradient for ever paying for sex, although in the last 5 years those in social classes I and II are more likely to have paid for sex than those in other social classes. This may be linked with the finding that those whose work takes them away from home are more likely to have paid money for sex than those whose does not (Table 5.7).

A 2.5-fold increase in the proportions ever paying for sex was found among men who have ever had a male partner. This excess remains when payment for sex in the last 5 years is considered. Among men who reported ever paying for sex, 38.5% had one paid partner, 50.5% had two to nine paid partners and 10.9% reported paying for sex with 10 or more women. The proportions of men reporting ever paying for sex increases with the number of female partners ever (Table 5.8), rising from 1.7% of men with two lifetime partners to 17.0% of men with 10 or

Table 5.8. Proportions of men who have paid for sex with a woman by number of heterosexual partners ever
[Source: booklet, question 7a; 13]

Number of partners	All partners		All unpaid partners*	
	(%)	Base	(%)	Base
			100.0	13†
0	0.1	527	1.6	535
1	0.2	1617	1.6	1640
2	1.7	829	3.8	847
3–4	4.7	1445	4.8	1446
5–9	7.9	1539	7.4	1532
10+	17.0	1941	11.7	1824

* Difference between total partners and paid partners.
† Fewer partners in total than paid partners.

more lifetime partners. By subtracting the number of partners who have been paid for sex from the total number of female partners reported, an estimate of the number of unpaid female partners can be derived. At first sight, this calculation yields a somewhat unexpected distribution. It suggests that some men did not count their prostitute partners among their total partners, since they reported greater numbers of paid partners than total partners. The size of this discrepancy is likely to be small, since only 2.7% of those who reported any paid partners reported fewer total partners than paid partners. The discrepancy may not necessarily be illogical, since men may have paid for sexual experiences, such as non-penetrative sex with women, which would not be included in the definition of a sexual partner in question 7. The relationship between the total number of partners and experience of paying for sex is not simply a function of additional commercial partners, since the proportion of men who have ever paid for sex also increases with the numbers of unpaid partners (Table 5.8) to 11.7% of those with 10 or more unpaid partners.

The factors associated with ever paying for sex in bivariate analysis were examined in a logistic regression model that included age, marital

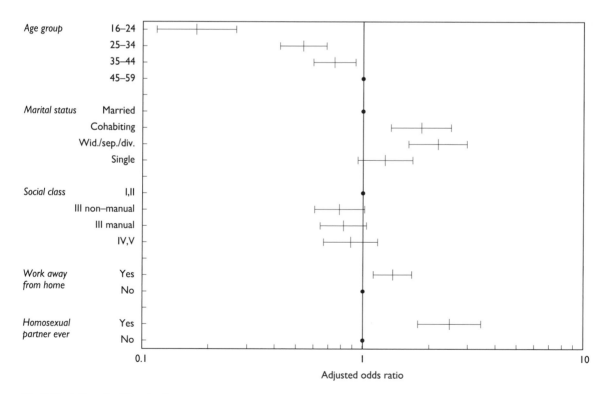

Fig. 5.10. Adjusted odds ratios for ever paying for sex with a woman.
[Source: booklet, question 13]

status, social class, work away from home and a homosexual partner ever. The results are shown in Fig. 5.10. Age and marital status exerted the dominant effects in the model, with the odds ratio for commercial sex increasing rapidly with age. Men who were cohabitees or widowed, separated or divorced were significantly more likely than married men to report contact with prostitutes. After controlling for other variables, single men did not differ significantly from married men in the odds of reporting experience of commercial sex. This contrasts with the bivariate analysis, which suggest a lower prevalence amongst single men. The difference in effect is due to confounding by other variables, particularly age. Working away from home was sustained as an independent effect in the model. A history of a homosexual partner ever was associated with significantly raised odds of commercial sex contact. The implication of this finding is that women in the sex industry may encounter a disproportionate number of bisexual men as clients (Day et al., 1993). Such a finding is not novel, and Bell & Weinberg (1978) found that 13% of homosexual men interviewed by them had paid for sex with a woman at least once (reanalysis of data in Reinisch et al. (1990)).

Travel and sexual partnership

Increasing attention has been paid to the potential role of sex tourism, and the adoption of new sexual partners while travelling, as a source of both STDs and HIV infection. All respondents were asked whether their work ever took them away from home overnight. This was used as a proxy indicator for travel, which might provide opportunities for forming new sexual partnerships. Table 5.9 shows the distribution of the number of sexual partners for those who gave a history of travelling away from home for work, as compared with those who did not. For men there is little difference in the overall frequency distribution between the two groups, apart from the finding that a higher proportion of those who do not travel for work reported no partners.

For women, there are quite marked differences in the distribution of partners between the groups, although the proportion of women working away from home is very much smaller than for men. The causal chain in this relationship for women is unclear. As well as the many influences that determine whether a woman is able to work away from home, travel away from home may afford opportunities for new sexual relationships. This has been explored further in Table 5.10, which examines the relationship between types of sexual partnership and work away from home. For men, those with concurrent partnerships were more likely to work away from home than those who reported one partner or serial relationships. The effects are different for women, indicating, as in Table 5.9,

Table 5.9. Distribution of number of heterosexual partners in the last 5 years by experience of work away from home
[Source: interview classification section 9c; booklet, question 7b]

Number of heterosexual partners in the last 5 years	Men		Women	
	Work away from home (%)	No work away from home (%)	Work away from home (%)	No work away from home (%)
0	2.9	10.9	6.0	9.4
1	60.6	54.9	56.6	68.3
2	11.1	9.6	16.4	10.6
3–4	12.4	11.9	14.1	7.5
5–9	8.1	7.9	5.0	3.5
10+	4.9	4.8	2.0	0.7
Base	2 175	5 826	779	9 230

Table 5.10. Proportion of respondents whose work takes them away from home by types of sexual partnerships in the last 5 years
[Source: interview classification section, question 9c; booklet, questions 10–12]

	Men		Women	
	Work away from home (%)	Base	Work away from home (%)	Base
Monogamous	26.4	5 144	6.3	7 636
Serial partners	26.8	1 079	13.5	1 005
Concurrent partners	36.3	996	16.3	636
All	27.8	7 219	7.8	9 277

that women with multiple partners of any type are more likely than those with one partner to report working away from home.

Any interpretation is complex, but the findings may reflect the marked difference in mobility between men and women. It appears that social constraints may have a greater effect on women than men. Causality cannot be attributed, because age, marital status, domestic responsibility and work opportunities are likely to confound the relationship.

Johnson, A.M., Wadsworth, J., Wellings, K., Bradshaw, S. & Field, J. (1992) Sexual behaviour and HIV risk. *Nature*, **360**, 410–12.

Kinsey, A.C., Pomeroy, W.B. & Martin, C.E. (1948) *Sexual Behaviour in the Human Male*. W.B. Saunders, Philadelphia.

Klassen, A.D., Williams, C.J., Levitt, E.E., Rudkin-Mincot, L., Miller, H.G. & Gunjel, S. (1989) Trends in premarital sexual behaviour. In Turner, C.F., Miller, H.G. & Moses, L.E. (eds) *Sexual Behaviour and AIDS*, pp. 548–67. National Academy Press, Washington.

Mant, D., Vessey, M. & Loudon, N. (1988) Social class differences in sexual behaviour and cervical cancer. *Community Medicine*, **10**, 52–6.

May, R.M. & Anderson, R.M. (1987) Transmission dynamics of HIV infection. *Nature*, **326**, 137–42.

Padian, N.S. (1988) Prostitute women and AIDS: epidemiology. *AIDS*, **2**, 413–19.

Pankhurst, C. (1913) *The Great Scourge: London*.

PHLS (1992) Sexually transmitted diseases in England and Wales: 1981–1990. *Communicable Diseases Report*, **2**, R1–R12.

Piot, P., Plummer, F.A., Rey, M.A. *et al.* (1987) Retrospective seroepidemiology of AIDS virus infection in Nairobi prostitutes. *Journal of Infectious Diseases*, **155**, 1108–12.

Potts, M., Anderson, R. & Boily, M.-C. (1991) Slowing the spread of human immunodeficiency virus in developing countries. *Lancet*, **338**, 608–12.

Quinn, T.C., Mann, J.M., Curran, J.W. & Piot, P. (1986) AIDS in Africa: an epidemiologic paradigm. *Science*, **234**, 955–63.

Reinisch, J.M., Ziemba-Davis, M. & Sanders, S.A. (1990) Sexual behaviour and AIDS: lessons from art and sex research. In Vocher, B., Reinisch, J.M. & Gottlieb, M. (eds) *AIDS and Sex: An Integrated Biomedical and Biobehavioural Approach*, pp. 37–80. Oxford University Press, Oxford.

Serwadda, D., Wawer, M.J., Musgrave, S.D. *et al.* (1992) HIV risk factors in three geographic strata of rural Rakai District, Uganda. *AIDS*, **6**, 983–9.

Smith, T.W. (1991) Adult sexual behaviour in 1989: number of partners, frequency of intercourse and risk of AIDS. *Family Planning Perspectives*, **23**, 102–7.

Smith, T.W. (1992) A methodological analysis of the sexual behaviour questions on the general social surveys. *Journal of Official Statistics*, **8**, 309–25.

Spencer, L., Faulkner, A. & Keegan, J. (1988) *Talking about Sex*. SCPR, London.

Turner, C.F. (1989) Research on sexual behaviors that transmit HIV: progress and problems. *AIDS*, **3**, S63–S69.

Wadsworth, J. & Johnson, A.M. (1991) Measuring sexual behaviour. *Journal of the Royal Statistical Society Series A*, **154**, 367–70.

Wadsworth, J., Wellings, K., Johnson, A.M. & Field, J. (1993) Sexual behaviour. *British Medical Journal*, **306**, 582–3.

Ward, H., Day, S., Mezzone, J. *et al.* (1993) Prostitution and risk of HIV: female prostitutes in London. *British Medical Journal*, **307**, 356–8.

Weeks, J. (1981) *Sex, Politics and Society: The Regulation of Sexuality since 1800*. Longman, New York.

Zelnick, M. & Kantner, J.F. (1983) First intercourse among young Americans. *Family Planning Perspectives*, **15**, 64–70.

Chapter 6
Heterosexual Practices

ANNE JOHNSON & JANE WADSWORTH

Heterosexual relationships include a range of practices that are a source of sexual pleasure. In addition to penile–vaginal intercourse, practices such as orogenital contact, anal intercourse and manual genital stimulation have been part of the repertoire of human sexual behaviour throughout history. These practices may be a prelude to, in addition to, or an alternative to, coitus. Little is known about the pattern, frequency or variability of this repertoire in contemporary British society.

Different sexual activities were frequently depicted in the erotic art of antiquity. Reinisch documents the practice of orogenital contact and anal intercourse in the art and literature of ancient Greek and Roman cultures (Reinisch *et al.*, 1990). Similar material survives from prehistoric Peru (Gebhard, 1970), and later material abounds from China, Japan, Africa and Europe. Reinisch (1990) and others have argued that Christianity severely curtailed the acceptance of sexual pleasure and its expression in erotic art. Sex became increasingly dominated by its procreative function while the expression of sexual pleasure became associated with lust and immorality (Wilson, 1973).

In the second half of the 20th century, sexual expression has become increasingly separated from its reproductive function through the availability of effective contraception and treatment for sexually acquired infections. At the same time, sex research has focused on the important pleasurable nature of the human sexual response (Masters & Johnson, 1966).

While art and literature provide evidence of the occurrence of a wide range of sexual practices in many human populations, the frequency and extent of these practices are not known. The prevalence, or at least the acceptability, of practices must have been influenced by differing cultural norms between societies and throughout history (Weeks, 1981).

The Kinsey studies (Kinsey *et al.*, 1948, 1953) provide detailed accounts of the variety of human sexual practices but, because of the lack of representativeness of the samples (see Chapter 1), are not suitable for comparison with the prevalence of different activities reported from the present survey. Gorer (1971) provided some indication of the frequency of intercourse within and outside marriage in his 1969 random sample survey of nearly 2000 English men and women, but did not report on specific sexual practices. Little is known about sexual practices other than intercourse from probability samples, although some inconclusive data can be obtained from studies carried out in clinic, quota and magazine surveys (Gorer, 1971; Simon *et al.*, 1990; Voeller, 1990).

The potential range of questions that might be asked in this context is wide, but the objectives of the study served to focus the enquiry on practices of particular relevance to contemporary concerns. An understanding of the range and prevalence of experience was required for the design of sexual health promotion programmes. The practices selected were those which are particularly relevant to the transmission of sexually acquired organisms, such as vaginal and anal intercourse, and to the occurrence of unwanted pregnancy and also included were those forms of sexual expression that have a low risk in this context, such as mutual masturbation and orogenital contact, and which may be regarded as safer sexual practices. Paradoxically, the behaviour that has received the greatest approval in Christian teaching for procreation, unprotected vaginal intercourse, has come to be seen as one of the most problematic, in terms of potential health risk, for both unwanted pregnancy and STD.

Reluctantly, questions on masturbation were excluded from the survey, because discussion of this practice had met with both distaste and embarrassment from respondents involved in the qualitative work on question design (Spencer *et al.*, 1988). It appeared unwise to prejudice response to questions of greater relevance to public health policy in order to obtain data on this undoubtedly important area of sexual expression.

As with other aspects of behaviour, the questions on sexual practices were designed to assess whether behaviour patterns are associated with particular demographic or social characteristics of respondents, how prevalent are the behaviours and to what extent these may have varied over time.

Methodological aspects

Question format

All questions on frequency and type of sexual practice were asked in the self-completion booklet. (The rationale for this approach is discussed in Chapter 2.) This chapter focuses on heterosexual practices reported in questions 1, 2 and 3 of the booklet. These covered the frequency of heterosexual sex in the last 4 weeks and the last 7 days, the most recent occasion of vaginal intercourse, active (by you to a partner) and passive (by a partner to you) oral sex, anal sex and non-penetrative sex. All the terms used were defined in a glossary at the beginning of the question-naire, as well as in the questions themselves.

The preference that emerged from the qualitative research for more formal terms describing sexual practices guided the decision to use precise and neutral language (Spencer *et al.*, 1988). Decisions on questionnaire design are more fully discussed in Chapter 2. While using formal language rather than the vernacular, highly technical scientific language that might be misunderstood was avoided. The questionnaire contained relatively simple descriptions of the behaviour of interest. In presenting the data, more technical language is used in order to simplify data presentation without repetition of cumbersome terms.

Response assumptions

In calculating prevalence estimates for different behaviours, certain strict assumptions were made about the experience of those who did not complete the booklet (see Chapter 3, p. 55). Those who reported never having experienced heterosexual intercourse and those who reported no intercourse after age 13 were counted as never having had vaginal, oral or anal sex. The assumption that the respondent had no experience of genital contact that had not led to intercourse (non-penetrative sex) could only be made for those who reported in face-to-face interview that they had no heterosexual experience at all (interview, question 31d).

The self-completion questionnaire included a number of 'skips', where subsequent questions were asked only when an affirmative answer was given to a stem question. For example, those who reported (booklet, question 1a) that they had never had vaginal, oral or anal sex with an opposite-sex partner (213 men, 208 women) skipped subsequent questions on practices and frequency. For prevalence estimates of vaginal, oral and anal sex (booklet, question 3a–d), these respondents were assumed never to have experienced these practices. No assumptions could be made about non-penetrative sex for this group of respondents.

Item non-response on frequency and type of sexual practice varied from question to question, depending upon the content and complexity of the enquiry. Overall item non-response for sexual practices was approxi-mately 6–7% of the total sample for most questions. This was made up of those who declined to complete the booklet (3.7% of men and 4.0% of women) (see Chapter 3), as well as those who, for whatever reason, failed to complete a particular question, whether due to refusal, inability to understand the question or inadvertently skipping questions.

Results

The frequency of heterosexual sex

The frequency of sexual contact may be influenced by a number of factors. Apart from the many emotional, psychological and physical factors which may determine frequency, other influences include the availability of partners, the stability of the sexual relationship, whether the partners live together and the age of the partners. Rates might also be expected to vary with the length of the relationship and with the number of recent sexual partners reported. All these factors were explored from the responses to the question on frequency of heterosexual intercourse, 'On how many occasions in the last 4 weeks have you had sex with a man (woman)?' (booklet, question 2a). 'Sex' was defined as vaginal intercourse, oral sex or anal sex. In addition, a question was asked about frequency of sex in the last 7 days (booklet, question 2e). The analysis here focuses on frequency in the last 4 weeks, since the longer time scale more readily captures the considerable variability in activity. Although the 4-week time scale may be affected by greater difficulties of recall, it provides a more realistic period for behavioural estimates. Frequency measured over only 7 days may be influenced by factors such as temporary absence of a partner or menstruation.

The overall distribution of reported frequency of heterosexual sex by age is shown in Fig. 6.1, expressed as centiles by age for men and women. In contrast to gender differences in reporting numbers of partners (see Chapter 5), men and women show high levels of consistency in the overall pattern of reported frequency of heterosexual sex. The distribution is highly skewed, indicating considerable variability in frequency of occasions. The median of the distribution never exceeds five acts of heterosexual sex in the last month at any age, while the 95th centile of the distribution for women reaches 25 acts in the last 4 weeks. Above this a small proportion of respondents reported very high frequencies, up to a maximum of 130 occasions in the last 4 weeks. The mean frequency of heterosexual sex thus exceeds the median at all ages (Table 6.1).

Age and frequency of heterosexual sex

The frequency of sex varies substantially with age for both men and women (Fig. 6.1 & Table 6.1). The reported median rises to a maximum of five times per month for women aged 20–29 and for men aged 25–34, thereafter declining to a median of two for men aged 55–59, with more than 50% of women in this age group reporting no sex in the last month. In general, men and women were very consistent in reporting, but where

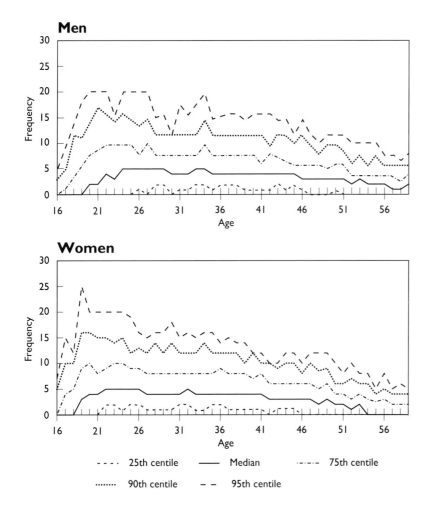

Men

Women

Fig. 6.1. Frequency of heterosexual sex in the last 4 weeks, centiles by age. (Each centile gives the proportion of respondents reporting frequency of intercourse at or below the level indicated, e.g. the bottom line (25th centile) indicates that 25% of respondents report frequency of intercourse at or below this level for each age.) [Source: booklet, question 2]

gender differences occur in frequency of sex this is most striking at the extremes of the age distribution. Women aged 16–24 reported higher frequencies than men of the same age, but after the age of 50 the median frequency is lower for women than for men.

These small age-related differences can be explained by the patterns of age mixing between couples discussed in Chapter 5. This showed the tendency for men to form relationships with woman younger than themselves so that young women should report similar frequencies to those of men a few years older than themselves. Amongst those over 50, women are more likely than men to be widowed, separated or divorced and therefore to be without a regular sexual partner, accounting for the lower rates amongst older women. Conversely, men of this age have younger partners on average than at an earlier age (see Chapter 5). The

Table 6.2. Frequency of heterosexual sex in the last 4 weeks by age and marital status
[Source: booklet, question 2]

| Age | Centiles | | | Base |
	25th	Median 50th	75th	
Men				
Single				
16–24	0	0	4	1 588
25–34	0	0	5	533
35–44	0	0	1	170
45–59	0	0	0	99
All	0	0	4	2 390
Divorced, separated				
16–24	0	3	15	16†
25–34	0	2.5	8	101
35–44	0	2	6	119
45–59	0	0	5	133
All	0	1	6	369
Widowed				
16–24	—	—	—	0*
25–34	—	—	—	0*
35–44	0	0	2	6*
45–59	0	0	0	40
All	0	0	0	46
Married				
16–24	4	7	10	155
25–34	3	6	10	1 166
35–44	3	5	8	1 475
45–59	1	3	6	1 591
All	2	4	8	4 387
Cohabiting				
16–24	5	8	15	144
25–34	4	6	12	241
35–44	3	6	10	132
45–59	2	3	8	82
All	3	6	12	599

continued

Table 6.2. *Continued*

Age	Centiles			Base
	25th	Median 50th	75th	
Women				
Single				
16–24	0	0	6	1 475
25–34	0	0	5	460
35–44	0	0	1	108
45–59	0	0	0	91
All	0	0	5	2 134
Divorced, separated				
16–24	0	2.5	8	33
25–34	0	2	8	222
35–44	0	0	4	273
45–59	0	0	1	283
All	0	0	4	810
Widowed				
16–24	—	—	—	1*
25–34	—	—	—	3*
35–44	0	0	0	26
45–59	0	0	0	161
All	0	0	0	191
Married				
16–24	4	6	10	319
25–34	3	5	8	1 716
35–44	2	5	8	1 832
45–59	1	2	4	1 858
All	2	4	8	5 724
Cohabiting				
16–24	3	7	12	297
25–34	3	6	10	301
35–44	2	5	10	141
45–59	0	4	6.5	57
All	3	6	10	797

* Base <10.
† Note small base.

Table 6.3. Frequency of heterosexual sex in the last 4 weeks by age and social class
[Source: booklet, question 2]

Social class	16–24				25–34				35–44				45–59				All ages			
	25th	50th	75th	Base	25th	50th	75th	Base	25th	50th	75th	Base	25th	50th	75th	Base	25th	50th	75th	Base
Men																				
I	0	1.5	8	34	0	3	6	203	2	4	8	165	0	3	6	159	1	4	6	561
II	0	4	10	172	2	5	8	646	2	4	8	767	1	3	6	613	1	4	8	2 198
III NM	0	3	10	239	2	5	8	455	2	4	8	359	1	3	6	351	1	4	8	1 404
III M	0	2	7	345	1	5	9	574	1	4	8	422	0	2	4.5	460	0	3	7	1 801
IV	0	2	8	224	0	4	9	211	0	4	8	183	0	2	4	204	0	3	7	822
V	0	1	4	49	0	2	8	70	0	3	6	51	0	0	3	44	0	1	6	214
Other	0	0	2	358	0	1	6	75	0	0	5	49	0	0	2	69	0	0	2	551
Women																				
I	3	6	10	26	2	4	8	203	2	4	8	189	1	3	6	156	2	4	8	574
II	2	5	10	215	2	4	8	903	2	4	8	910	0	2	4	851	1	4	7	2 879
III NM	0	4	8	507	1	5	8	655	1	3	7	525	0	2	4	556	0	3	7	2 243
III M	1.5	5	9	212	3	6	9	577	2	5	8	374	0	2	4	475	1	4	8	1 638
IV	0	3.5	8	284	0	3	8	296	1	3	7	172	0	0	3	285	0	3	6	1 037
V	2	6	10	27	0	5	9	67	0	4	6	53	0	0	2	71	0	3	7	218
Other	0	0	5	514	0	2	8	356	0	0	4	197	0	0	0	277	0	0	4	1 344

are means-related, while sexual practice may be both culturally and biologically determined (Cox *et al.*, 1987). Perhaps the most striking feature about the data presented in Table 6.3 is the absence of any strong trend in the reported frequency of sex between the different class groups.

There is a weak trend for those in social classes IV and V to report a lower frequency of sex in the last 4 weeks compared to that reported by those in social classes I, II and III, but in turn this may be influenced by marital status and age within class groups. The finding is similar to that in Chapter 5, where the relationship with social class was weak in comparison with the strong relationships with age, marital status and numbers of partners. The independent influence of social class is examined in a multivariate model later in this chapter.

One possible influence on this relationship may be the nature of work itself, with those in manual occupations being more likely to take on shift work, overtime and more unsocial hours, as well as doing physically demanding work. All these might be expected to influence coital frequency.

Table 6.4. Frequency of heterosexual sex in the last 4 weeks by age and length of marriage or cohabitation*
[Source: booklet, question 2]

Age and length of marriage or cohabitation	Centiles 25th	Median 50th	75th	Base
Men				
16–24				
<2 years	5	10	14	166
2–5 years	3	6	10	126
6+ years	—	—	—	5†
25–34				
<2 years	4	8	12	217
2–5 years	3	6	10	563
6+ years	3	6	9	602
35–44				
<2 years	4	9	15	68
2–5 years	3	6	10	162
6+ years	3	5	8	1 353
45–59				
<2 years	4	7.5	12	34
2–5 years	2	4	7	73
6+ years	1	3	5	1 552
Women				
16–24				
<2 years	4	8	12	274
2–5 years	3	6	10	309
6+ years	3	5	8	26
25–34				
<2 years	4	8	12	220
2–5 years	3	5	8	631
6+ years	3	5	8	1 147
35–44				
<2 years	6	10	14	51
2–5 years	3	6	10	180
6+ years	2	4	8	1 721
45–59				
<2 years	3	6	8	24
2–5 years	2	4	7.5	59
6+ years	0	2	4	1 808

* Analysis restricted to those currently married or cohabiting with an opposite-sex partner.
† Base <10.

Length of relationship and frequency of sex

In addition to the influence of chronological age, and the availability of a
regular partner, the frequency of sex may be influenced by the length of a
relationship. This factor was examined for those who were currently
married or cohabiting with a heterosexual partner. In this group, the data
are not confounded by the variability introduced by the absence of a
regular and available partner. Data on the lengths of relationships
were derived from classification question 1, which records the length of
marriage or cohabitation, although not necessarily the time from first
intercourse in that relationship.

Table 6.4 shows the relationship between length of marriage or
cohabitation and the reported frequency of sex in the last 4 weeks
stratified by age group. For all age groups and for men and women there
is a clear trend of reducing frequency of sexual intercourse with increasing
length of relationship. When account is taken of the length of relationship, the age effects are less marked than those apparent in Tables 6.1
and 6.2. For those who have been married or cohabiting for less than 2
years and are under the age of 45, no age-related trend is discernible. For
those in longer-established relationships (6 or more years), age effects are
relatively small below the age of 45.

Length of relationship appears to be closely associated with the frequency of sex and partly accounts for the observed association between
age and frequency, suggesting that the notion of declining sexual activity
or appetite with age is too simple an explanation for the observed decline
in frequency of sexual activity with advancing years. The excitement of a
relatively new partnership presumably has a role to play in the increased
frequency of activity in the early years of a relationship. As relationships
mature, other responsibilities such as child care, work and familiarity may
influence the frequency of sexual contact.

Number of partners and frequency of heterosexual sex

Since frequency of sex is influenced by the availability of a regular
partner, it may also be influenced by the number of partners with whom
sexual intercourse occurs. The net result of these two influences is by
no means obvious. Those with many partners may engage in frequent
short-term serial relationships and in the absence of a regular partner
experience relatively low rates of intercourse. This possibility must be
balanced against the observed higher rates of intercourse apparent in
new relationships, the higher rates of intercourse and the greater numbers of partners reported by younger age groups, as well as the greater
opportunities offered by concurrent relationships with more than one
partner.

Table 6.5. Frequency of heterosexual sex in the last 4 weeks by numbers of sexual partners in the last 5 years
[Source: booklet, questions 2 & 7b]

| Number of partners | Centiles | | | | | | | |
| | Men | | | | Women | | | |
	25th	50th	75th	Base	25th	50th	75th	Base
Married or cohabiting								
0	0	0	0	32	0	0	0	64
1	2	4	8	3838	2	4	8	5513
2	3	5	10	418	3	6	10	524
3–4	4	6	12	380	4	7	12	283
5–9	4	8	12	188	3.5	8	12	103
10+	6	9	15	105	8	17	25	21
Not married or cohabiting								
0	0	0	0	669	0	0	0	850
1	0	0	3	528	0	0	3	921
2	0	0	4	368	0	3	7	552
3–4	0	2	6	553	0	3	8	497
5–9	0	2	7	431	0	2	8	253
10+	2	5	12	267	0	2.5	10	61

Table 6.5 shows the relationship between the number of heterosexual partners reported in the last 5 years and the reported frequency of intercourse, separating those who are married and cohabiting from those who are not. Once the data are stratified in this way, the frequency of intercourse for men and women increases with increasing numbers of sexual partners, although this effect is least evident in women who are not married or cohabiting. The relationship is consistent for those who are married or cohabiting and those who are not, although overall rates are much higher in the former group. It is important to appreciate in this analysis that current sexual activity (last 4 weeks) has been analysed in relation to numbers of partners over the longer time period of 5 years. To this extent the observed relationship is simply an indicator of levels of sexual activity in relation to partner numbers. Although a relationship between frequency and numbers of partners can be demonstrated, it is noteworthy that amongst those who are not married or cohabiting, current levels of activity are only at a similar level to those of married or cohabiting individuals, even for those who reported 10 or more partners in the last 5 years. Availability of a regular partner in this analysis continues to be a dominating influence on coital frequency.

As the data presented in Chapter 5 indicate, many of the demographic characteristics associated with numbers of partners are also associated with frequency of heterosexual sex, although the effects are not necessarily in the same direction; for example, the single have more sexual partners but lower sexual frequency. In order to assess fully the relationship between numbers of partners and frequency of intercourse, multivariate models are required that take account of the various possible influences on the frequency of heterosexual activity.

Multivariate analysis of frequency of heterosexual sex

In order to examine the independent influence of factors associated with the frequency of heterosexual sex in the last 4 weeks in bivariate analysis, a simple linear model (Appendix 3, Table A6.5) was developed. Gender, age, marital status, social class and the number of heterosexual partners in the last 5 years were entered into the model. All these factors, with the exception of gender, contributed significantly to the reported frequency of sexual intercourse in the last 4 weeks. Frequency of intercourse was significantly lower in those in social classes IV and V and significantly higher with increasing number of partners after controlling for other variables in the model. The lack of influence of gender on reported frequency confirms the consistency between men and women in reporting the frequency of sexual contact.

Partner's age might influence the frequency of intercourse and a further model was developed to include age of partner, with the analysis restricted to those who have been sexually active in the last year. In this model, social class no longer exerted a significant effect, while partner's age was significantly associated with frequency of intercourse, confirming the influence of age of both partners on recent frequency of contact.

By confining the model to those who were married or cohabiting, the length of the current relationship and the age of the partner could be included in the analysis. On this reduced sample, the model was broadly similar. The influence of age of spouse or cohabitee and length of relationship was significant, but there was no significant contribution from gender or social class. This multivariate model confirms the initial bivariate findings, and underlines the remarkably similar patterns of reporting between men and women.

Age and marital status are thus confirmed as significantly related to frequency of contact, but unlike the data on number of partners (see Chapter 5), frequency of activity is greater amongst the married and cohabiting. As with partner numbers, associations with social class are weak. Within the model a significant association with numbers of partners is found, but the practical importance of this effect must be interpreted with care, in view of the overwhelming influence of partner availability as measured by marital status.

The repertoire of heterosexual practices

In addition to the frequency of sex, the enquiry focused attention on the repertoire of heterosexual practices of particular interest in sexual health issues. The range of experience was explored in a series of questions that invited the respondent to report the last time that (s)he experienced different sexual practices (if ever) (booklet, question 3). Six possible options were offered for the most recent occasion, which ranged from 'in the last 7 days' to 'more than 5 years ago', with a final option of reporting 'never'.

The enquiry encompassed a number of practices (question 3a–e). Vaginal sexual intercourse was defined as a man's penis entering a woman's vagina. Oral sex (oral sexual intercourse) was defined as a man's or woman's mouth on a partner's genital area. Respondents were asked to discriminate between active ('by you to a partner') and passive ('by a partner to you') oral sex. For the purposes of analysis, these have been termed cunnilingus (oral stimulation of the female genitals) and fellatio (oral stimulation of the male genitals). Anal sex (anal sexual intercourse) was defined to respondents as a man's penis entering a partner's anus (rectum or back passage).

A measure of the practice of sexual stimulation without intercourse (non-penetrative sex) between couples was included because of its potential importance as a means of sexual outlet avoiding pregnancy and the risk of STD. The qualitative work for the survey revealed a poor understanding of the terms 'non-penetrative sex' and 'mutual masturbation' as well as a distaste for the latter term (Spencer et al., 1988). The question was one of the most difficult to design. The form of words finally chosen was 'genital contact with a man (woman) not involving intercourse (for example, stimulating sex organs by hand but not leading to vaginal, oral or anal intercourse)'. Despite the long-winded terminology, this description appeared to be well understood by respondents, particularly after the explanation in parentheses was added to the question.

Figure 6.2 shows the overall proportions of the population reporting different sexual activities in different time periods, presented as cumulative percentages. Women and men reported broadly similar patterns. There were, however, marked differences in the proportions of the population who reported experience of different practices.

All but 6.3% of women and 7.3% of men reported experience of vaginal intercourse at some time in their life so far, with 56.2% of men and 56.6% of women reporting this activity in the last week (Table 6.6).

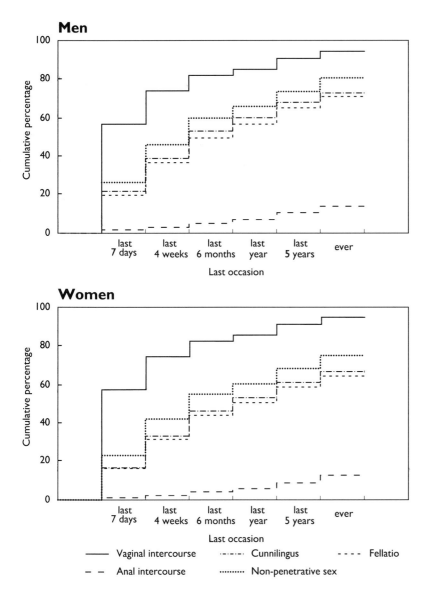

Men

Women

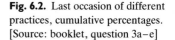

Fig. 6.2. Last occasion of different practices, cumulative percentages. [Source: booklet, question 3a–e]

After vaginal intercourse, non-penetrative sex was the most frequently reported activity. Seventy-five per cent of women and 82% of men had experience of genital stimulation that did not result in intercourse (non-penetrative sex) at some time, and one in four had experienced this in the last 7 days.

Cunnilingus and fellatio were common experiences, although both genders reported slightly greater experience of cunnilingus than fellatio (72.9% vs 69.4% for men, 66.2% vs 64.0% for women). Some experience

Table 6.6. Distribution of recency of different sexual practices
[Source: booklet, question 3a–e]

Recency of sexual practice	Men				Women			
	Vaginal intercourse (%)	Oral sex* (%)	Anal sex (%)	Non-penetrative sex† (%)	Vaginal intercourse (%)	Oral sex* (%)	Anal sex (%)	Non-penetrative sex† (%)
In the last 7 days	56.2	24.5	1.7	26.4	56.6	19.9	1.2	23.1
7 days–4 weeks ago	16.6	17.5	1.1	18.9	17.1	17.1	1.2	19.0
4 weeks–6 months ago	8.8	13.7	2.0	13.9	7.9	12.7	1.9	12.8
6 months–1 year ago	3.9	6.7	1.7	6.4	3.1	6.6	1.6	5.3
1–5 years ago	4.7	8.0	3.4	7.7	5.3	7.5	3.0	7.9
>5 years ago	2.4	4.8	4.0	6.9	3.7	5.3	3.9	6.9
Never	7.3	24.8	86.1	17.9	6.3	30.8	87.1	25.0
Base	7870	7814	7828	7490	9789	9654	9721	9257

* Cunnilingus or fellatio.
† See response assumptions p. 147.

Table 6.7. Proportions of respondents reporting orogenital sexual contact reported in the last year
[Source: booklet, question 3b,c]

Orogenital sexual contact	Men (%)	Women (%)
Cunnilingus only	6.4	5.5
Fellatio only	2.7	3.3
Both cunnilingus and fellatio	46.5	40.7
Any orogenital contact	55.6	49.5
No orogenital contact	44.4	50.5
Base	7747	9434

of either cunnilingus or fellatio was reported by 75.2% of men and 69.2% of women, while 24.5% of men and 19.9% of women reported cunnilingus or fellatio in the last week (Fig. 6.2 & Table 6.6).

A lower proportion of respondents reported oral sex than vaginal intercourse in the last week, despite the fact that a high proportion of individuals have some experience of the practice. This indicates that oral sex is a rather less frequent practice than vaginal intercourse. There was a

Table 6.8. Prevalence of different sexual practices in the last year and ever by sex and age group
[Source: booklet, question 3a–e]

	Vaginal intercourse			Oral sex*			Anal sex			Non-penetrative sex		
	Last year (%)	Ever (%)	Base	Last year (%)	Ever (%)	Base	Last year (%)	Ever (%)	Base	Last year (%)	Ever (%)	Base
Men												
16–17	40.1	42.5	361	30.5	32.0	360	7.4	7.7	363	57.1	61.5	210
18–24	78.7	86.9	1 540	69.6	76.7	1 533	8.1	11.0	1 542	75.7	85.3	1 427
25–34	90.8	96.6	2 069	77.0	87.8	2 058	6.6	16.1	2 053	75.3	86.4	2 015
35–44	91.4	97.6	1 934	68.1	82.5	1 912	6.2	16.5	1 913	66.6	83.7	1 896
45–59	87.9	97.5	1 969	41.7	61.8	1 951	5.1	12.3	1 958	47.7	68.3	1 942
All ages	85.5	92.7	7 870	62.4	75.2	7 814	6.5	13.9	7 828	65.5	80.1	7 490
Women												
16–17	38.0	39.4	442	32.1	32.8	442	5.4	5.6	446	65.4	66.7	236
18–24	84.4	88.6	1 712	69.8	75.8	1 706	8.6	13.9	1 709	78.2	84.8	1 570
25–34	92.2	97.5	2 747	73.3	83.2	2 706	6.6	14.4	2 726	68.1	81.1	2 666
35–44	91.5	100.0	2 411	59.0	74.6	2 374	4.8	13.1	2 390	60.6	76.7	2 368
45–59	78.4	97.5	2 476	29.8	50.2	2 426	4.3	11.6	2 450	39.0	61.2	2 417
All ages	84.7	95.7	9 789	56.3	69.2	9 654	5.9	12.9	9 721	60.2	75.0	9 257

* Either cunnilingus or fellatio.

Age and sexual practices

Both frequency of sex and numbers of partners have been shown to be related to current age, and here the relationship between age and sexual practices is examined. The data for the last year and ever are shown in Table 6.8. While experience of vaginal intercourse is a nearly-universal experience for men and women by the age of 25, there are marked age differences in other practices, most notably for oral sex (either cunnilingus or fellatio) (Table 6.8). More than 60% of men and women aged 18–44 reported oral sex in the last year, but this declined to less than 30% of women and 42% of men aged 45–59. This might be explained partly by diminishing availability of partners in the older age group; however, the relationship is sustained for experience of oral sex 'ever'. Half the women and nearly two-thirds of the men over the age of 45 reported ever having oral sex, compared with over four-fifths of those aged 25–34. The last in turn exceed the older cohort aged 35–44 in their experience of oral sex. Even amongst the youngest group aged 18–24, who have relatively few years of sexual experience, women and men exceed those older than 45 in the proportion reporting any experience of oral sex. In the age group 16–24, amongst those who had *ever* had vaginal intercourse, 79% reported oral sex in the last year and 85% ever, suggesting that this practice may be becoming particularly prevalent amongst those embarking on their sexual careers.

The data indicate that there are generational changes in the practice of oral sex and that this has become an increasingly common practice in recent decades. Gagnon & Simon (1987) provide supporting evidence for this view from the Kinsey data and from a subsequent survey of young college-educated men and women in the 1960s. Because of the lack of sample representativeness, it is difficult to compare these studies directly, but there is evidence of increasing experience of orogenital contact amongst US men and women born in the first 30 years of the 20th century in the early Kinsey data. Gagnon & Simon also conclude that 'in the 1967 cohort about 80% of both men and women with frequent coitus had oral sex, a substantial increase from the 45% amongst comparably coitally experienced women in the Kinsey *et al*. studies'. They also argue that in 1967 orogenital contact was still largely practised by those who had already experienced coitus.

More recent data, however, suggest that in a proportion of young people, experience of oral sex may precede coitus (Coles & Stokes, 1985). Newcomer & Udry (1985), in a survey of US teenagers from a Southern US city, found that 25% of virgin boys and 15% of virgin girls had given or received orogenital stimulation. Cunnilingus was more frequently reported than fellatio. In our data, amongst those over 18 who had not yet experienced vaginal intercourse, but reported that they had had some sexual experience, 6.3% of men and 3.4% of women reported experience of fellatio and 5.2% of men and 4.4% of women reported experience of cunnilingus.

The data from the survey, together with those from other sources, support the view that orogenital contact, though a well-recognized form of sexual expression throughout history, has become more widely practised through the 20th century. Earlier in this chapter, attention was drawn to the Christian focus on sex only for procreation as an influence which, in the past, may have decreased the prevalence of other forms of sexual expression, or at least the reporting of them. Simon *et al*. (1990) have argued that the practice may have become more common as sexual activity in the 20th century became viewed as a 'positive experience, rather than as a matter of obligation or reproductive responsibility'. Improved hygiene may also have had a role to play.

Evidence is emerging that orogenital contact may be experienced by increasing proportions of those who have not yet had vaginal intercourse.

heterosexual anal intercourse may detract from the importance of vaginal intercourse as a means of transmission.

In considering education strategies, it is of concern that the highest prevalence of recent anal intercourse (in the last year) is occurring amongst those aged 16–24 who have experience of vaginal intercourse. This is also the group experiencing the highest rate of partner change and who are passing through a sexually experimental phase of their lives (see Chapter 5). However, in interpreting data on the influence of age on sexual practices, account must also be taken of sexual careers. Older people may have practised anal intercourse at an earlier time in their lives, but no longer include it in their current sexual repertoire. Nevertheless, as Fig. 6.2 indicates, the majority of those who have ever had anal intercourse have experience of this in the last 5 years.

Analysis of reporting non-penetrative sex by age group also showed age differences in behaviour (Table 6.8). For both men and women aged 18–59, the proportion reporting non-penetrative sex in the last year and

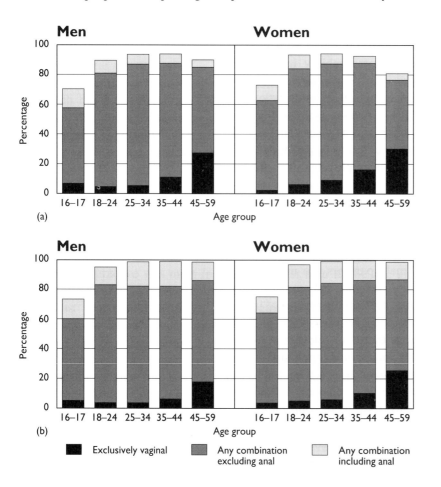

Fig. 6.5. Patterns of sexual practices by age group.
[Source: booklet, question 3a–e]

ever declined with increasing age. Over 75% of men and women aged 18–24 reported this activity in the last year, but this proportion fell to 47.7% of men and 39.0% of women amongst the over 45s. Nevertheless, this was a common activity in all age groups. The data suggest that such activity may also have increased with successive generations, since 68.3% of men and 61.2% of women over 45 reported ever having experience of non-penetrative sex not leading to intercourse, compared with 85.3% of men and 84.8% of women in the youngest age group (18–24). At first sight, these findings may appear surprising, since the group aged 45–59 became sexually active in the era before the availability of reliable contraception. They might be expected to have relied to a greater extent on non-penetrative sex as a means of sexual expression in order to avoid unwanted pregnancy. Balanced against this is the greater discussion, education and openness in sexual matters in later generations, which may have led to greater knowledge and the practice of a wider sexual repertoire. It is possible that the question on non-penetrative sex was less well understood by older respondents than younger respondents, leading to under-reporting, but this in turn would lend support to an explanation involving generational changes in knowledge of possible modes of sexual expression.

Age differences in the overall pattern of behaviour are shown in Fig. 6.5 for the last year and ever. It is evident that the proportion reporting only vaginal intercourse in the last year increases with age. These age effects are less marked in the data for patterns of sexual practices ever, the most marked pattern being the large increase in those over 45 reporting only vaginal intercourse in their lifetime. This suggests both ageing and age cohort effects in the data. Both these effects are less evident for the practice of anal intercourse.

Secular trends in sexual practices

The foregoing discussion has commented in some detail on the age effects on both recent and lifetime experience of sexual practices. It is evident from this that, in addition to possible ageing effects in the frequency and variety of sexual practices, there have also been marked secular trends in patterns of behaviour. These are summarized in Fig. 6.6, where reporting of sexual practices ever and in the last year are presented by year of first intercourse. For both men and women, experience of oral and non-penetrative sex appears to have increased through the 1950s and 1960s, reaching a steady level of more than 80% of those who experienced their first sexual intercourse in the 1970s onwards.

By contrast, there is very little in the way of a secular trend in the reporting of anal intercourse, other than a slight tendency for the most

Table 6.10. *Continued*

	Vaginal intercourse		Oral sex		Anal sex		Non-penetrative sex	
	(%)	Base	(%)	Base	(%)	Base	(%)	Base
Women								
Married								
16–17	—	2*	—	2*	—	2*	—	2*
18–24	99.2	332	78.3	332	8.4	330	81.9	330
25–34	99.3	1751	77.4	1722	6.5	1732	71.9	1715
35–44	98.4	1853	61.5	1825	4.6	1832	63.0	1827
45–59	91.0	1893	32.7	1847	4.7	1867	44.8	1851
All ages	96.3	5832	58.0	5728	5.4	5764	60.9	5725
Cohabiting								
16–17	—	7*	—	7*	—	7*	—	5*
18–24	100.0	290	84.2	286	14.1	287	83.4	285
25–34	99.4	304	83.2	302	7.9	303	75.1	301
35–44	98.0	146	71.8	142	4.0	146	79.0	140
45–59	91.5	55	46.3	56	8.6	55	44.6	55
All ages	98.6	802	78.7	794	9.9	798	76.8	787
Widowed, separated, divorced								
16–17	—	0	—	0	—	0		
18–24	88.5	35	77.9	35	10.3	35	58.6	35
25–34	81.2	224	65.2	222	7.6	222	58.6	222
35–44	62.9	301	45.3	297	5.7	299	43.6	299
45–59	34.7	435	19.2	428	3.0	434	18.6	432
All ages	55.6	995	39.6	983	5.1	990	36.6	988
Single								
16–17	37.0	432	31.3	432	4.2	436	64.8	228
18–24	75.4	1054	62.9	1052	7.1	1056	76.0	919
25–34	66.5	468	55.3	461	5.8	470	53.0	429
35–44	45.8	111	37.7	110	7.5	112	41.5	102
45–59	18.8	92	12.0	92	0.0	92	11.1	77
All ages	61.8	2158	51.4	2147	6.0	2167	64.1	1755

* Base <10.
† Note small base.

For the practice of anal sex, perhaps surprisingly, consistently higher rates are observed amongst the cohabiting men and women and widowed, divorced and separated men than amongst married respondents, a point discussed later in relation to number of sexual partners.

Amongst single people, the proportion reporting anal intercourse is similar to that reported by married people, despite the fact that a high proportion do not report vaginal intercourse in the last year. While higher proportions of those in married or cohabiting relationships report non-penetrative sex in the last year than those without such partnerships, this remains a common practice regardless of marital status.

Table 6.10 also shows the proportion of respondents reporting different sexual practices in the last year stratified by age and marital status.

Table 6.11. Prevalence of other sexual practices in the last year reported by respondents who have had vaginal intercourse in the last year by age and marital status [Source: booklet, question 3b–e]

	Oral sex		Anal sex		Non-penetrative sex	
	(%)	Base	(%)	Base	(%)	Base
Men						
Married						
16–17	—	0	—	0	—	0
18–24	87.7	157	6.9	155	76.9	156
25–34	82.3	1171	5.3	1164	79.5	1161
35–44	71.4	1464	5.7	1458	70.3	1460
45–59	43.4	1501	5.0	1503	51.2	1497
All ages	65.2	4293	5.4	4280	66.3	4274
Cohabiting						
16–17	—	1*	—	1*	—	1*
18–24	89.1	138	12.7	138	85.5	138
25–34	92.0	233	10.2	233	84.1	233
35–44	92.8	126	9.0	126	78.1	126
45–59	70.6	76	4.4	75	66.8	74
All ages	88.7	574	9.8	574	80.9	573
Widowed, separated, divorced						
16–17	—	0	—	0	—	0
18–24	91.4	16†	13.8	16†	83.2	16†
25–34	86.6	92	19.1	92	72.3	92
35–44	82.3	85	13.3	85	75.8	85
45–59	75.4	101	12.4	101	61.1	101
All ages	81.8	294	14.9	293	70.1	293
Single						
16–17	75.0	141	16.5	141	81.6	141
18–24	85.7	895	10.6	893	84.8	895
25–34	84.6	373	8.4	372	83.0	374
35–44	73.6	78	7.2	77	67.7	78
45–59	58.7	27	7.1	27	61.9	27
All ages	83.3	1514	10.3	1510	82.8	1515

continued on p. 174

Table 6.13. Proportion of respondents reporting different sexual practices in the last 5 years by number of partners in last 5 years and age group
[Source: booklet, questions 3a–e, 7b]

Sexual practice and age group	Number of partners											
	0		1		2		3–4		5–9		10+	
	(%)	Base	(%)	Base	(%)	Base	(%)	Base	(%)	Base	(%)	Base
Men												
Vaginal intercourse												
16–17	0.0	207	100.0	51	100.0	20	100.0	33	100.0	34	100.0	15†
18–24	0.0	193	98.4	326	99.1	202	98.8	344	99.2	274	97.8	197
25–34	2.4	94	99.4	1 069	98.6	257	99.4	329	99.8	196	100.0	120
35–44	0.5	87	99.0	1 403	99.2	182	99.0	143	100.0	83	96.8	31
45–59	4.2	113	98.7	1 576	97.4	129	97.3	94	98.7	38	100.0	15†
All ages	1.1	693	98.9	4 425	98.7	791	98.9	943	99.5	625	98.6	378
Oral sex												
16–17	0.0	207	62.4	51	70.6	20	80.6	32	84.2	34	97.4	15†
18–24	1.2	193	77.8	324	79.0	201	90.4	341	92.6	272	96.5	197
25–34	1.0	93	85.0	1 065	88.0	256	94.1	327	96.3	195	97.7	120
35–44	2.9	83	76.8	1 389	86.6	181	91.4	143	96.6	83	93.0	31
45–59	2.8	111	49.8	1 561	70.7	129	91.1	94	91.4	38	90.5	14†
All ages	1.3	688	69.1	4 390	82.1	788	91.6	937	93.7	622	96.4	377
Anal sex												
16–17	0.0	207	13.3	54	31.6	21	21.0	32	13.0	34	19.3	14†
18–24	0.0	193	5.4	325	10.5	205	8.8	343	13.0	273	31.6	197
25–34	0.0	94	6.6	1 061	12.2	255	20.0	326	15.2	195	36.7	120
35–44	0.0	85	8.4	1 387	16.1	181	15.5	145	25.1	83	25.9	31
45–59	0.4	113	6.4	1 567	9.2	129	16.2	93	20.4	38	20.8	14†
All ages	0.1	692	7.1	4 394	12.7	793	14.9	939	15.7	622	31.9	377
Non-penetrative sex												
16–17	0.0	56	71.3	51	94.1	21	93.9	32	86.9	34	86.5	15†
18–24	3.0	77	85.5	325	87.3	205	90.0	342	93.1	275	87.5	197
25–34	12.3	58	81.6	1 060	88.1	254	86.0	326	92.2	196	89.0	119
35–44	4.5	66	74.6	1 386	84.9	182	81.4	145	85.4	83	82.9	31
45–59	11.2	104	56.1	1 563	61.0	129	73.9	93	75.5	36	92.7	14†
All ages	6.7	362	70.5	4 385	82.9	792	85.7	939	90.4	624	87.7	377

continued

Table 6.13. *Continued*

Sexual practice and age group	Number of partners											
	0		1		2		3–4		5–9		10+	
	(%)	Base	(%)	Base	(%)	Base	(%)	Base	(%)	Base	(%)	Base
Women												
Vaginal intercourse												
16–17	0.0	268	100.0	69	100.0	34	100.0	40	100.0	29	—	2*
18–24	0.0	188	99.0	634	98.7	317	100.0	325	100.0	196	100.0	52
25–34	4.6	87	99.4	1846	99.4	396	99.8	282	100.0	107	100.0	23
35–44	3.0	81	99.3	1979	98.3	222	99.1	102	100.0	21	—	4*
45–59	2.0	280	98.4	2019	98.2	125	100.0	42	—	6*	—	1*
All ages	1.3	904	99.0	6546	98.8	1094	99.8	792	100.0	358	99.4	82
Oral sex												
16–17	0.0	268	77.1	69	76.6	33	85.2	40	100.0	31	—	2*
18–24	0.0	188	77.3	628	85.4	317	90.4	325	95.7	196	100.0	52
25–34	3.2	86	80.3	1817	86.0	391	93.7	275	97.3	107	95.9	23
35–44	1.7	81	66.9	1947	87.3	219	91.9	100	100.0	21	—	4*
45–59	2.7	278	40.2	1968	78.8	125	76.2	44	0	6*	—	1*
All ages	1.3	900	63.6	6430	85.0	1084	90.7	784	96.9	360	98.8	82
Anal sex												
16–17	0.0	268	8.5	72	20.4	34	11.8	40	22.1	31	—	2*
18–24	0.0	188	12.2	630	17.2	316	14.7	326	17.4	197	23.5	52
25–34	0.0	87	8.7	1827	14.0	392	18.3	283	21.7	107	26.5	23
35–44	0.6	81	6.7	1958	7.2	222	27.4	102	25.6	21	—	4*
45–59	0.2	279	5.9	1991	10.3	125	17.0	44	—	6*	—	1*
All ages	0.1	903	7.6	6477	13.3	1089	17.6	794	19.6	361	27.0	82
Non-penetrative sex												
16–17	0.0	58	85.9	72	95.9	34	84.6	40	90.5	31	—	2*
18–24	0.0	51	83.4	627	86.1	316	91.1	327	90.6	197	94.3	52
25–34	13.1	52	75.8	1810	81.8	389	83.0	279	90.8	107	95.6	23
35–44	8.9	72	67.6	1953	82.9	219	79.6	98	72.7	21	—	4*
45–59	5.0	264	53.2	1976	64.8	123	64.4	43	—	6*	—	1*
All ages	5.3	496	67.2	6437	81.8	1081	85.0	786	89.2	361	94.6	82

* Base <10.
† Note small base.

For anal intercourse, the differential reporting between social classes is less clear. Overall there is no class trend in the reporting of anal intercourse at any time, although reporting over the last year shows an increased proportion reporting anal intercourse amongst those in lower social classes.

Perhaps the most remarkable finding is in the similarities rather than the dissimilarities across the groups. Given the strong age effects that have been observed in sexual practices, which suggest that there have been rapidly changing fashions in sexual behaviour over the last few decades, our evidence suggests that these have been widely adopted throughout different social groups. In view of the relationships between age, marital status and social class, these bivariate relationships are examined further in a multivariate model.

Numbers of partners and sexual practices

The sexual repertoire may be influenced by previous sexual experience as well as by other identified variables such as age and marital status. Table 6.13 shows the relationship between numbers of partners in the last 5 years and sexual practices over the same time period. There is a clear trend of increasing proportions reporting oral, anal and non-penetrative sex with increasing numbers of partners. While this relatioship may be confounded by age (which is associated both with types of sexual practice and with numbers of partners), stratifying the data by age (Table 6.13) shows that the trend holds true within age groups for both men and women. Those with greater numbers of partners may have a greater repertoire of practices. This may result either from greater experience of learning different techniques from different partners or because preference for sexual variety provides motivation to seek larger numbers of partners.

This finding may help to explain the data in Table 6.11 demonstrating the greater range of sexual practices amongst those who are sexually active but not currently married, since these respondents are amongst those known to report greater numbers of partners (see Chapter 5).

Multivariate analysis

In order to examine the interactions between the various factors shown to be associated with different sexual practices in the last year, a series of logistic models was constructed. Variables included in the models were age group, marital status, social class and number of partners in the last year.

The results of the models are presented as adjusted odds ratios with 95% confidence intervals in Fig. 6.7. All respondents were included in the

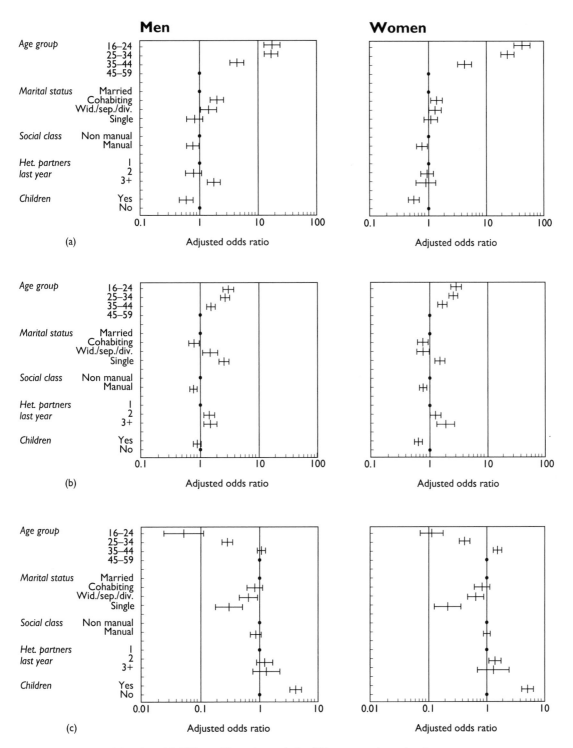

Fig. 6.7. Adjusted odds ratios with 95% confidence intervals for different sexual practices in the last year: (a) oral sex, (b) anal sex, (c) non-penetrative sex.
[Source: booklet, question 3b–e]

models. Oral and non-penetrative sex remained strongly related to age, marital status and numbers of partners in the last year. Social class exerted a relatively weak effect, with those in manual classes (III manual, IV, V) being less likely to report oral and non-penetrative sex in the last year than those in non-manual classes, after adjusting for other variables in the model. The effects were similar for women and men.

Anal sex showed a slightly different pattern, as suggested by the bivariate analysis. It was not significantly associated with age for men and only weakly associated with age for women, with younger women being more likely to report anal sex in the last year. Marital status exerted a weak effect in the model. The adjusted odds ratio for anal sex amongst those with two or more partners in the last year remained significantly raised (in excess of two for women and in excess of three for men). Social class exerted a significant but small effect in the model, but in the opposite direction from that for oral and non-penetrative sex, with those in manual social classes being more likely to report anal intercourse in the last year.

Summary

This chapter has examined the frequency of heterosexual sex and the repertoire of heterosexual practices. Men and women were very consistent in their reporting of both the frequency of sex and the pattern of practices.

The frequency of heterosexual sex (defined as acts of oral, vaginal and anal intercourse) showed very wide variability as measured by the number of occasions in the last 4 weeks, with a small proportion of the population reporting a very high frequency of sexual contact. Age was closely related to number of acts, with frequency peaking in the mid twenties and thereafter showing a gradual decline, more marked for women than men. This gender difference is probably a result of men adopting younger female partners as they grow older.

Not surprisingly, partner availability strongly influenced the frequency of sex, which was highest in the married and cohabiting groups of all ages. There was only a very weak relationship between social class and frequency of sex.

There was a strong association in all age groups between length of relationship and frequency of sex, with number of occasions in the last 4 weeks being much lower in longer relationships. It appears that the lower frequency of sex amongst older respondents is partly related to their longer relationships.

Within marital status categories, frequency of sex in the last 4 weeks increased with increasing numbers of partners in the last 5 years. However, amongst those outside married or cohabiting relationships, even those with high numbers of partners only achieved rates of heterosexual intercourse similar to those of the married. The bivariate findings in relation to frequency of sex were largely confirmed in multivariate analysis.

Respondents reported a varied repertoire of sexual practices. While vaginal intercourse predominated as the most prevalent practice, more than three-quarters of the sample had experience of non-penetrative sex not leading to intercourse and 70% had some experience of either cunnilingus or fellatio. In contrast, any experience of anal intercourse was reported by only 13.9% of men and 12.9% of women.

A number of factors are identified as influencing the repertoire of sexual practices. Recent and lifetime experience of oral and non-penetrative sex increased with decreasing age, indicating evidence of both age and age cohort effects. The data are consistent with other sources, indicating a considerable increase in popularity of orogenital contact. There was evidence of orogenital contact occurring as a prelude to first intercourse in a minority of respondents. Oral and non-penetrative sex in the absence of vaginal intercourse appeared to be unusual, although they were reported most frequently in those aged 18–24. There was, however, little evidence of widespread adoption of these activities as alternatives to vaginal intercourse in order to reduce the risks of unwanted pregnancy or STD. In contrast to oral and non-penetrative sex, there was little evidence of an increase in the practice of anal sex over recent decades. However, recent experience of anal intercourse was most frequent amongst young respondents and those with multiple partners.

Oral, anal and non-penetrative sex were reported at consistently higher rates amongst those who were not married, and who had had vaginal intercourse in the last year, than amongst the married, indicating that this group may have a wider repertoire than those in more stable relationships. This effect appears to be related to the relationship between the number of partners and practices. The prevalence of oral, anal and non-penetrative sex all increased with numbers of partners.

As with other areas of behaviour, social class had only a weak relationship with reported patterns of behaviour. In a multivariate analysis that controlled for the factors evident in bivariate analysis, those in non-manual classes were more likely to report oral and non-penetrative sex while those in manual classes were more likely to report anal sex. These effects were weak compared with the influences of age, marital status and the number of partners.

As with the number of partners, there is wide variability in the frequency of sex and patterns of sexual practices. Those outside married or cohabiting relationships may experience less frequent sex overall, but they are more likely to have multiple partners, to experience a wider range of practices and to have recent experience of more risky practices, such as anal intercourse. At the same time, this is a group who also have a wider experience of non-penetrative and oral sex, implying skills for the adoption of lower-risk sexual practices and for expressing sexual pleasure through a range of different activities.

References

Bungay, G.T., Vessey, M.P. & McPherson, K. (1980) Study of symptoms in middle life with special reference to the menopause. *British Medical Journal*, **281**, 181–3.

Coles, R. & Stokes, G. (1985) *Sex and the American Teenager*. Harper, New York.

Cox, B.D., Blaxter, M., Buckle, A.L.J. *et al.* (1987) *The Health and Lifestyle Survey*. Health Promotion Research Trust, London.

European Study Group (1989) Risk factors for male to female transmission of HIV. *British Medical Journal*, **298**, 411–5.

Gagnon, J.H. & Simon, W. (1987) The sexual sampling of orogenital contacts. *Archives of Sexual Behaviour*, **16**, 1–25.

Gebhard, P.H. (1970) Sexual motifs in prehistoric Peruvian ceramics. In Bowie, T. & Christiansen, C.V. (eds) *Studies in Erotic Art*, pp. 109–44. Basic Books, New York.

Gebhard, P.H. & Johnson, A.B. (1979) *The Kinsey Data: Marginal Tabulations of the 1938–1963 Interviews Conducted by the Institute of Sex Research*. W.B. Saunders, Philadelphia.

Gorer, G. (1971) *Sex and Marriage in England Today*. Nelson, London.

Johnson, A.M. (1988) Social and behavioural aspects of the HIV epidemic – a review. *Journal of Royal Statistical Society Series A*, **151**, 99–114.

Kinsey, A.C., Pomeroy, W.B. & Martin, C.E. (1948) *Sexual Behaviour in the Human Male*. W.B. Saunders, Philadelphia.

Kinsey, A.C., Pomeroy, W.B., Martin, C.E. & Gebhard, P.H. (1953) *Sexual Behaviour in the Human Female*. W.B. Saunders, Philadelphia.

Masters, W. & Johnson, V. (1966) *Human Sexual Response*. Churchill, London.

Newcomer, S.F. & Udry, J.R. (1985) Oral sex in an adolescent population: *Archives of Sexual Behaviour*, 41–6.

Osborn, M., Hawton, K. & Gath, D. (1988) Sexual dysfunction among middle aged women in the community. *British Medical Journal*, **296**, 959–62.

Padian, N., Marquis, L., Francis, D.P. *et al.* (1987) Male-to-female transmission of human immunodeficiency virus. *Journal of American AIDS*, **258**, 788–90.

Reinisch, J.M., Ziemba-Davis, M. & Sanders, S.A. (1990) Sexual behaviour and AIDS: lessons from art and sex research. In Vocher B., Reinisch J.M. & Gottlieb M. (eds) *AIDS and Sex: An Integrated Biomedical and Biobehavioural Approach*, pp. 37–80. Oxford University Press.

Simon, W., Kraft, D.M. & Kaplan, H.B. (1990) Oral sex: a critical overview. In *AIDS and Sex: An Integrated Biomedical and Biobehavioural Approach*, pp. 257–75. Oxford University Press.

Spencer, L., Faulkner, A. & Keegan, J. (1988) *Talking about Sex*. SCPR, London.

Starr, B.D. & Weiner, M.B. (1981) *The Starr–Weiner Report on Sex and Sexuality in the Mature Years*. McGraw-Hill, New York.

Voeller, B. (1990) Heterosexual anal intercourse: an AIDS risk factor. In *AIDS and Sex: An Integrated Biomedical and Biobehavioural Approach*, pp. 276–310. Oxford University Press.

Weeks, J. (1981) *Sex, Politics and Society: The Regulation of Sexuality Since 1800*. Longman, New York.

Wilson, S. (1973) Short history of Western erotic art. In Melville, R. (ed.) *Erotic Art of the West*, pp. 11–31. G.P. Putnam & Sons, New York.

Chapter 7
Sexual Diversity and Homosexual Behaviour

KAYE WELLINGS, JANE WADSWORTH
& ANNE JOHNSON

The aim of this chapter is to map the extent and range of patterns of sexual diversity. A major problem for scientific investigation in this area is that the choice of gender of sexual partner is not neutral; different social and moral values are attached to particular preferences. Diversity of sexual orientation may be universal in human societies (Ford & Beach, 1952), but the level of approval varies markedly and in most Western societies homosexual preference is tolerated but stigmatized.

Only in very recent times has there been a shift away from the treatment of homosexuality as sickness or sin. Until 1967 male homosexuality was a criminal offence in Britain, and only in 1974 was it removed from the list of psychiatric disorders by the American Psychiatric Association (to be replaced by the diagnosis 'sexual orientation disturbance' (Bayer, 1981)). Also, only comparatively recently have social scientists come to view homosexuality as other than clinical or social deviance (Weeks, 1986).

The emerging perspective in the latter part of the 20th century is that homosexuality is part of a broad spectrum of sexual expression. The origins of this view are to be found partly in Freud's concept of the 'polymorphous perverse' sexuality of infancy (although Freud was inclined to see this more as an innate capacity than as a social or psychological norm (Freud, 1953)). Empirically, the perspective owes much to the work of Kinsey, who for the first time designed a research instrument to represent sexual orientation as a continuum rather than two fixed and dichotomous points (Kinsey *et al.*, 1948).

If the scientific community has been slow to accept sexual diversity, the general public has shown even greater resistance. Public attitudes to homosexuality are still characterized by a deep ambivalence (see Chapter 8). The growing acceptance of same-gender sexual relations in the 1970s suffered a setback in the 1980s with the emergence of AIDS, which seemed to precipitate a resurgence of anti-gay sentiment (Wellings & Wadsworth, 1990). Socially acceptable sexual behaviour is still predominantly heterosexual. We have not yet moved into a culture which tolerates sexual variety.

Implications for research

Public and professional attitudes to homosexuality are not merely of academic or sociological interest but of direct *practical* relevance to the conduct of research. Researchers cannot escape locating themselves within a particular paradigm, which is reflected in the research instrument. It is perhaps worth stating at the outset the assumptions which guided the construction of the questions relating to sexual orientation in this survey.

1   The polarity 'homosexual–heterosexual' is an inadequate categorization of the population; same- and opposite-gender sexual expression are better represented as a continuum than as a pair of fixed-point response options. The Kinsey scale – rating same- and opposite-gender sexual attraction and experience on a seven-point rating scale – has been adapted for this survey as a five-point scale (see below).

2   The terms heterosexual and homosexual were not used within the research instrument for the following reasons.

(a)   The use of the term 'homosexual' might invite a low rate of reporting, on the assumption that a respondent is less likely to ascribe to him or herself a stigmatizing identity than to report a particular practice.

(b)   The use of a term denoting a sexual identity is irrelevant in the context of HIV and STD, since it is sexual practice and not identity which is relevant to understanding the dynamics of transmission.

(c)   Development work for the survey revealed some lack of understanding of the term 'homosexual' (Spencer *et al.*, 1988), which was confirmed in the British Social Attitudes survey (Wellings & Wadsworth, 1990). Possibly because of a misunderstanding over the Greek root 'homo' meaning 'same', a sizeable majority believed homosexuality to refer to sex between two men, whilst only a minority believed it to refer also to sex between two women.

Thus although the terms homosexual and heterosexual are used throughout this chapter to describe sexual activity with same- and opposite-gender partners respectively, these terms did not feature in the questionnaire. Respondents were simply asked to report attraction and experience, with men and with women (see below).

How homosexual behaviour is viewed socially influences not only the kinds of questions asked and the way in which they are phrased, but also responses to them and even the uses to which the data might be put. An important caveat here is that since homosexual sex is stigmatized in Britain, it can be expected to be under- rather than over-reported. For the same reason, it is possible that some people who had experienced homosexual sex would be less willing to participate in the survey. Because of possible reporting and response bias, all prevalence figures relating to homosexual activity should be regarded as minimum estimates.

In terms of the use of the data, the prevalence of same-gender sexual practice is clearly of central significance as a public health question in the AIDS era. Where transmission of a virus is linked with particular sexual practices it is important to estimate their prevalence. At the same time, political use of these data cannot be ignored. According to some observers, one of the most important contributions a survey of sexual behaviour can make is to provide the empirical framework for a recognition of sexual diversity (Gagnon & Simon 1973). Statistical and moral deviance tend to be equated in this context. Whilst deviation from a statistical norm might properly be termed *diversity*, relating to a continuum of behaviours in which no more value is attached to one point than another, deviation from a moral norm denotes *perversion* – a term highly laden with opprobrium. Statistics have political significance in so far as they have the potential to normalize particular practices. For this reason Kinsey's findings (Kinsey *et al.*, 1948, 1953), indicating a larger than expected prevalence of same-gender sexual practice, were greeted enthusiastically by the homosexual community.

Question formulation

Two questions relating to sexual orientation were asked in the face-to-face interview, and the self-completion booklet contained questions on homosexual behaviour. The first of these (question 31), in the face-to-face part of the schedule, requested respondents to locate themselves in terms of both sexual attraction and experience on a five-point rating scale. At this point, sexual experience was self-defined (see below). Show-cards were used, enabling respondents to read the statements themselves and to respond using only a letter of the alphabet. The questions were worded as follows for men; for women the terms male and female were transposed.

Card K

I have felt sexually attracted . . .

. . . *only to females, never to males*	*(K)*
. . . *more often to females, and at least once to a male*	*(C)*
. . . *about equally often to females and to males*	*(F)*
. . . *more often to males, and at least once to a female*	*(L)*
. . . *only ever to males, never to females*	*(D)*
I have never felt sexually attracted to anyone at all	*(N)*

Table 7.2. Orientation of sexual experience and attraction: male respondents
[Source: interview, question 31a,b]

| Experience | Attraction | | | | | |
	Only to women (%)	Mostly to women (%)	Equally to women and men (%)	Mostly to men (%)	Only to men (%)	No attraction (%)
Only with women	90.19	2.01	0.15	0.02	0.03	0.37
Mostly with women	1.96	1.82	0.09	0.04	0.04	0.00
Equally with women and men	0.00	0.08	0.20	0.02	0.02	0.00
Mostly with men	0.08	0.01	0.02	0.35	0.10	0.00
Only with men	0.02	0.01	0.00	0.10	0.26	0.00
No experience	1.56	0.05	0.02	0.02	0.01	0.37

Base = 8335.

Table 7.3. Orientation of sexual experience and attraction: female respondents
[Source: interview, question 31a,b]

| Experience | Attraction | | | | | |
	Only to men (%)	Mostly to men (%)	Equally to women and men (%)	Mostly to women (%)	Only to women (%)	No attraction (%)
Only with men	92.42	2.44	0.08	0.02	0.07	0.74
Mostly with men	0.78	1.38	0.02	0.05	0.03	0.00
Equally with women and men	0.03	0.01	0.04	0.02	0.03	0.00
Mostly with women	0.02	0.00	0.01	0.10	0.03	0.00
Only with women	0.01	0.00	0.00	0.01	0.10	0.00
No experience	1.02	0.01	0.01	0.00	0.03	0.50

Base = 10412.

sex. 2.2% of men reported having felt attracted to, but having no experience with, someone of their own gender, and for women the comparable figure 2.6%. Conversely, 2.1% of men and 0.8% of women reported homosexual experience but exclusively heterosexual attraction.

Prevalence of homosexual experience

The answer to the question, 'What is a reasonable estimate of the prevalence of homosexual experience among British men and women?', depends largely on the context in which the question is posed and the purposes for which the data are collected. As stated above, it is both possible and desirable to produce several estimates of prevalence depending on the criteria used to define homosexual activity (Fig. 7.1 & Table 7.4). In the context of the HIV/AIDS epidemic, a definition which includes genital contact will clearly be important, since this describes the practices which could lead to the exchange of body fluids. If we are concerned with *currently practising* homosexuals then a definition must incorporate some measure of recency.

Responses to all questions relating to same-gender sexual contact were used to provide prevalence estimates for several same-gender experiences that are summarized in Table 7.4. It should be emphasized that no one of these individually can be taken as a single prevalence estimate of homosexual orientation.

It will be recalled that the first question on same-gender experience was asked in the face-to-face interview, whilst all others relating to sexual orientation were contained within the self-completion booklet. The use of show-cards and letters of the alphabet indicating particular responses allowed respondents to avoid audibly disclosing personal information. Even so, respondents might still have felt more at ease reporting under conditions of greater privacy. This was provided by the self-completion booklet: higher levels of reporting of homosexual activity could be expected in questions within the booklet than within the questionnaire.

The repetition of the question asking about any homosexual contact within the booklet (question 4a) allowed respondents a further opportunity to report such experience and also permitted direct comparisons to be made between responses to the two. Since the main difference between these questions lies in the manner of data collection (face-to-face in the case of the one, self-recorded in the other), any reporting variation might be attributed to this difference. In fact, as Fig. 7.2 shows, for women of all ages, and for men older than 19, the proportion reporting same-gender sexual contact in the booklet was higher than in the face-to-face interview. Among men (but not so notably among women), the

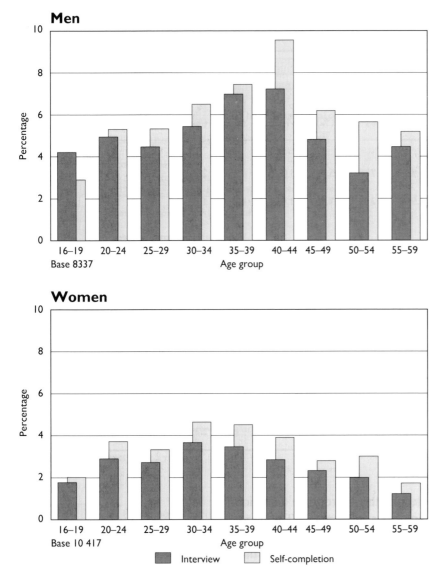

Fig. 7.2. Homosexual experience reported at interview and self-completion, by age. [Source: interview, question 31b; booklet, question 4a]

three contemporary national surveys in the USA, derive lifetime prevalence estimates of male–male experience within the range 4.8%–4.9%. Prevalence estimates for male–male contact within the last year lie within the range 1.2%–2.4%.

The French national survey of sexual lifestyles found that 4.1% of men reported at least one occurrence of intercourse with a person of the same sex during their lifetime (ACSF Investigators, 1992). Sundet *et al.* (1988), from a random sample survey of the Norwegian population aged 18–60, reported that 3.5% of men and 3.0% of women claim to have had at least one same-gender sexual partner, which again is consistent with the British data for men. Sundet *et al.* also asked about same-sex partners in the last 3 years, a time period which is not directly comparable with the time periods of 2 and 5 years in this survey, and derived figures of 0.9% for men and 0.9% for women.

The aggregate figures show a marked difference in the prevalence of same-sex experience between men and women. While 6.1% of men have had some kind of homosexual experience, only 3.4% of women have done so, and this ratio of roughly 2:1 is consistent across all definitions despite the similarity in the prevalence of same-sex attraction. This is in contrast to the Norwegian data, in which no difference was found between men and women (Sundet *et al.*, 1988).

Analysis by age however, does, show signs of some convergence between the sexes in terms of reporting same-gender experience. The ratio of men to women reporting at least one lifetime homosexual partner is 1.9:1, 1.8:1, 2.3:1 and 2.5:1 for the four successive age bands 16–24, 25–34, 35–44 and 45–59. It may be that the social pressures on women that contribute to the greater difference between attraction and experience are weakening with successive generations.

Sociodemographic variation in prevalence

To date it has been difficult to draw general conclusions from research on homosexuality because of non-random sampling procedures and the problems involved in finding representative samples of those who have same-gender sex. Most recent studies have tended to use volunteer samples, obtaining respondents through gay and lesbian bars, social and friendship networks, organizations and clubs.

While these samples are essential to an understanding of homosexual behaviour and relationships, they do not constitute representative samples of men with same-sex experience. Gay bar samples draw heavily on individuals in particular social environments, and are skewed towards urban, young, self-identified homosexuals, and those seeking partners. Homosexual organizations are likely to attract those who feel able to be more open about their sexual orientation.

Focused or purposive samples of homosexual men have tended to be middle class and urban. They are also biased towards younger and more highly educated men who are in employment (Hunt *et al.*, 1991). This survey provides an opportunity to explore to what extent some of these attributes are inherent characteristics of people who have same-gender sex. Since the sample is randomly selected, it can be expected to contain more of those who do not self-identify as gay than purposive samples.

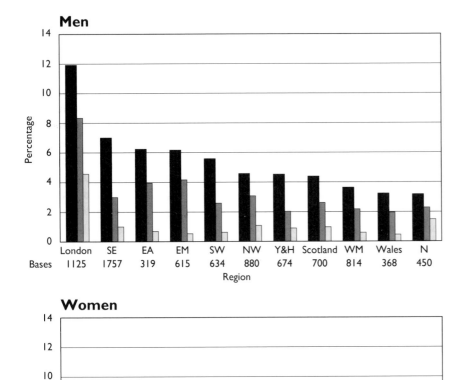

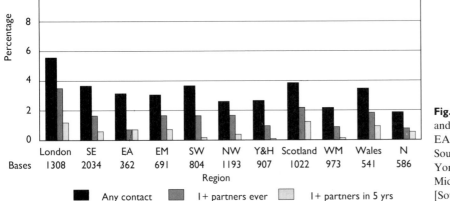

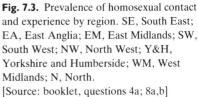

Fig. 7.3. Prevalence of homosexual contact and experience by region. SE, South East; EA, East Anglia; EM, East Midlands; SW, South West; NW, North West; Y&H, Yorkshire and Humberside; WM, West Midlands; N, North.
[Source: booklet, questions 4a; 8a,b]

Again, the possibility of a reporting bias operating here cannot be ruled out, since the more hospitable environment which attracts men who have sex with men to London might also make it easier to report such relationships. Our data suggest that the advantages of living in the capital in terms of acceptance and anonymity may be more real for men than for women, for whom the regional variation is less marked (Fig. 7.3).

Table 7.6. Residence and mobility by homosexual activity
[Source: booklet, question 8b]

Homosexual partner in last 5 years	Men		Women	
	Yes (%)	No (%)	Yes (%)	No (%)
London always	8.3	2.6	1.8	2.1
Moved to London	35.2	10.4	22.2	10.4
Moved (not to London)	48.7	64.4	54.4	64.7
Didn't move (not in London)	7.8	22.6	21.7	22.8
Base	118	8 189	65	10 333

Age-related variations in same-gender sexual experience

Clear age-related patterns emerge from the data on sexual orientation. In response to the question about same-gender attraction, members of the youngest age group of male respondents aged 16–24 (though not female respondents in this age group) are more likely to report having been attracted to someone of the same gender compared with other age groups (Table 7.4). In terms of lifetime experience, the age-related pattern differs markedly for men and women. The proportion of male respondents who report ever having had same-gender sexual experience peaks for the 35–44 age group (Fig. 7.4 & Table 7.4). For women, no such peak occurs amongst 35–44 year olds, and prevalence is lowest for women aged 45 and over. This is a consistent result across responses relating to lifetime experience of any form of sexual contact but it does not apply to more recent practice – see below.

The atypical position of 35- to 44-year-old men is particularly clear in Fig. 7.5, showing cumulative percentages for age at first homosexual experience for men and women by age group. (The booklet asked those who reported ever having any kind of sexual experience or sexual contact with someone of the same gender as themselves, 'How old were you the first time that ever happened?') Again, men aged 35–44 years are distinct from all other age groups. They are more likely to report homosexual experience at some time in their lives, compared with those younger and older than themselves, and more than twice as likely to report having a homosexual experience before the age of 16 as those 20 years younger than themselves (Table 7.7 & Fig. 7.5).

This pattern is not the same for women. One of the noticeable features

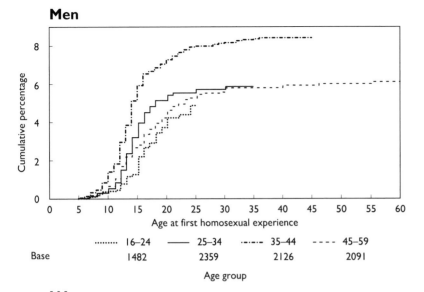

Men

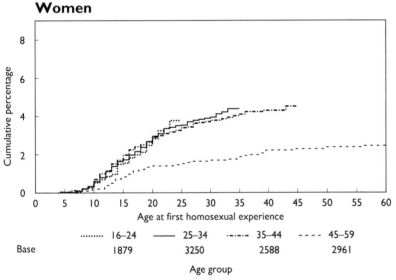

Women

Fig. 7.5. Age at first homosexual experience by age group.
[Source: booklet, question 4b]

Women from their mid-twenties to their mid-forties are more likely than those either younger or older than this to report ever having had homosexual experience.

   The age pattern, however, seems more to reflect a general liberalizing effect of the early 1960s following the deliberations of the Wolfenden Committee's Report on Homosexuality (1957), which culminated in the 1967 Act, than an effect of the Act itself. There is little evidence that the 1967 legislation *per se* had any major impact on behaviour. There is no

Men

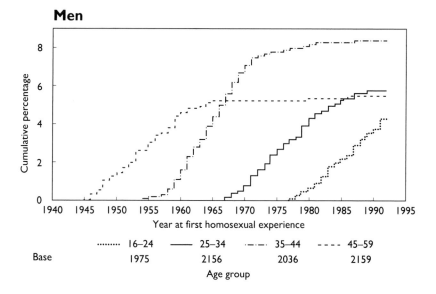

Year at first homosexual experience

	········ 16–24	—— 25–34	—·— 35–44	– – – – 45–59
Base	1975	2156	2036	2159

Age group

Women

Year at first homosexual experience

	········ 16–24	—— 25–34	—·— 35–44	– – – – 45–59
Base	2231	2878	2557	2742

Age group

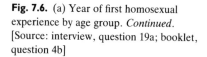

Fig. 7.6. (a) Year of first homosexual experience by age group. *Continued.* [Source: interview, question 19a; booklet, question 4b]

marked increase in the proportions reporting homosexual experience after the age of 21, the age at which homosexual relations became legal between consenting men, and the slope of the curve for 35- to 44-year-old men shows no obvious change immediately before or after 1967 (Fig. 7.6a).

The year in which laws are actually enacted is relatively arbitrary. Legal reform both responds to, and accelerates the process of, social change, and it is the underlying social trends which are probably more

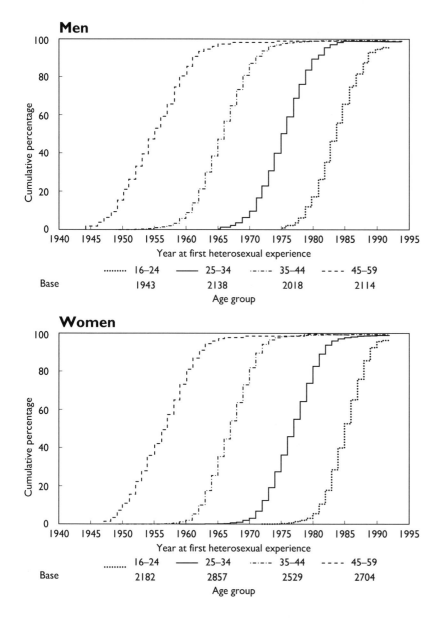

Fig. 7.6. *Continued.* (b) Year of first heterosexual experience by age group. [Source: interview, question 19a; booklet, question 4b]

important in explaining behaviour. Shortly after the Wolfenden Committee, a contemporary poll showed nearly a quarter of British people to be in favour of a change in the law; 8 years later the proportion had increased to nearly two-thirds (Bancroft, 1989). The 1967 Act both reflected and furthered a social climate in which the gay population was able to be less covert, but it seems likely that it was this social climate rather than the specific legislation that had a major impact on behaviour.

If this hypothesis provides the explanation for the different pattern in those aged 35–44, at first sight it is curious that the trend does not seem to have been sustained in the younger age groups. The pattern for first homosexual experience amongst men younger than 35 follows that of men aged 45–59 rather than those aged 35–44. There seems no reason to suppose that the trend initiated in the 1970s should not have continued, had it not been halted by other circumstances. One explanation might be that the upward trend in homosexual activity with successive age groups was reversed by the AIDS epidemic. Those in the 25–34 age group would have been between the ages of 16 and 25 in 1981 when the first case of AIDS was recorded in Britain, and those aged 16–24, 15 or younger.

The age-related pattern for lifetime experience described above does not apply to accounts of more recent practice (Table 7.4 & Fig. 7.4). Reports of same-gender partners in the most recent periods, 5 years, 2 years and 12 months, decrease with increasing age for all but the youngest age group. For women, the likelihood of having had a female sexual partner in the recent past decreases steadily with current age. In general, the older the respondent, the less likely it is that recent same-gender partners will be reported, and this age profile is consistent for all but the youngest age group of men.

It is not clear what might account for the slight reduction in recent experience among 16- to 24-year-old men. In the case of recent practice, age-related trends must clearly be interpreted in the context of lifecourse factors and secular change, although there will be interplay between the two. Some men in this age group may have yet to experience same-gender sex. A further explanatory factor might be that since the age of homosexual consent is 21, young men under that age may be under-reporting.

The apparent restraint amongst younger men might also reflect concerns brought about by the AIDS epidemic or, indirectly, AIDS-related changes in the social climate surrounding male homosexuality, particularly since it does not feature in the data for women. The exact balance of these different factors in terms of their influence on behaviour remains a matter for conjecture.

Stability of orientation

The extent to which the recording procedures used in the questionnaire can measure change in sexual orientation over time is limited. The fact that reports of lifetime same-gender experience are cumulative rather than relating to discrete time periods in the past restricts analysis in terms of life history. There is no opportunity for measuring the duration of relationships (except those involving a same-gender partner in the last 5 years) or the point in people's lives at which they occurred.

The difference in prevalence between lifetime and current homosexual experience points to the likelihood that homosexual experience is often a relatively isolated or passing event. Almost certainly, respondents who report having had some homosexual experience but no genital contact (2.4% of men and 1.7% of women) are predominantly those for whom the same-gender experience was a transient part of their sexual development. For the majority of respondents reporting same-gender genital contact, the event took place more than 5 years ago.

The proportion of respondents reporting *ever* having a same-gender sexual partner is higher than in more recent time periods, for both men and women. Ever having had a male sexual partner was reported by 3.5% of men, 1.4% in the last 5 years and 1.1% in the last year. For women, the comparable figures are 1.7%, 0.6% and 0.4% respectively (Table 7.4). This 'seemingly episodic character' of same-gender sexual contacts is noted by Rogers & Turner (1991) for men, and our data seem to confirm this for women too.

Some observations can be made on homosexual behaviour through the lifecourse, from the relationship between the time of first homosexual experience and subsequent experience. Fewer questions were asked about first homosexual experience compared with first heterosexual experience, and they were asked within the self-completion component of the questionnaire rather than face-to-face. Homosexual experience occurring for the first time in the early teens is unlikely to lead on to more consistent homosexual behaviour. Men and women whose first experience of same-gender sex occurred before the age of 16 were less likely to have had genital contact, and less likely to report having had a same-gender sexual partner within the last 5 years (Fig. 7.7) than those for whom this experience occurred at the age of 16 or later. Other sources suggest that later homosexual experiences are more important in predicting more persistent homosexual orientation (Dank, 1971).

These findings at least support the view that for some, sexual development is characterized by a labile stage of orientation preceding a later state of greater stability. A form of bisexuality prevalent in early adulthood may represent a transitional phase in which preferences are tested through experimentation with different lifestyles and relationships. Kinsey *et al.* (1948) interpreted their data as showing that homosexuality peaks in the early teens and declines slowly with increasing age. Using data from the 1970 Kinsey Institute survey, Rogers & Turner (1991) estimate that of more than 20% of US men who reported sexual contact to orgasm with another man at some time in their life, only a third reported such contact occurring after the age of 20.

It has been observed that homosexual acts may occur in situations where the sexes are segregated – in prisons, for example, and in the

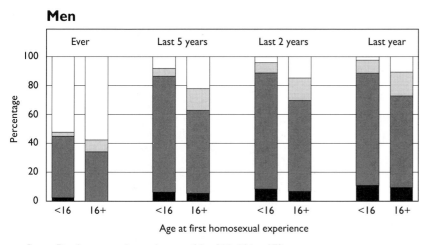

Men

Base   First homosexual experience: <16 = 311; 16+ = 179

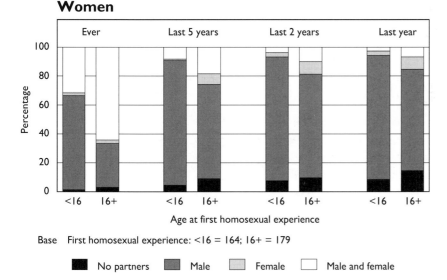

Women

Base   First homosexual experience: <16 = 164; 16+ = 179

█ No partners   ▓ Male   ░ Female   ☐ Male and female

Fig. 7.7. Gender of partners in different time intervals by age at first homosexual experience.
[Source: booklet, questions 4b; 7a–d; 8a–d]

armed forces – where same-gender contact might be exploited in the absence of opportunities for contact with members of the opposite sex (Bancroft, 1989). Implicit in this is the notion of a so-called 'facultative' homosexuality, according to which homosexual expression borne out of coexistence with people of the same gender is more likely to be opportunistic.

Our data afford an oportunity for investigating this phenomenon, in the context of single-sex boarding schools. The data have been analysed by attendance at such schools for men and women. If 'facultative' homo-sexual expression occurred more frequently in a single-sex environment,

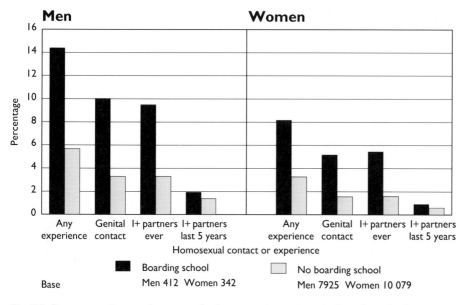

Fig. 7.8. Percentage of respondents reporting homosexual experience by boarding school attendance.
[Source: booklet, questions 4a,c; 8a,b]

a higher proportion of those who attended boarding school might be expected to report homosexual experience *ever* compared with those who did not, but the effect of institution would not be expected to be sustained up to the most recent period of reporting. As Fig. 7.8 shows, the data are entirely consistent with this hypothesis. For the questions asking about any same-gender sexual contact, genital contact and sexual partnerships, those who had a boarding school education are more likely to have had homosexual experience than those who did not . The findings are broadly similar for both men and women. In the more recent time period, however, there is little difference between the two groups. Thus although boarding school education seems to provide greater opportunities for same-gender experience, it seems to have little or no effect on homosexual practice later in life.

Multivariate analysis

Drawing age, schooling, social class and region together in logistic regression models (Figs 7.9 & 7.10), there are clearly different associations for men and women and for experience ever and in the last 5 years, but these influences are not necessarily mutually independent. Schooling has an important influence on whether someone has ever had a homosexual

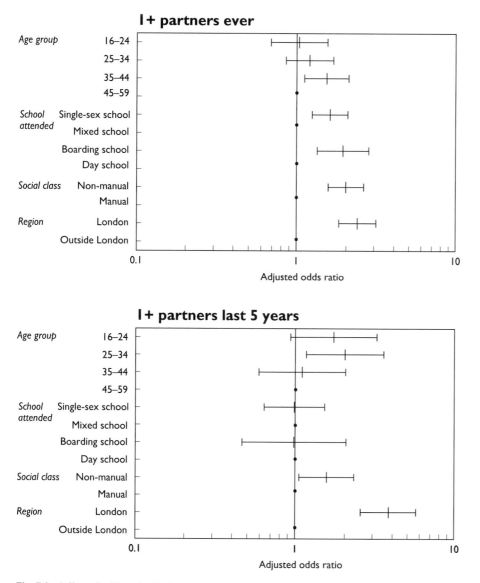

Fig. 7.9. Adjusted odds ratios for homosexual behaviour: men.
[Source: booklet, questions 8a,b]

partner, but no significant impact on homosexual partnerships in the last 5 years. Social class also shows a stronger effect on partners ever than partners in the last 5 years. In contrast, for men the effect of region increases as the time interval decreases. This is consistent with the concept of migration to London to seek a more favourable environment for a homosexual lifestyle. The effect of age is not clear-cut and exerts a stronger influence on recent behaviour of women than men.

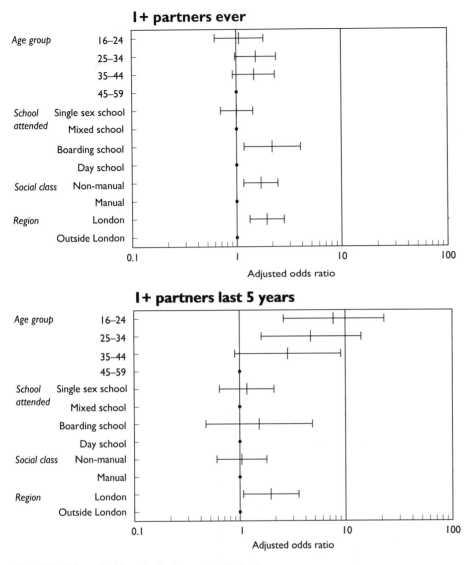

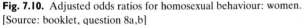

Fig. 7.10. Adjusted odds ratios for homosexual behaviour: women. [Source: booklet, question 8a,b]

Exclusivity of same-sex experience

Exclusively homosexual behaviour appears to be rare. Table 7.8 and Figs 7.11 & 7.12 illustrate the mixing of male–male, female–female and male–female sex reported by British men and women. It can be seen that very substantial proportions of those reporting same-sex partners also report opposite-sex partners. The majority of those who have had some homosexual experience have had sex with both men and women. Of men who report having ever had a male sexual partner in their lifetime, 90.3%

Table 7.8. Gender of partners in different time intervals
[Source: booklet, questions 7a–d, 8a–d]

	Time periods for sexual partner reporting			
	Ever (%)	In last 5 years (%)	In last 2 years (%)	In last year (%)
Men				
Exclusively female	90.1	90.5	88.8	86.5
Exclusively male	0.3	0.6	0.6	0.7
Male and female	3.4	0.8	0.5	0.4
No partners	6.2	8.1	10.1	12.4
Base	8 009	8 044	8 039	8 047
Women				
Exclusively male	92.7	90.4	88.1	86.0
Exclusively female	0.1	0.2	0.2	0.2
Male and female	1.7	0.5	0.2	0.2
No partners	5.6	9.0	11.4	13.6
Base	10 040	10 055	10 048	10 057

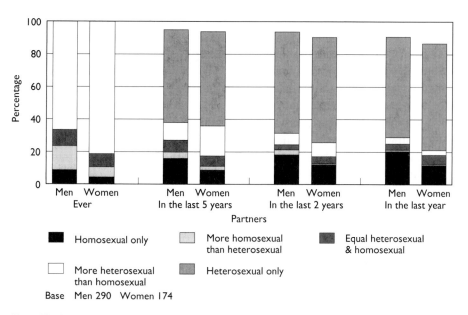

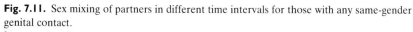

Fig. 7.11. Sex mixing of partners in different time intervals for those with any same-gender genital contact.
[Source: booklet, questions 4c, 7a–d; 8a–d]

demonstrate that 'very substantial proportions of men who report male–male sexual contacts in adulthood also report male–female sexual contacts'. At least one female sexual partner was reported by 92.3% of men who had one male sexual partner in adulthood, and by 86.4% of those with more than one male sexual partner (Rogers & Turner, 1991). Data from the French survey of sexual lifestyles show that 82% of men and 78% of women who had had homosexual intercourse at least once, had also had heterosexual intercourse (ACSF Investigators, 1992). From the Norwegian national survey, Sundet *et al.* (1988) report that of men and women reporting same-gender practice, 83% and 75% respectively also reported opposite-gender practices.

These findings have important implications for HIV-preventive strategies, since they suggest that the proportion of men who have sex with both men and women may be larger than indicated in surveys using purposive samples. If the hypothesis is correct, these men may be covert in their homosexual practice, and they may represent a hard-to-reach population in terms of health education and prevention.

Number of partners

There is a prevailing view that men who have sex with men have far larger numbers of sexual partners than those who have sex with women (Bancroft, 1989). As far as women are concerned little seems to be known or surmised, but what empirical work there is points to a tendency of lesbian women to experience relatively stable, long-term relationships (Bell & Weinberg, 1978). Of interest in these data is the extent to which they support this stereotypical image.

Looking at the aggregate data for responses to the question asking about numbers of same-gender partners (Table 7.10), roughly half of all men and two-thirds of women who report having had a same-gender partner in their lifetime have had only one. At the opposite end of the spectrum, 11.4% of men had 20 or more male sexual partners and 3.9% had 100 or more. No woman had more than 20 female partners. (A male sexual partner, it will be recalled, was defined as someone with whom a man has had oral sex or anal intercourse, or with whom other forms of genital contact had taken place, and a female partner one with whom a woman has had oral sex or other forms of genital contact. This differs from the definition of a heterosexual partner, which includes acts of vaginal intercourse, oral or anal sex and does not include non-penetrative sex.)

It would, of course, be quite misleading to base any assumptions about homosexual behaviour in general on these figures, since the proportion reporting a same-sex partner includes a number of respon-

Table 7.10. Heterosexual and homosexual partners ever and in the last 5 years
[Source: booklet, questions 7a,b; 4c; 8a,b]

	Men		Women	
	Homosexual (%)	Heterosexual (%)	Homosexual (%)	Heterosexual (%)
Partners ever				
1	50.4	22.0	67.4	41.7
2–9	32.6	51.9	30.6	51.1
10–19	5.6	14.5	2.0	5.3
20–99	7.5	10.8	0.0	1.8
100+	3.9	0.8	0.0	0.1
Base	286*	7 489†	174*	9 471†
Partners: last 5 years				
0	61.8	2.3	64.1	3.6
1	16.3	60.5	22.4	71.4
2–9	12.8	32.0	13.0	24.0
10–19	4.9	3.5	0.5	0.7
20–99	3.2	1.7	0.0	0.2
100+	1.0	0.01	0.0	0.01
Base	290*	7 484†	175*	9 459†

* Any same-gender sexual contact.
† Any opposite-gender partner.

dents for whom the experience was a single, possibly youthful and experimental, occurrence and for whom a homosexual inclination was not a lasting orientation. Figure 7.13 shows that the likelihood of having a recent partner of the same gender decreases markedly with age. Yet looking at the more recent time period of 5 years, 61.8% of men and 64.1% of women who ever had genital contact with someone of the same gender had no partner in the last 5 years. In contrast, 2.3% of men and 3.6% of women had no heterosexual partner in the last 5 years (Table 7.10).

Marked differences can be seen in the pattern of numbers of same-gender compared with opposite-gender partners (Fig. 7.14). Broadly speaking, the proportion reporting large numbers of sexual partners in the last 5 years is higher for men reporting homosexual partners than it is for men reporting heterosexual partners. However, as Hunt *et al.* (1991) argue, the proper comparison to be made is between the median number of lifetime *penetrative* homosexual partners (in the Sigma study this was

Table 7.11. Proportion of men and women reporting ever having had a homosexual partner by number of heterosexual partners
[Source: booklet, questions 7a, 8a]

Number of heterosexual partners	Men (%)	Men Base	Women (%)	Women Base
0	4.7	523	1.5	569
1	2.2	1647	0.4	3952
2	3.9	850	0.8	1700
3–4	2.9	1476	1.3	1832
5–9	3.9	1559	3.6	1310
10+	4.8	1955	10.2	678
Total with at least one heterosexual partner	3.6	7486	1.8	9473
Total	3.7	8009	1.7	10042

more female partners are more likely to have had a male sexual partner than are those with one (4.8% vs 2.2%), but women with this number of male partners are considerably more likely to have had a female partner than are those with only one male partner (10.2% vs 0.4%). Thirty-nine per cent of women who have had sex with a woman are in the subgroup of those with 10+ opposite-gender partners. There may be grounds for suggesting a consistent profile of experience-seeking amongst a small minority of women – those who seek diversity in terms of *numbers* of partners also do so in terms of the gender of those partners.

Homosexual practices

Questions were asked about sexual practices relating to their same-gender partners in particular periods. Thus, male respondents were asked to provide information on whether or not they had experienced oral and anal sex, and genital stimulation with a man, and female respondents on whether they had experienced oral sex and genital stimulation with a woman.

There is marked evidence of a broad repertoire of sexual acts amongst those with same-gender partners. There is certainly less emphasis on penetrative intercourse (anal in this case) amongst those with homosexual

Table 7.12. Reporting of same-gender sexual practices in different time intervals: men by age group
[Source: booklet, questions 4c; 6a−e]

	16–24 (base = 48)				25–34 (base = 80)				35–44 (base = 105)				45–59 (base = 67)			
	<1 yr (%)	1–5 yr (%)	>5 yr (%)	Never (%)	<1 yr (%)	1–5 yr (%)	>5 yr (%)	Never (%)	<1 yr (%)	1–5 yr (%)	>5 yr (%)	Never (%)	<1 yr (%)	1–5 yr (%)	>5 yr (%)	Never (%)
Receptive anal	21.0	3.6	12.6	62.8	16.3	14.4	17.4	51.9	9.7	1.8	15.2	73.3	10.0	1.4	21.4	67.2
Insertive anal	25.1	6.6	3.2	65.1	24.8	11.6	9.5	54.1	8.7	2.3	17.3	71.6	8.8	2.3	15.6	73.3
Receptive oral	34.1	16.0	17.9	32.0	35.0	12.1	24.9	28.1	9.5	6.3	29.1	55.1	16.6	4.5	27.9	51.0
Insertive oral	37.7	11.4	14.5	36.4	35.4	11.5	18.9	34.2	12.4	5.1	21.5	61.0	15.1	1.6	27.8	55.4
Non-penetrative	33.8	27.2	33.0	6.1	33.9	10.1	43.4	12.6	16.5	4.1	68.8	10.6	16.3	6.2	66.5	11.0

Base: men reporting same-gender genital contact.

experience compared with those with heterosexual experience. This is of particular interest in the context of HIV, since homosexual anal sex has been so heavily implicated in transmission of the virus, and safer-sex strategies directed towards male homosexuals constantly stress the wisdom of adopting alternative forms of sexual expression. As Table 7.12 and Figs 7.16 & 7.17 show, oral sex and non-penetrative sex are more commonly reported by men with recent homosexual contact, than are receptive and insertive anal sex. Only 10.5% of men with some same-gender genital contact report never having experienced non-penetrative sex, compared with 66.3% who report no insertive anal sex, and 64.6% no receptive anal sex.

The proportions of men reporting same-gender sexual contact who report anal sex are lower for our sample than for other samples of homosexual men. Surveys based on focused samples of gay men show that the prevalence of penetrative sex is lower in homosexual than in heterosexual relationships. Reporting Project Sigma data, Hunt *et al.* (1991) show that the median number of male sexual partners reported is four times as large as the median number of penetrative partners in the past year, and Davies *et al.* (1992) that fewer than half (46%) of gay men interviewed had engaged in anal sex in the month before interview. The survey reported here shows the proportions to be considerably lower even for the longer time period of 1 year (Table 7.12), and this adds to the evidence of differences in the composition of this randomly selected sample of men with some homosexual experience, and samples based on men who self-identify as gay.

A common belief relating to homosexual relationships is that they mimic heterosexual patterns of sexual activity, adopting complementary

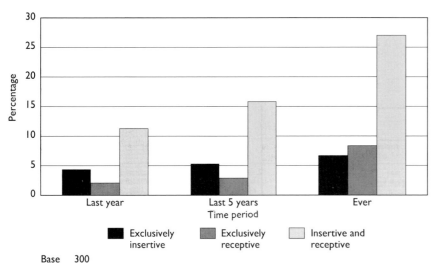

Fig. 7.18. Modality of anal sex: men reporting homosexual genital contact. [Source: booklet, questions 4c; 6c,d]

Table 7.13. Reporting of same-gender sexual practices in different time intervals: women [Source: booklet, questions 4c; 6a,b,c]

	16–24 (base = 30)				25–34 (base = 54)				35–44 (base = 53)				45–59 (base = 36)			
	<1 yr (%)	1–5 yr (%)	>5 yr (%)	Never (%)	<1 yr (%)	1–5 yr (%)	>5 yr (%)	Never (%)	<1 yr (%)	1–5 yr (%)	>5 yr (%)	Never (%)	<1 yr (%)	1–5 yr (%)	>5 yr (%)	Never (%)
Passive oral	42.3	25.7	12.1	19.9	20.3	7.8	31.9	40.0	9.0	2.7	40.1	48.2	3.0	3.9	30.5	62.7
Active oral	30.0	28.6	9.1	32.2	23.4	8.7	25.6	42.3	9.0	4.2	40.4	46.3	3.0	2.5	29.2	65.3
Non-penetrative	30.6	38.2	17.5	13.7	28.8	7.4	53.3	10.5	11.3	9.1	70.0	9.6	5.6	2.7	78.6	13.1

Base: women reporting genital contact.

of its lower risk, and the 'higher prestige assigned to it in the gay community'. This differential might also be a function of age mixing.

For the sample of women who have had same-gender sexual contact, activities investigated included passive and active oral sex, and mutual masturbation (Table 7.13, Figs 7.17 & 7.19). Using differences between age groups to detect trends over time, the practice of oral sex can be seen to have increased recently, a trend which was also apparent in heterosexual relationships (see Chapter 5). Whilst women in the oldest age group 45–59 reporting non-penetrative sex in the last year outnumbers those reporting oral sex in this period by roughly 3:2, the ratio narrows with decreasing age and is ultimately reversed for the 16–24 age group, so that reports of oral sex outnumber those for non-penetrative

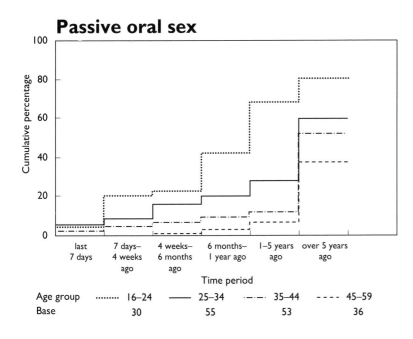

Passive oral sex

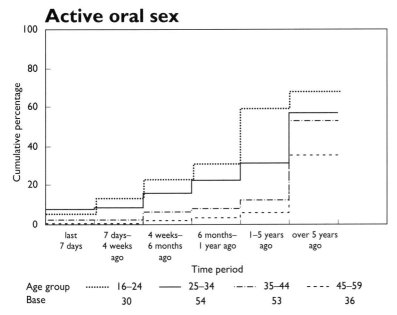

Active oral sex

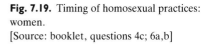

Fig. 7.19. Timing of homosexual practices: women.
[Source: booklet, questions 4c; 6a,b]

sex (mutual masturbation). As Figs 7.17–7.19 show, the age group that reports the highest levels of sexual activity (as measured by most recent experience of particular sexual practices) is that of 25–34 year olds. This is nearly a decade later than for those reporting on heterosexual partnerships, and is consistent with later age at first experience.

Spencer, L., Faulkner, A. & Keegan, J. (1989) *Talking about Sex*. SCPR, London.

Sundet, J.M., Kvalem, I.L., Magnus, P. & Bakketeig, L.S. (1988) *Global Impact of Aids Conference*. Alan R. Liss, London.

Weatherburn, P., Davies, P.M., Hunt, A.J., Coxon, A.P.M. & McManus, T.J. (1990) Heterosexual behaviour in a large cohort of homosexually active men in England and Wales. *AIDS Care*, **2**(4), 319–24.

Weatherburn, P., Hunt, A.J., Hickson, F.C.I. & Davies, P.M. (1992) *The Sexual Lifestyles of Gay and Bisexual Men in England and Wales*. Project Sigma, London.

Weeks, J. (1986) *Sexuality*. Tavistock Publications, London.

Weinberg, M.S. & Williams, C.J. (1974) *Male Homosexuals: Their Problems and Adaptations*. Oxford University Press, New York.

Wellings, K. & Wadsworth, J. (1990) AIDS and the Moral Climate. In Jowell, R. *et al.* (eds) *British Social Attitudes; The 7th Report*. Gower, London.

Wolfenden Report (1957) *Report of the Committee on Homosexual Offences and Prostitution*, Cmnd 247. HMSO, London.

Chapter 8
Sexual Attitudes

KAYE WELLINGS, JULIA FIELD
& LUKE WHITAKER

Sex is heavily regulated in all societies (Ford & Beach, 1952). One measure of the strength of this regulation is the extent to which social rules governing sexual conduct are internalized into public attitudes and opinion. This chapter looks at moral values associated with, and attitudes towards, sexual behaviour during the course of life. Many of the conventions governing sex in our society can be traced to their religious origins. The equation of sex with procreation and its containment within marriage are central to the Judaeo-Christian religions (Russell, 1929), and though less strongly expressed than hitherto, still colour our moral judgement. Even in secular societies, we can see a legacy of the traditional Christian view that sexual intercourse should take place within marriage for the purpose of reproduction.

Sexual relations that take place between those in monogamous, heterosexual and procreative couples are almost universally accepted in every culture. Social disapproval tends to be reserved for relationships which occur outside this dyad, the degree of disapproval depending on the strength of taboos in particular cultures. Generally, the strongest regulation extends to those sexual relationships and practices that are not capable of being reproductive or in which reproduction is considered socially inappropriate. Sex between two people of the same sex is an obvious focus for opprobrium, but the stigma also extends to precocious sex, sex before and outside marriage, and to non-exclusive sexual relationships, and so on.

Constraints usually take the form of social sanctions, but in some instances the law is invoked to uphold and underpin moral norms. In England and Wales, anal sex between a man and a woman is legally prohibited, for example, and sex between two men is heavily legally circumscribed. Sexual relations before an age judged to be socially appropriate are legally regulated and sexual non-exclusivity still features among legal grounds for divorce. Abortion, the ultimate expression of the severance of sex from its reproductive consequences, although legalized more than 25 years ago, is still the subject of constant public debate.

Opinions were sought on the strength of marriage as an institution, as measured by views on the age at which it should be entered and the ease with which it should be dissolved, on the age before which sexual intercourse should not occur, on sex before and outside marriage, and attitudes towards sexual exclusivity and homosexuality. Opinions on abortion are also included here – an important measure of the degree to which people are prepared to tolerate sex being separated from procreation.

A considerable body of data on sexual attitudes already exists. This survey is unique in providing an opportunity to explore how attitudes correspond with behaviour. The exact nature of the relationship between the two must remain a matter for conjecture. The assumption that attitudes might predict behaviour needs to be viewed with caution. Attitudes may influence behaviour but it is equally plausible that those with experience of a particular pattern of behaviour will adopt an attitude in keeping with their experience.

Some insight into the relationship between the attitudes and behaviour is useful though, particularly in the context of advice on risk reduction in relation to sexual health. It is sometimes assumed that a change in attitudes is a necessary prerequisite to any modification in behaviour. Whether or not this is the case, there is a more important sense in which a knowledge of sexual attitudes can aid sexual health promotion. Plainly, health educational advice, if it is to be adopted, must contain messages that are acceptable to the audience, and consistent with their sexual preferences. For example, there would seem little point in urging monogamy and sexual restraint on a population heavily committed to polygamy and sexual licence. Thus for health educators the value of insights into attitudes lies not in the possibility of manipulating attitudes to modify behaviour, but in selecting and harnessing those attitudes most likely to support sexually healthy behaviour.

Methodological note

Many of the questions used in this survey are taken from the stock of questions included in the annual British Social Attitudes Survey (Airey, 1984; Airey and Brook, 1986; Brook, 1988; Harding, 1988; Wellings & Wadsworth, 1990). A similar set is asked in the US General Social Survey (Smith, 1990). This decision was made partly on the grounds of expediency, since such questions have been extensively piloted and also because their repeated use has resulted in a good deal being known about the associations of their responses. Because they have been asked at regular intervals since their introduction to the British Social Attitudes Survey in 1983, they have the additional advantage of allowing trends to be discerned.

Possible sources of response bias, such as social desirability, may be exacerbated and accentuated in the investigation of attitudes. Since the attitudinal questions were asked in the face-to-face section of the questionnaire, and since the topics are so value laden, there might have been considerable scope for the intrusion of this bias. In formulating these questions, every effort was made to avoid any form of labelling with moral connotations. Terms such as adultery, infidelity and promiscuity convey such strong moral reprobation that it is difficult to imagine responses not being influenced by their use in a question, and so these words were deliberately avoided in order to minimize the effect of a social desirability response (see also Chapter 2, p. 25). Instead, questions simply stated what was involved in practice. Fluency of style may sometimes have suffered as a result, but in the interests of validity and reliability neutral and accurate phraseology was used. A further preventive measure adopted in this context was the use of show-cards, allowing respondents to provide answers without having to verbalize them.

Another response bias which applies particularly to attitude-scale items has been described as 'acquiescence' or 'agreement' bias, a general tendency toward assent rather than dissent with an expressed viewpoint. This applies particularly to the use of Likert-type scales in which subjects are asked to place themselves on a five-point scale for each statement — running from 'strongly agree' to 'agree', 'uncertain', 'disagree' and 'strongly disagree'. Where the opportunity arises, responses to statements expressing opposite points of view on the same issue have been checked for consistency in an attempt to determine the extent of such bias (see p. 252).

Attitudes, beliefs and knowledge

For ease of understanding, social psychologists make a rough distinction between opinions, attitudes and beliefs according to the strength of conviction, whether they are chiefly cognitive or emotional in origin, and the extent to which they are related to action. Attitudes are reinforced by beliefs (the cognitive component) and often attract strong feelings (the emotional component) that will lead to particular forms of behaviour (the action tendency component).

The boundary between attitude and knowledge measurement is both fine and blurred, and it has to be said that we cannot always know whether respondents interpreted particular questions as attempts to test knowledge or elicit attitudes. A case in point is the example of sex before the age of 16. If a man has sexual intercourse with a woman under this age, he is acting unlawfully, and so a recommendation of a later age as the minimum for first intercourse may be influenced by both knowledge and opinion. In the case of any legally sanctioned activity, the choice of the response option 'sometimes wrong' may thus be more a reflection of knowledge of the law than personal opinion.

Views on age at first intercourse

All respondents were asked for their views on a minimum age for first sexual intercourse. The question asked was, 'In general, is there an age below which you think young people nowadays ought not to start having sexual intercourse . . . first, for boys? . . . and for girls?' Response options permitted respondents to cite a specific age, or to express the view 'Depends on the individual' or 'Not before marriage'. Of particular interest with respect to these data is the extent to which public opinion on a minimum age at first intercourse is in line with, first, legally imposed age limits and, secondly, the actual age at which this occurred for respondents and at which it occurs for most people today. Of interest too is the question of whether views on an appropriate age differ for men and women.

Recommended minimum age compared with legal age

Roughly one in eight respondents took the view that an appropriate age at first intercourse would depend on individual readiness and gave no specific age (Table 8.1). Considerably fewer, around 4% of the sample, believed that, irrespective of age, intercourse should not occur before marriage. This view was some four times more likely to be volunteered by the oldest respondents (45–59) than by the youngest (16–24). This reflects age-related patterns of pre-marital experience described in Chapter 4.

Table 8.1. Views on minimum age for first sexual intercourse. '*In general, is there an age below which you think young people nowadays ought not to start having sexual intercourse?*' [Source: interview, question 34a,b]

Views of . . .	. . . on ideal age for	Age					Depends on individual not age	Not before marriage	Other	No view/don't know	Base
		Under 13	13–15	16–17	18–19	20+					
Men	Boys (%)	0.7	15.6	48.6	11.8	1.8	13.8	3.2	0.9	3.7	8268
Men	Girls (%)	0.5	13.5	51.0	13.1	1.9	12.6	3.5	0.8	3.1	8262
Women	Boys (%)	0.3	9.6	48.0	18.8	2.5	12.4	4.3	0.9	3.2	10349
Women	Girls (%)	0.3	8.4	49.5	20.3	2.7	11.2	4.9	1.0	1.9	10348

According to the law governing the age of sexual consent, it is an offence for a man to have sex with a woman aged under 16 in Britain, although the woman commits no offence in participating. The age at which a man is permitted to have sex, or a woman to have sex with him, is not legally regulated, and the law is also silent on the matter of sex between two women. There seems to be no evidence from these data of widespread support for a lowering of the age of sexual consent (Tables 8.1 & 8.2). Only a minority of people – in the region of one in eight of the sample as a whole – are in favour of sexual intercourse being permitted before the age of 16 for boys or girls (Table 8.2). Marginally fewer women than men favour intercourse under 16 and there is a tendency for both men and women to believe that under 16 is more appropriate for boys than girls. The proportion of men believing it acceptable for boys to have sexual intercourse before the age of 16 is 16.3%, whilst only 9.9% of women do so; 13.9% of men view this to be right for girls, compared with 8.7% of women.

Views differ markedly with the age of the respondent. Looking at responses for different age groups (Table 8.2), younger people are more likely than older ones to be in favour of intercourse occurring before the present legal age of sexual consent. The proportion of 16–24 year olds

Table 8.2. Views on minimum age for first sexual intercourse. '*In general, is there an age below which you think young people nowadays ought not to start having sexual intercourse?*' [Source: interview, question 34a,b]

Views of . . .	. . . on age for	Proportion of respondents in each age group citing this age to be under 16				
		16–24	25–34	35–44	45–59	Total
Men	Boys					
	%	24.3	19.2	12.7	9.5	16.3
	Base	1 951	2 139	2 019	2 159	8 268
Men	Girls					
	%	21.0	15.9	11.5	7.9	13.9
	Base	1 949	2 138	2 016	2 159	8 262
Women	Boys					
	%	16.2	10.6	7.6	6.2	9.9
	Base	2 207	2 862	2 538	2 741	10 348
Women	Girls					
	%	14.4	9.2	6.6	5.5	8.7
	Base	2 207	2 863	2 538	2 741	10 349

who favour a minimum age for sexual intercourse before the age of 16 is more than twice that among 45- to 59-year-olds, irrespective of whether the respondent is a man or a woman or whether the response relates to boys or girls. However, even among the young this is still a minority view.

Knowledge of the law relating to the age of sexual consent

The knowledge that it is unlawful for a man to have sex with a young woman aged under 16 is virtually universal (95.7% of men and 96.8% of women know this to be so). However, almost as large a majority (92.2% of men and 92.5% of women) mistakenly believe that the woman herself is committing an offence by having sex under the age of 16. Furthermore, a majority (69.0% of men and 67.6% of women) wrongly believe that it is against the law for a man aged under 16 to have sex, and that a *woman* who has sex with a *man* under 16 is also committing an offence (76.0% of men and 73.3% women) (Fig. 8.1).

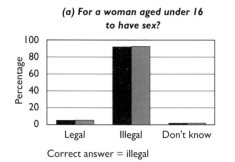

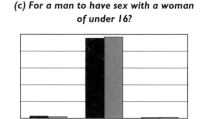

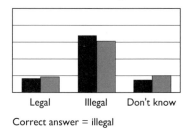

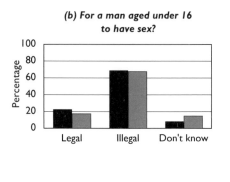

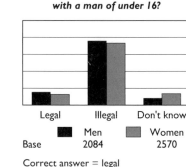

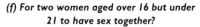

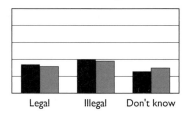

Fig. 8.1. Men's and women's knowledge of the law relating to age of sexual consent. '*Would you tell me whether you think each of these things is legal or illegal under the law . . .*' [Source: interview, question 35]

Considerable uncertainty also surrounds the legal age of sexual consent for same-gender sex. The 1967 Act made it lawful for two men over the age of 21 to have sexual relations together in private and with mutual consent. Sex between two women is neither legislated for nor against. One in three women and one in four men did not know the legal position on sexual relations between two women, and 20.1% of women and 15.1% of men lack information on the law relating to men. Sixty-eight per cent of men and 61.3% of women know that sex between two men under the age of 21 is illegal. Only a third of the sample were aware that sex between two women is not legislated against.

Ideal age in relation to actual age

In general, views on a minimum age for first sexual intercourse correspond fairly closely to current behavioural norms. Recalling Chapter 4, the median age at first intercourse for 16- to 24-year-old respondents was 17, and this is also the age at which the majority of respondents find it acceptable for first intercourse to have occurred (Table 8.1). Older respondents favour a later age than do younger ones, but even so, the majority of those aged 45–59 who specify a minimum age for sexual intercourse see no objection to its occurrence at or before the age of 17. It seems then as if people are providing responses more in line with present-day norms than with those which prevailed in their own youth. The median age at first intercourse for men aged 45–59, for example, was 20, yet 73.9% of men in this age group believe it acceptable for young men below that age to be having sexual intercourse.

Views on an appropriate minimum age for sexual intercourse are related to personal experience none the less. Predictably, those who themselves experienced first intercourse at a younger age were more likely to favour a lower age limit for others, and those who first experienced sexual intercourse at an older age were more likely to recommend a higher minimum age for others. The difference between actual age at first intercourse and recommended minimum age for young people of the same gender was calculated for each respondent and these results are summarized in Table 8.3. The proportion of people who themselves had intercourse before the age they regard today as the minimum, varies with a number of factors, several of which are clearly related. Number of sexual partners, for example, varies with current age and also the age at which intercourse first takes place.

Overall, this analysis shows that those who experienced intercourse themselves before the minimum they now recommend for others are a minority. Women are less likely than men to do so, but the gender differences are not marked. Fewer than one in five women aged 16–24

Table 8.3. Proportion of people who had intercourse before the age they would recommend for young people today
[Source: interview, questions 19a; 34a,b; booklet, questions 7a; 8a]

	Men		Women	
	(%)	Base*	(%)	Base*
Age				
16–24	17.8	1 199	18.9	1 454
25–34	19.4	1 699	13.9	2 374
35–44	15.8	1 563	10.9	2 021
45–59	12.4	1 573	6.5	2 070
Married	15.3	3 709	9.8	5 020
Cohabiting	19.7	481	15.0	698
Widowed, separated, divorced	21.0	335	16.4	854
Single	16.7	1 510	16.3	1 346
Social class				
I/II	11.1	2 165	7.7	2 824
III NM	15.0	1 197	10.7	1 804
III M	21.1	1 515	14.2	1 475
IV, V, other	21.4	1 154	18.6	1 812
Education				
Degree	7.1	715	4.9	618
A level	13.6	2 043	8.6	1 778
O level	17.4	1 773	12.2	3 021
Other	11.9	146	11.7	121
None	24.6	1 349	16.5	2 377
Homosexual partners ever	16.4	5 818	12.0	7 773
1+ homosexual partners ever	15.1	201	19.8	139
Heterosexual partner ever				
1	3.8	1 243	5.9	3 155
2	8.7	680	13.1	1 408
3–4	13.9	1 184	14.6	1 510
5–9	17.7	1 259	19.8	1 103
10+	30.2	1 502	23.0	533
Overall	16.3	6 035	12.1	7 920

* Includes only those who have had sexual intercourse and who specify a minimum age for sexual intercourse.

were experienced at a younger age than they now see as ideal, but this proportion is nevertheless nearly three times higher than amongst women aged 45–59. The age gradient for men is less clear.

The number of heterosexual partners is a very important influence, as shown in Table 8.3, those with large numbers being much more likely to recommend a later starting age for others than they experienced themselves. Educational level also plays an important role, those with no qualifications being more than twice as likely to have had intercourse themselves, at an age they now feel to be premature, than those with education to A level or beyond. The social class effect is slightly weaker than that of educational level for men and slightly stronger for women. Logistic regression was used to identify which of the factors mentioned above were significant. In order of importance of influence, the variables significantly associated with the tendency to recommend a later age for first intercourse than self-experienced were number of heterosexual partners, educational level, current age, social class, marital status and whether or not the respondent had had any homosexual partners.

Reasons for choice of age

Respondents who gave a minimum age for first intercourse were asked to give the main reason for their choice from a pre-formulated list, and these are summarized in Fig. 8.2. By far the most common reason identified (by 57.8% of women and 54.0% of men) was that, before the age given, young people are not sufficiently emotionally mature. Men were more likely than women to feel that those younger than the minimum age they stated had not learnt enough about sex. Women were slightly more likely to mention risks to health, but these accounted for responses from fewer than 10% of respondents. Even smaller proportions mentioned lack of physical maturity and that sex before the stated age was morally wrong. Older respondents were more likely to cite risks to health than were younger respondents, but they were no more likely to state that sexual intercourse before a certain age was morally wrong.

A good age for marriage

Respondents were asked what they thought was a good age for marriage for both men and women and their responses were notable more for their similarity than their differences. Twenty-five was the age given for both sexes by more than a quarter of men and women (Table 8.4). However, about equal proportions of men thought under 25, 25 or over 25 was an appropriate age for men, while women tended on average to favour a slightly older age for men. Men and women were more in accord about a 'good' age for women to marry, but on average it was a younger age than was thought appropriate for men: nearly half of both men and women thought an age below 25 was most appropriate.

How does this pattern of opinions about a good age for marriage

marital sex, for example, vary markedly from those towards extra-marital sexual relationships. Three-quarters of the sample consider sex before marriage not wrong at all (or only rarely so), whilst a similar and slightly higher proportion – nearly 80% – consider sex outside marriage to be always or mostly wrong.

It seems clear that the necessity of marriage as a precondition of sex is becoming very much a thing of the past. Acceptance of sex before marriage is now nearly universal, with nearly three-quarters of men and two-thirds of women condoning it as not wrong at all. Fewer than one in 10 respondents (8.2% of men and 10.8% of women) believe it to be always or mostly wrong. Women are marginally less tolerant than men,

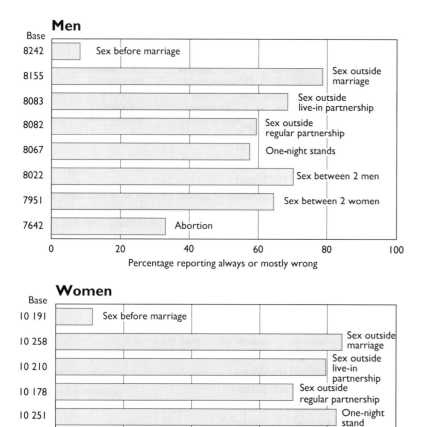

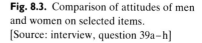

Fig. 8.3. Comparison of attitudes of men and women on selected items. [Source: interview, question 39a–h]

Table 8.5. Views on selected sexual relationships and encounters
[Source: interview, question 39a–h]

	Always wrong (%)	Mostly wrong (%)	Sometimes wrong (%)	Rarely wrong (%)	Not wrong at all (%)	Base
Sex before marriage						
Men	4.7	3.5	10.7	7.6	73.5	8 242
Women	5.8	5.0	15.0	8.1	66.1	10 191
Sex outside marriage						
Men	47.0	31.8	17.4	1.1	2.7	8 155
Women	55.6	28.6	13.7	0.9	1.2	10 258
Sex outside live-in relationship						
Men	35.8	32.7	19.6	2.9	9.0	8 083
Women	46.9	32.7	14.3	1.6	4.5	10 210
Sex outside regular relationship						
Men	28.9	30.6	22.5	5.5	12.6	8 082
Women	37.6	32.4	18.2	3.9	8.1	10 178
One-night stand						
Men	35.8	21.7	17.8	6.5	18.2	8 067
Women	62.4	20.3	10.6	2.3	4.4	10 251
Sex between two men						
Men	60.8	9.4	6.4	3.9	19.6	8 022
Women	46.2	11.7	10.7	6.1	25.3	9 629
Sex between two women						
Men	51.2	13.3	9.2	4.7	21.7	7 951
Women	46.6	12.2	10.2	5.9	25.0	9 667
Abortion						
Men	16.8	16.3	41.2	8.0	17.7	7 642
Women	17.7	19.9	42.1	7.5	12.8	9 458

but the disparity diminishes with decreasing age. Age has a bearing on attitudes, though it is weaker than might be expected (Fig. 8.4). Not surprisingly, pre-marital sex is viewed with greatest leniency in the age group in which it is most likely to occur. Only one in 20 men and women aged between 16 and 24 consider pre-marital sex to be wrong, compared with nearly three times as many men and more than four times as many women in the oldest age group, 45–59. Yet even amongst the oldest age group, those who disapprove are still in a minority.

of women aged 16–24 compared with 82.0% and 87.2% respectively amongst 45- to 59-year-olds. There is no clear age-related trend in these data (Fig. 8.5). Neither the return to more traditional moral values documented in the trend literature of the mid 1980s (Airey, 1984; Harding, 1988) nor the slight reversal of this trend apparent towards the end of the decade (Wellings & Wadsworth, 1990) are evident from an analysis of these data by age.

In terms of *marital status*, those who are married or widowed have a greater commitment to the institution of marriage. They are more likely to see sex before and outside marriage as wrong than are those who are cohabiting or divorced and separated, though the differences are not great (Appendix 3, Table A8.2A). Bivariate analysis shows views on the value of exclusiveness in sexual relationships to vary with social class, those in lower social strata being more censorious than those in higher ones, although the gradient is clearer for women than for men.

What do these results tell us about sex in relation to marriage as an institution in contemporary Britain? It seems clear that marriage as a necessary precondition to having sex is a thing of the past. Yet these findings give little support to the assertion that marriage is losing its importance in Britain. Whilst it is clear that it is no longer seen as the starting point of sexual relationships, once entered into it is certainly viewed by the majority of the population as an exclusive relationship for men and women alike. Care needs to be taken here in distinguishing attitudes from behaviour. Disapproval of behaviour does not mean that people refrain from it. Adultery is still one of the most widely cited grounds for divorce in Britain. But practice aside, the principle of monogamy is held in very high regard.

Casual sex

One of the health promotion messages formulated for risk reduction in relation to HIV and sexual health generally has been to avoid casual sex. A question was therefore included to elicit opinions on 'one-night stands', which are commonly equated with casual sex (Spencer *et al.*, 1988). As with other attitude questions, whether the respondent should answer these questions in relation to him or herself, or to some generalized other, was not specified.

The answers showed that the level of opprobrium attached to one-night stands is high. Not only is it high, but it is also the issue on which the views of men and women are most divided. On all questions relating to exclusivity, women are less tolerant than men of people having sexual relationships with partners in addition to their marital, cohabiting or regular partners, but they are especially censorious on the topic of one-night stands. Whilst 35.8% of men view this as always wrong, 62.4% of women do so (Table 8.5 & Fig. 8.5).

Ideals of monogamy seem to be more strongly held by women than men. This gender difference has been found to be common to many other societies (Foa *et al.*, 1987). Views on why this may be so will depend on the particular theory of sexuality held. Those who subscribe to sociobiological theories of sexuality may see it as a biologically driven commitment on the part of women to monogamy and men to polygamy, tracing it back to the seeking of reproductive advantages by males and females in the distant past. Those favouring a Marxist feminist perspective may see it as a reflection of the power base of our society, in which male economic power and a property view of women nurture and permit a double standard (Brunt, 1982). Whatever the explanation, there seems little doubt that British women have a greater commitment to monogamy than men.

Homosexuality

In the late 20th century, depending on the social circles one moves in, homosexuality may be viewed as a proud source of identity, a more or less tolerated 'alternative lifestyle', or as a perverse and bestial crime against God and nature (Scull, 1989). This attitudinal eclecticism is reflected in our data. Views are more strongly polarized on these kinds of sexual relationships than on any other. More of the responses fall into the 'not wrong at all' category at the extreme end of the scale compared with those on the issue of exclusivity; one in five respondents believe sex between people of the same gender to be not at all wrong (Table 8.5).

However, despite the spread of opinion, homophobic attitudes are widespread in Britain. More than two-thirds of men (70.2%) and more than half of women (57.9%) believe sex between two men to be always or mostly wrong, and there is only marginally less condemnation of sex between two women (which 64.5% of men and 58.8% of women see as always or mostly wrong). Younger respondents are not markedly more tolerant than older ones (Fig. 8.6). Acceptance of homosexuality is scarcely greater in British society than it is in the USA, where the practice of homosexual acts is still illegal in some States. Three-quarters of US respondents in the 1989 General Social Survey judged such practice to be always or almost always wrong (Smith, 1990).

In comparing attitudes towards sexual exclusivity and homosexual relations, the pattern of the disparity between men and women is reversed (Fig. 8.3). Women tend to be more accepting than men of same-gender relationships, and this is more marked in attitudes towards sexual relations between two men than in attitudes towards sexual relations between two women. It has been noted that most researchers fail to

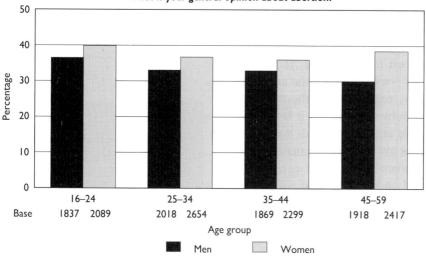

Fig. 8.7. Views on abortion: proportion stating abortion is always or mostly wrong. [Source: interview, question 39h]

is Roman Catholic are very much more likely to oppose abortion than those of another affiliation or of no affiliation. Abortion was believed to be mostly or always wrong by 58.9% of women reporting Roman Catholic affiliation, compared with 33.7% of Anglicans and 31.7% of those with no affiliation; for men the comparable figures are 58.8%, 29.3% and 28.0% (Appendix 3, Table A8.2A). Respondents of non-Christian and 'other' Christian denominations were also more likely to oppose abortion, although the difference for these groups is less marked. These findings are not consistent with those from other surveys, which have shown that only a small percentage of Roman Catholics follow their Church's position, a total ban on abortion with the exception, nowadays, of cases which save the woman's life (Francome, 1988).

Relationship between attitudes and behaviour

Table 8.6 shows the associations between attitudes and the behaviours that most closely correspond to them. In general, those without experience of behaviours on which views are sought are more likely to perceive them as wrong. This is especially marked in the case of pre-marital sex. Respondents who themselves had had no sexual intercourse before marriage were nearly 10 times as likely to frown on this practice as those who had. The association was also marked for homosexual experience. Men who, in the self-completion component of the questionnaire, reported never having had sexual experience with a man were more than three times as likely to view such relationships as wrong as were those

Table 8.6. Concordance of sexual attitudes and sexual experience: proportions reporting behaviour as always or mostly wrong
[Source: interview, question 39a–h]

	Men				Women			
	Experience		No experience		Experience		No experience	
	(%)	Base	(%)	Base	(%)	Base	(%)	Base
Sex before marriage (respondents ever married‡	5.1	1 138	46.2	115	4.2	1 428	38.2	374
Sex outside marriage (respondents married 5+ years)	47.7	354	80.7	3 371	50.0	198	84.9	4 832
Sex outside cohabitation (respondents cohabiting 5+ years)	44.9	30	66.5	125	61.2	25	80.2	211
Sex outside regular partnership (single or w/s/d for 5+ years)*	53.7	1 014	63.8	748	61.6	544	73.4	1 067
One-night stands (2+ partners last 5 years)†	38.0	1 450	51.4	882	63.7	941	73.9	892
Sex between two men	19.3	301	69.3	7 997				
Sex between two women					11.0	197	55.1	10 205
Abortion					12.0	1 229	36.7	8 603

* Comparison between those who have had sex with at least one non-regular partner and those who only had sex with regular partners in the last 5 years.
† For those who have had two or more partners in the last 5 years, comparison between those who have had sex once only with any partner and those who have had sex more often.
‡ Only includes respondents who completed the long questionnaire.

who had done so, and women who reported no sexual experience with a woman were five times as likely to see such behaviour as wrong.

Attitudes to non-exclusive sexual relationships – sex outside marriage, sex outside a cohabiting relationship and sex outside a regular partnership – varied less markedly with reporting of experience, but nevertheless a tendency towards greater lenience can be seen amongst those with some experience of the behaviours they were judging. Again it must be stressed that any direction of causal influence is unclear. In terms of chronological order, the experience – where it has occurred – clearly predates the attitudinal statement, which could suggest that attitudes are expressed to support the behaviour reported. However, it is also possible that respondent's attitudes have been constant over time and that particular views have led to certain types of behaviour.

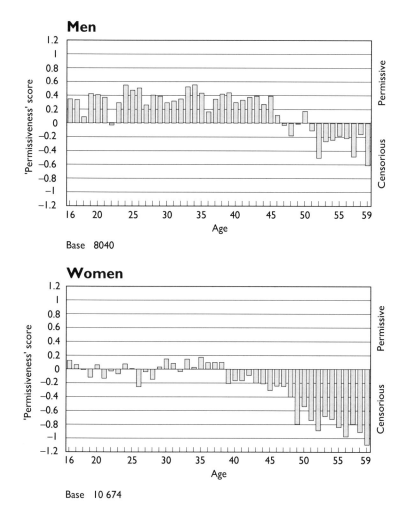

Base   8040

Base   10 674

Fig. 8.8. Relationship between 'permissiveness' and age. [Source: interview, question 39a–h]

The first two principal components together account for 58.0% (37.2% for the first and 20.8% for the second) of the total variation in people's views on sexual morality, and only these two of the eight possible components are considered further.

In general, men's scores for permissiveness are higher (more liberal) than women's and this difference is reversed for attitudes towards homosexuality. The level of permissiveness as shown in Fig. 8.8 highlights striking differences between men and women as well as age trends. Men under 45 show a relatively constant level of permissiveness that reverses sharply after the age of 50. In contrast, women under 45 seem relatively neutral as far as a general attitute of sexual permissiveness can be measured on this scale, but become increasingly censorious with increasing years after the age of 45.

Attitudes towards homosexuality, while showing no marked age trends, do show contrasting patterns for men and women. Men in general are quite intolerant of homosexuality while women are more tolerant, particularly those in their twenties and thirties.

General permissiveness and attitudes towards homosexuality could be expected to vary with a number of characteristics, the most obvious of which are shown in Table 8.7. Not surprisingly, education is strongly associated with permissiveness and also with tolerance of homosexuality. The higher the level of education the more liberal the attitudes of both men and women, and this gradient is particularly steep for women. The mean permissiveness score for women rises from −0.68 for those with no qualification to 0.85 for those with a degree, a difference of almost one standard deviation. For men, the strongest relationship is between

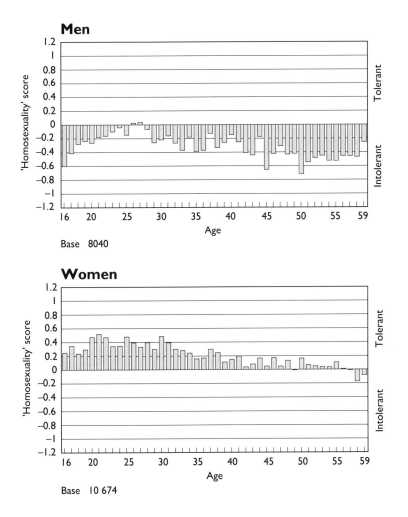

Fig. 8.9. Relationship between attitude to homosexuality and age.
[Source: interview, question 39a–h]

permissiveness and homosexual experience, though clearly there is no indication here to what extent homosexual experience is the cause or the consequence of a general permissiveness trait.

The variables shown do not necessarily have independent effects on the two scores. Analysis of variance was carried out for men and women separately to assess the combined effects of age, marital status, social class, education, region of residence and homosexual experience. For men, all variables except region of residence had a significant effect on both permissiveness and attitudes towards homosexuality. For women, a broadly similar pattern was seen except that region of residence remained significant for the permissiveness score.

Other studies suggest a number of antecedent variables associated with attitudes towards homosexuality. Data from the 1981 European Values Study show that in all countries, approval of homosexuality was greater among the young and better educated (Jensen *et al.*, 1988). US research shows a higher prevalence of negative attitudes towards homosexuals in men than women, amongst older people and those of lower educational level (Hong, 1983, 1984; Herek, 1984; Kite, 1984; Kurdek, 1988). These findings are confirmed in our data.

We cannot tell to what extent these effects (Figs 8.8 & 8.9) can be attributed to cohort or lifestage effects. Attitudes towards moral issues are shaped by an individual's social and personal experiences – those in certain age bands share a common experience, having been brought up in a particular moral climate, but views on sexual behaviour will also vary with different stages of life. These data do, however, testify to a strong influence of age on attitudes held.

Opinions on the significance of sex

In order to minimize the intrusiveness of the survey, no questions were asked about personal sexual satisfaction, the quality of sexual relationships or the importance attached to sex, in the behavioural section of the questionnaire. Instead, these areas were explored by means of attitudinal questions probing general opinions rather than personal experience. These questions were asked only in the long questionnaire so that data are available for the quarter of the sample who completed this part of the interview schedule.

The importance of sex within marriage

Two statements were included in the set relating to the importance of sex within a marriage or relationship. These were: 'Companionship and

Table 8.8. '*Now please would you say how far you agree or disagree with each of these things . . .*'
[Source: interview, question 40a–h]

	Agree strongly or agree (%)	Neither agree/ disagree (%)	Disagree or disagree strongly (%)	Base
'It is natural for people to want sex less often as they get older'				
Men	37.9	28.3	33.8	2 082
Women	37.7	28.5	33.7	2 567
'Having a sexual relationship outside a regular one doesn't necessarily harm that relationship'				
Men	17.2	11.6	71.2	2 079
Women	13.2	8.2	78.6	2 566
'Companionship and affection are more important than sex in a marriage or relationship'				
Men	67.2	22.0	10.8	2 079
Women	68.4	21.7	9.9	2 563
'Sex without orgasm, or climax, cannot be really satisfying for a man'				
Men	48.7	17.4	33.9	2 077
Women	43.3	27.3	29.4	2 557
'Sex without orgasm, or climax, cannot be really satisfying for a woman'				
Men	37.4	27.7	34.9	2 078
Women	28.6	21.5	49.9	2 562
'A person who sticks with one partner is likely to have a more satisfying sex life than someone who has many partners'				
Men	50.4	28.9	20.8	2 080
Women	51.6	30.0	18.5	2 552
'Sex is the most important part of any marriage or relationship'				
Men	16.9	20.9	62.2	2 078
Women	16.4	15.8	67.8	2 560
'Sex tends to get better the longer you know someone'				
Men	68.6	21.8	9.6	2 080
Women	69.9	19.3	10.9	2 560

affection are more important than sex in a marriage or relationship', and 'Sex is the most important part of any marriage or relationship'.

Most noteworthy perhaps, given the emphasis placed on the importance of sex in some sections of the media (Brunt, 1982), is the sizeable majority of respondents who do not see sex as the most important part of a marriage or relationship. Two out of three respondents agree that companionship and affection are more important than sex in a marriage or relationship and only one in 10 disagree (Table 8.8). Reactions to a statement expressing the opposite view, that sex is the most important

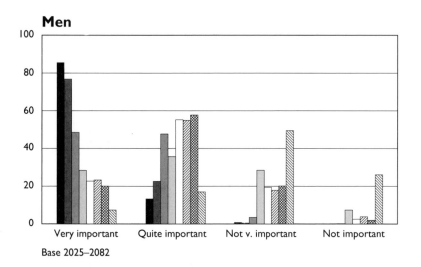

Men

Base 2025–2082

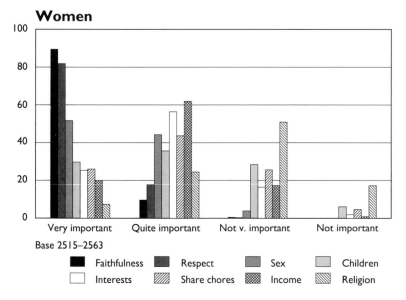

Women

Base 2515–2563

Faithfulness Respect Sex Children
Interests Share chores Income Religion

Fig. 8.10. Factors associated with a happy marriage.
[Source: interview, question 37a–h]

part of any marriage or relationship, are generally consistent, though interestingly the proportion agreeing, 16.9% of men and 16.4% of women, is higher than the 10.8% of men and 9.9% of women who disagree with the converse. Since agreement with the first statement is inconsistent with agreement with the second, a comparison of responses to this pair of statements provided an opportunity to gauge the extent of agreement or acquiescence bias. Logically consistent responses were given by 58.4% of men and 60.1% of women, that is their agreement or disagreement with the first statement was matched by the opposite response to the second.

Included in the attitudinal component was also a question seeking views on the importance of various factors in the making of a successful marriage (Fig. 8.10). Responses showed that faithfulness and mutual respect ranked higher than all other factors. Sex emerged as the third most commonly mentioned in the rank order, followed by having children, shared interests, shared chores, adequate income and shared religious beliefs.

The changing importance of sex

With age

The statement, 'It is natural for people to want sex less often as they get older', was intended to assess perceptions of the importance of sex with advancing years. It elicited neither strong disagreement nor agreement and responses were fairly evenly distributed across the scale. Young people with no first-hand experience were predictably more likely to report that they 'didn't know' than were those in the oldest age group (10.8% of men and 8.1% of women aged 16–24 compared with 2.1% of men and 2.8% of women aged 45–59).

At the aggregate level, the views of men and women correspond well: almost 38% of both men and women agreed or agreed strongly with the statement and 33.8% of both men and women disagreed. These broad findings conceal some variations between the sexes with marital status and age. Women who are married or living with a man are more likely to agree than men in these categories.

Differences between the marital status groups – married and widowed people are more likely to hold that sexual appetite is dulled with age, those who are single and cohabiting less so – may well reflect age differences (Table 8.9). Contrary to the commonly held view that young people see themselves as having a monopoly on sex, and have difficulty in imagining older people having sexual needs, these data show few signs of ageism in the views of the younger respondents. More than half of all 45–59 year olds agree that it is natural for people to want sex less often as

Table 8.9. Proportion of respondents agreeing or agreeing strongly with the statement '*It is natural for people to want sex less often as they get older*'

	Men		Women	
	(%)	Base	(%)	Base
Age group				
16–24	35.7	508	28.0	531
25–34	30.3	543	27.8	720
35–44	36.1	536	38.1	634
45–59	50.6	494	55.5	682
Marital status				
Married	39.6	1 162	43.1	1 567
Cohabiting	26.9	134	31.7	198
Widowed	30.8	15*	46.6	49
Separated, divorced	38.0	103	31.0	212
Single	37.4	669	25.7	539

* Note small base.

they get older, compared with fewer than a third of under 35s, and this difference is more marked for women than men.

With the length of the relationship

Two statements sought to elicit views relating to the effect of the duration and nature of relationships upon sexual satisfaction: 'A person who sticks with one partner is likely to have a more satisfying sex life than someone who has many partners', and 'Sex tends to get better the longer you know someone'.

   Both of these statements are of significance in the context of health education advice in relation to HIV/AIDS and sexual health. Those seeking to promote monogamous and long-term relationships can be heartened by the fact that the majority view on both is that exclusivity and familiarity are more likely to lead to satisfying sex lives than short-term, multiple sexual partnerships. Half of the sample agreed or agreed strongly with the statement to the effect that monogamy brings greater sexual satisfaction than having multiple partners, and more than two-thirds that the quality of sexual satisfaction increases with the duration of the relationship (Table 8.8 – the views of men do not differ greatly from those of women on these issues). In view of the higher level of support for the second statement compared with the first, it might be productive for health educators, and those concerned with effective communication aimed at stemming the spread of HIV and other sexually transmitted infections, to harness this support in their efforts to secure healthier lifestyles.

The importance of monogamy

The statement, 'Having a sexual relationship outside a regular one doesn't necessarily harm that relationship', required respondents to focus more on the consequences of infidelity than on its intrinsic morality. The nature of the relationship – whether it was marital, cohabiting or simply regular – was not specified. The pattern of responses varied little with the relationship status, except in so far as respondents were less likely to choose the extreme response option 'Disagree strongly'. None the less, aggregating the responses 'Disagree' and 'Disagree strongly', the majority of respondents, 71.2% of men and 78.6% of women, do not agree that no harm would be done to a regular sexual relationship by straying outside it.

Those who are married are more likely to regard sexual infidelity as potentially harmful than those who are single. Interestingly, among respondents who are cohabiting with a partner of the opposite sex, the pattern of responses by women is more similar to that of married women than single women; the same proportion of married as of cohabiting women (81%) disagree with the statement, compared with 74% of single women. For men the reverse is true – 65% of cohabiting men are in disagreement, compared with 75% of married men and 68% of those who are single – revealing greater discordance between the sexes in couples who live together outside marriage.

The role of orgasm in sexual satisfaction

No questions were asked about orgasm or sexual satisfaction in the behavioural component of the questionnaire. Attitudes relating to a generalized 'other' rather than self were considered to be less intrusive. The question of whether and to what extent orgasm is necessary to sexual satisfaction is of interest because of the role of ejaculation in the transmission of HIV. However, in view of the proliferation of interest in and advice on how to achieve sexual satisfaction in women's journals and men's magazines, it is also of interest to investigate how highly the sexual climax is rated in terms of sexual satisfaction.

Respondents were asked to express agreement or disagreement with the statement, 'Sex without orgasm cannot be really satisfying for a man', and the statement was repeated in a subsequent version substituting 'for a woman'. Both were asked of both male and female respondents.

This is not, apparently, an issue on which people generally tend to feel vehemently. Only a small minority selected the response options that allowed them to express the strongest agreement or disagreement.

In terms of gender differences in responses, men attach greater importance to orgasm in sexual satisfaction for either sex than do women, and both men and women see orgasm as more essential to a man's sexual satisfaction than to that of a woman. However, neither of these two views was held quite as strongly or as universally as could have been anticipated.

Nearly half (48.7%) of all men agree or agree strongly that orgasm is necessary to male sexual satisfaction, compared with 43.3% of women who hold this view in relation to men, but a third of all men disagree with the statement expressing this view. Orgasm is clearly not universally conceived as a prerequisite to male sexual satisfaction. This tends to run counter to the popular stereotype of men as sexually goal seeking.

Moreover, whilst both men and women attach greater importance to the male orgasm than to the female orgasm in sexual satisfaction, the proportion of men who believe the female orgasm to be necessary to women's sexual satisfaction is higher than the proportion of women who themselves hold this view. Therefore, it appears that men do not put the achievement of their own satisfaction before that of their partners. The view that sex without orgasm cannot be really satisfying for women was given by 37.4% of men compared with 28.6% of women (Table 8.8).

Summary

The view that emerges predominantly from these data is one of a British nation strongly committed to the ideal of the heterosexual, monogamous union, but one of considerable relaxation in attitudes towards teenage sexuality and, in particular, sex before marriage. Although there is no widespread support for a lowering of the age of sexual consent, views on the age before which sexual intercourse is thought to be inadvisable accord remarkably well with current patterns of behaviour. Nor is there apparently widespread opposition to the idea of sexual intercourse occurring before marriage. Acceptance of pre-marital sex is now nearly universal, as indeed is its practice (see Chapter 4).

The pattern of response to questions relating to sexual exclusivity contrasts markedly. The consensus view of British people is that sex outside a regular relationship is wrong and the strength of disapproval increases only slightly with the extent to which the relationship is formalized by marriage or common residence. Disapproval of infidelity extends to all age groups, the young being only marginally more tolerant than older respondents.

Ideals of monogamy seem to be more strongly held by women than men. Women are generally less tolerant than are men of non-monogamous relationships. This is seen most clearly in relation to casual sex, the notion of which finds far greater acceptance among men than women.

Responses to attitudinal questions show widespread condemnation of homosexual relationships, and reporting of such relationships (see Chapter 7) must be seen in this context. Here the pattern of gender differences is reversed and greater tolerance towards homosexual relationships is found amongst women. The use of principal component analysis provides some evidence of an underlying attitudinal trait of permissiveness. It does not, however, account for all the differences in attitudes; people exhibit varying profiles on different issues.

Bringing together practices reported and attitudes towards them reveals some congruence between the two. Not surprisingly, those who practise particular behaviours are more likely to condone them, and the converse is also true.

Responses to the questions on sexual satisfaction and the importance of sex within a relationship reveal the majority view to be that sex is not considered the most important part of a relationship, that a monogamous relationship is more likely to lead to greater sexual satisfaction and that sexual appetite does not necessarily diminish with age.

References

Airey, C. (1984) Social and moral values. In Jowell, R. & Airey, C. (eds) *British Social Attitudes Survey: The 1984 Report*. Gower, Aldershot.

Annual Abstract of Statistics (1991) No. 128. HMSO, London.

Brook, L. (1988) The public's response to AIDS. In Jowell, R., Witherspoon, S. & Brook, L. (eds) *British Social Attitudes Survey: The 5th Report*. Gower, Aldershot.

Brunt, R. (1982) The immense verbosity: permissive sexual advice in the 1970s. In Brunt, R. & Rowan, C. (eds) *Feminism, Culture and Politics*, pp. 143–70. Laurence and Wishart, London.

Central Statistical Office (1991) *Social Trends 21*, 1991 Edition. HMSO, London.

Foa, U.G., Anderson, B., Converse, J. *et al.* (1987) Gender-related sexual attitudes: some crosscultural similarities and differences. *Sex Roles*, **16**(9/10), 511–9.

Ford, C.S. & Beach, F.A. (1952) *Patterns of Sexual Behaviour*. Eyre and Spottiswoode, London.

Francome, C. (1988) Public support for the right to choose abortion. *New Humanist*, **103**, 15–16.

Glenn, N. & Weaver, C.N. (1979) Attitudes towards premarital, extramarital, and homosexual relations in the US in the 1970s. *Journal of Sex Research*, **15**, 108–18.

Gorer, G. (1971) *Sex and Marriage in England Today*. Nelson, London.

Harding, S. (1988) Trends in permissiveness. In Jowell, R., Witherspoon, S. & Brook, L. (eds) *British Social Attitudes: The 5th report*. Gower, Aldershot.

Herek, G.M. (1984) Beyond 'homophobia': a social psychological perspective on attitudes toward lesbians and gay men. *Journal of Homosexuality*, **10**, 1–22.

Hong, S.M. (1983) Sex, religion and factor analytically derived attitudes toward homosexuality. *Australian Journal of Sex, Marriage and Family*, **4**, 142–50.

Question format

Questions about perceived health and chronic illness, alcohol consumption, smoking, height and weight were asked in the face-to-face interviews, and a question on injecting prescribed and non-prescribed drugs was completed in the booklet. Enquiry into sexual and reproductive health included questions on experience of fertility and infertility, and attendance at an STD clinic. Women only were asked about experience of miscarriage and termination of pregnancy (abortion). A question on HIV antibody testing was also included (booklet, question 20). This enquired not only whether the respondent had had such a test, but also the reason for testing. Men were also asked whether or not they were circumcised.

Reported health and sexual behaviour

Questions on health included an item on self-reported health status on a five-point scale (interview, question 2a). As in other surveys (Cox *et al.*, 1987), the majority of men and women of all ages described their health as fairly good or very good for their age (Fig. 9.1 & Appendix 3, Table A9.1). Age trends show only a moderate effect, with an increasing proportion reporting their health to be poor or very poor with increasing age, while at the same time the proportion reporting very good health ('for your age') also increased (Fig. 9.1). There were only minimal differences between men and women in self-reported health status.

Marital status was more closely related to reported health in bivariate analysis (Fig. 9.1). While the proportion reporting very good health was relatively stable across the marital status categories, there were quite marked differences in the proportion reporting poor or very poor health by marital status group. Divorced and separated respondents were more likely to report poor health than married people (Fig. 9.1). In a cross-sectional survey, the reasons for this association must remain speculative, since ill-health may influence the likelihood of marriage or marital break-down while the absence of a long-term relationship may in turn influence physical, economic or psychological well-being.

A more objective question on health was asked about disability, chronic medical conditions and illness or accident in the last 5 years affecting the respondent's health for at least 3 months (interview, question 2b–d) (Table 9.1). The percentage of respondents reporting a permanent disability or chronic condition increased quite markedly with age, although the age trend for reported 3-month illness was more marked for women than for men. This is similar to age trends in other surveys (OPCS, 1992). The relationship between these three measures and reported health is complex. Thirteen thousand one hundred and thirty

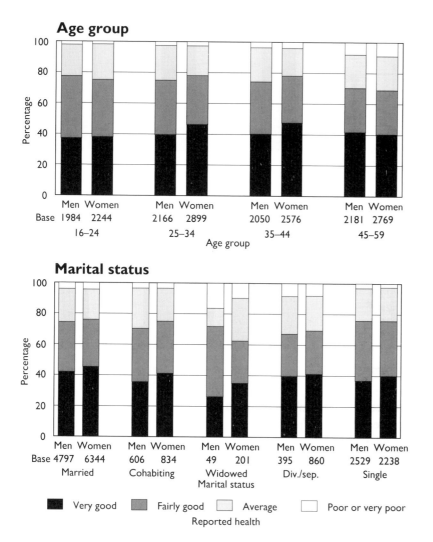

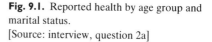

Fig. 9.1. Reported health by age group and marital status.
[Source: interview, question 2a]

respondents had no disability, no chronic condition and no illness whose effects lasted at least 3 months, and of these 81.6% felt their health was good or very good and less than 1% felt their health was poor or very poor. Permanent disability as well as a chronic condition and a 3-month illness were reported by 468 respondents; 50% of this group reported that their health was poor, while 23.9% felt their health was good or very good. In summary, most respondents with no identifiable serious medical problem felt that their health was good, while of those with problems, more than one in five took the view that their health was good.

Figure 9.2 illustrates the relationship between perceived health and sexual behaviour. Frequency of heterosexual intercourse was weakly re-

Table 9.2. Smoking behaviour by age group
[Source: interview, question 5]

Smoking	Men					Women				
	16–24 (%)	25–34 (%)	35–44 (%)	45–59 (%)	All ages (%)	16–24 (%)	25–34 (%)	35–44 (%)	45–59 (%)	All ages (%)
Non-smoker	53.1	43.0	36.7	27.0	39.7	52.7	47.0	42.5	43.5	46.2
Ex-smoker	6.3	15.4	25.4	39.7	22.0	6.4	14.3	20.8	22.5	16.4
Smokes <15 per day	22.8	15.8	11.7	9.5	14.8	25.5	16.9	13.1	11.5	16.4
Smokes 15+ per day	17.8	25.8	26.2	23.9	23.5	15.3	21.9	23.7	22.5	21.1
Base	1 963	2 151	2 031	2 161	8 306	2 215	2 874	2 544	2 739	10 372

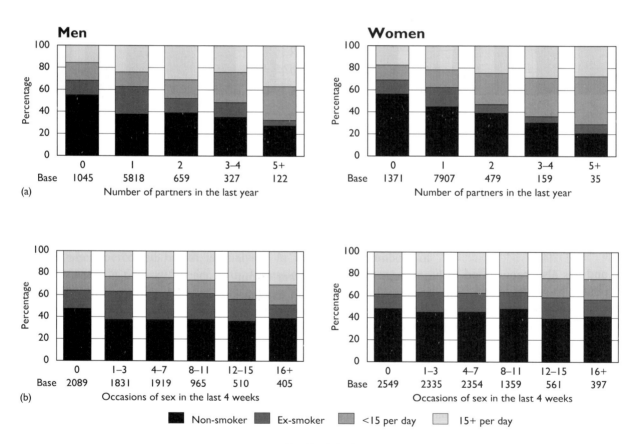

Fig. 9.3. Heterosexual behaviour by smoking: (a) number of heterosexual partners in the last year, (b) number of occasions of sex in the last 4 weeks.
[Source: interview, question 5a–c; (a) booklet, question 7d; (b) booklet, question 2a]

Table 9.2 shows the reported pattern of smoking by age group, which is similar to that reported in other surveys (Cox *et al.*, 1987; OPCS, 1991). The proportion of those who had never smoked declines with age, most markedly for men. Those under 35 were more likely to be current smokers than those over 35, reflecting the increasing proportion in older age groups who have given up smoking. The youngest age group (16–24) were the least likely to be heavy smokers (15 or more cigarettes per day).

Figure 9.3 illustrates the relationship between smoking and number of heterosexual partners reported in the last year, showing a striking trend of increasing prevalence of current smoking with increasing numbers of sexual partners. This finding is consistent with data from studies of contraceptive use and cervical cancer (Winkelstein, 1990). Such a bivariate relationship may be confounded by other influences on patterns of partnership formation and smoking, such as age (see Chapter 5), and this relationship is explored in greater detail below.

In addition to a relationship between smoking and sexual partnerships, there is also a weak relationship with the number of heterosexual acts in the last 4 weeks, those with a high frequency (12 or more) being more likely to smoke (Fig. 9.3). Both these relationships remained after adjustment for age and marital status.

Alcohol consumption and sexual behaviour

An association between alcohol consumption and sexual behaviour might be expected on a number of grounds, although the precise direction of the relationship may not be obvious. On the one hand, the social circumstances in which alcohol is consumed and the lessening of inhibition resulting from consumption might be associated with higher levels of sexual activity or new sexual partnership. Conversely, the depressant effect of large quantities of alcohol might be expected to have the reverse effect. Health educators have expressed concern that individuals may increase their risk-taking behaviour as a result of intoxication by alcohol. Recent studies, particularly among gay men, have found little evidence that alcohol intake is associated with more risky sexual behaviour at the time of consumption (Weatherburn *et al.*, 1993). There is no evidence from the present study that alcohol consumption has a major role to play in decisions about first intercourse (see Chapter 4). It is not possible to examine the immediate relationship between consuming alcohol and levels of sexual acitivity while under its influence, but overall patterns of alcohol consumption can be related to sexual behaviour. By so doing, it is not intended to impute a causal relationship between alcohol consumption and its immediate effects in sexual behaviour. Rather it is

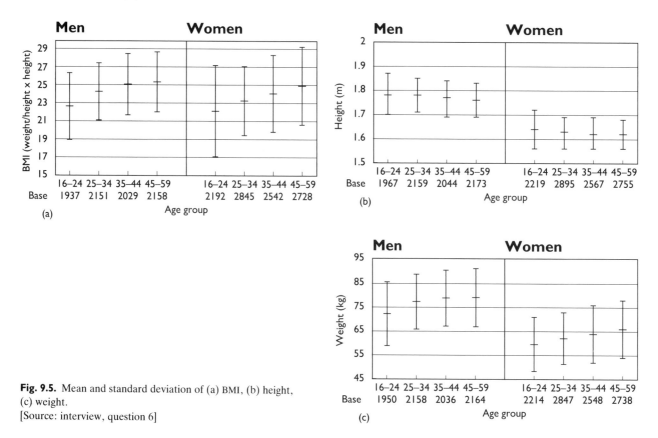

Fig. 9.5. Mean and standard deviation of (a) BMI, (b) height, (c) weight.
[Source: interview, question 6]

Figure 9.6 shows a strong relationship between the proportion of respondents reporting two or more partners in the last year and quartiles of BMI, with the likelihood of reporting two or more partners declining rapidly with increased BMI. This relationship is likely to be confounded by the relationship between BMI and age and is explored in greater detail in a logistic regression model.

The relationship between health-related behaviour and sexual behaviour

The foregoing analysis indicates that there may be complex relationships between health-related behaviour, demographic variables and sexual behaviour. The health-related factors found to be associated with sexual behaviour in bivariate analysis were examined in a logistic regression model. This model also took account of the demographic factors associated with reporting increased numbers of sexual partners that were identified in Chapter 5. Variables included in the model were age group,

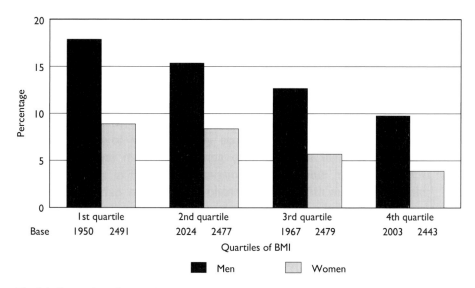

Fig. 9.6. Proportion of respondents reporting two or more partners in the last year by BMI. [Source: interview, question 6; booklet, question 7d]

social class, marital status, BMI, smoking and alcohol consumption. These were examined in relation to the likelihood of reporting two or more partners in the last year (Fig. 9.7). Results are expressed as adjusted odds ratios with their 95% confidence intervals. As discussed in Chapter 5, age group and marital status exert strong influences on patterns of sexual partnership, but after taking account of these variables, those who smoked or drank alcohol were significantly more likely to report multiple partnerships. (BMI was not a significant factor in the model, largely due to its strong association with age.)

The data are consistent with the well known association between smoking and drinking observed in other studies (Cox *et al.*, 1987). Our data clearly indicate a further association between smoking, drinking and multiple sexual partnerships, which confirms the suggestion that there is a relationship between a number of risk-taking behaviours. These effects appear to be independent of age and marital status. In the multivariate model, marital status remains the strongest effect, but the adjusted odds ratio for moderate or high alcohol consumption is in excess of 3 for both men and women for reporting two or more partners in the last year.

Table 9.4. Reported injecting drug use by age group
[Source: booklet, question 17]

Injected non-prescribed drugs	Men					Women				
	16–24 (%)	25–34 (%)	35–44 (%)	45–59 (%)	All ages (%)	16–24 (%)	25–34 (%)	35–44 (%)	45–59 (%)	All ages (%)
Ever	0.8	1.4	0.9	0.0	0.8	0.8	0.6	0.2	0.0	0.4
Last 5 years	0.8	0.7	0.3	0.0	0.4	0.8	0.3	0.1	0.0	0.3
Last year	0.2	0.6	0.2	0.0	0.3	0.3	0.1	0.0	0.0	0.1
Ever shared needles	0.3	0.6	0.7	0.0	0.4	0.4	0.4	0.1	0.0	0.2
Base	1640	2065	1914	1963	7582	1857	2742	2443	2479	9520

Table 9.5. Reported injecting drug use by geographical area
[Source: booklet, question 17]

	Greater London (%)	Rest of England and Wales (%)	Scotland (%)	Great Britain (%)
Ever				
Men	2.1	0.6	0.5	0.8
Women	0.8	0.3	0.6	0.4
In the last 5 years				
Men	1.4	0.3	0.3	0.4
Women	0.8	0.14	0.6	0.3
In the last year				
Men	1.0	0.15	0.0	0.3
Women	0.5	0.03	0.3	0.1
Base				
Men	993	5948	642	7582
Women	1165	7406	950	9520

respondent over the age of 44 reported injecting drug use. For the population under 45, the proportion reporting ever injecting was 1.0% for men and 0.5% for women. The low rates of injecting among those over 45 accord with studies indicating the rarity of drug injecting in Britain before the late 1960s (Stimson & Oppenheimer, 1982). Regional variations were detectable, with significantly higher rates of ever injecting among respondents in Greater London (2.1% of men, 0.8% of women)

(Table 9.5). The increased prevalence in London corresponds to the high proportion of Home Office notifications of drug addiction from the London area (Hartnoll *et al.*, 1985).

It should be emphasized that estimates of the prevalence of injecting drug use are likely to be minimum estimates for several reasons. Injecting illicit drugs is a both legally and socially censured behaviour that respondents might be particularly unwilling to report. Population estimates from the survey might also be lowered, since those injecting drugs are disproportionately represented amongst the homeless, who were not included in the sampling frame. Because of the rules about who should complete the booklet (see Chapter 3, p. 55), the question was not asked of a relatively high proportion of those aged 16–24, mainly the sexually inexperienced, so that population estimates for this group may be subject to greater error. Given these caveats, applying these rates to the population of England and Wales gives an estimate of 100 000 people injecting in the last 5 years and 175 000 ever. These figures are of a similar order of magnitude to Hillier's, who estimated 120 000 injecting drug users in England and Wales on the basis of scarce data from surveys of drug users and Home Office reports (Hillier, 1988).

Health service use and sexual behaviour

STD clinic attendance

Epidemiological studies indicate that the likelihood of acquiring an STD increases with the number of sexual partners with whom unprotected sexual intercourse takes place (Aral & Holmes, 1990). No direct questions were asked about specific sexually acquired infections because of the difficulties of defining these in terms comprehensible to respondents. Attendance at an STD (or special/venereal disease (VD)) clinic was used as a proxy indicator, since open-access clinics, free at the time of use, are available throughout Britain, and are widely used by all sectors of the sexually active population (Belsey & Adler, 1981). Routine statistics on STD diagnoses are collected from these clinics and up to 90% of STDs in the country are thought to be diagnosed and treated in these settings rather than in general practice (Department of Health, 1991; Catchpole, 1992).

Although not all those who attend STD clinics have a sexually acquired infection, the majority are likely to perceive themselves to be at risk of infection. The probability of attendance should therefore be associated both with numbers of partners and the demographic and other factors shown to be related to partner change (see Chapter 5). Routine STD clinic statistics have the disadvantage that they are based on 'episodes'

Table 9.6. STD clinic attendance by age group
[Source: booklet, question 16]

STD clinic attendance	Men					Women				
	16–24 (%)	25–34 (%)	35–44 (%)	45–59 (%)	All ages (%)	16–24 (%)	25–34 (%)	35–44 (%)	45–59 (%)	All ages (%)
In the last year	1.7	1.3	0.7	0.3	0.9	1.6	1.3	0.1	0.1	0.8
In the last 5 years	4.9	5.4	2.7	0.9	3.4	4.7	4.2	1.3	0.6	2.6
Ever	5.0	11.8	10.5	5.3	8.3	5.2	8.1	6.4	2.6	5.6
Base	1 644	2 072	1 939	1 977	7 632	1 867	2 757	2 461	2 499	9 584

of STD in a given time period rather than on the number of people with STD. Demographic data collected on attenders are restricted to age and gender and limited data on sexual orientation have only been collected recently (Belsey & Adler, 1981; Catchpole, 1992). No routine information is collected on the sexual behaviour of attenders.

At least one attendance at an STD clinic was reported by 8.3% of men and 5.6% of women and less than 1% reported attending in the last year (Table 9.6). STD clinic attendance was closely associated with age. Table 9.6 and Fig. 9.8 indicate that the likelihood of attendance in the last 5 years for women is highest in the youngest age group (16–24) but for men peaks in the 25–34 age group, thereafter declining in older age groups. This is consistent with data on age from STD clinic returns (KC60) for England and Wales, showing that for confirmed STD diagnoses, the average age is approximately 3 years younger for women (24) than men (27) (Department of Health, 1991). Similarly, the number of confirmed diagnoses in men exceeds those in women at all ages except for those under 25. The proportion of respondents reporting *ever* attending a clinic peaked in the 25–34 age group and rapidly declined with increasing age. This corresponds to what is known about changing patterns of partnership formation over the preceding decades (see Chapter 5), the increased incidence of STDs through the 1960s and the establishment of more STD clinics (Adler, 1982).

Substantial regional variation in frequency of STD clinic attendance in the last 5 years is also evident (Appendix 3, Table A9.1). These differences are most marked for residents of Greater London – 7.4% of men and 6.7% of women reported STD attendance in the last 5 years, compared with 3.4% of men and 2.6% of women for the entire sample. The lowest levels of attendance were reported by men and women from

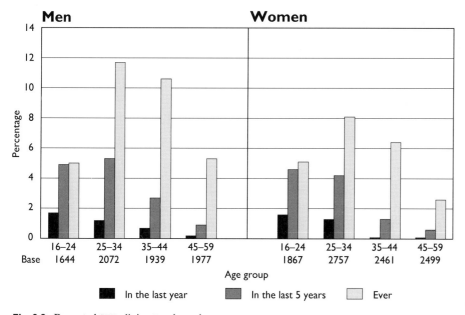

Fig. 9.8. Reported STD clinic attendance by age group.
[Source: booklet, question 16]

the northern region (1.3% and 0.8% respectively) and women in Wales (0.5%). These findings are again consistent with data from KC60 returns, which indicate the greatest number of attendances per head of the population in the Northern Thames Regional Health Authorities (Department of Health, 1991).

The proportion attending also varied markedly by marital status. Only 1.1% of married women and 1.5% of married men reported STD clinic attendance in the last 5 years, with substantially higher incidence in all other marital status categories with the exception of widowed women (Appendix 3, Table A9.1). This is entirely consistent with data on increased numbers of partners amongst those who are not married.

In 1978, Belsey & Adler attempted to assess the relationship between numbers of attenders and numbers of attendances by undertaking a survey of a representative sample of STD clinic attenders in England and Wales (Belsey & Adler, 1981). Attendances exceeded the number of attenders by a factor of 1.3 and this ratio varied both by region and by sexual orientation of the patient. They estimated that in 1978, 332 000 individuals attended clinics in England and Wales. The equivalent estimate from our data was 261 000 attenders in the last year and just under 900 000 in the last 5 years. As the number of STD clinic attendances (but not necessarily attenders) is known to have increased since 1978, this suggests that STD clinic attendance may be under-reported in the survey.

Other factors might also lead to different estimates, such as double-counting of individuals who attended more than one clinic and the inclusion of those not resident in Britain in the Belsey & Adler survey, as well as the substantial differences in methodology for deriving estimates.

STD clinic attendance and behaviour

The likelihood of attending an STD clinic increased markedly with increasing number of heterosexual partners (Table 9.7). Over one in seven of those with five or more heterosexual partners in the last 5 years had attended a clinic in that time and more than one in five of those reporting 10 or more lifetime partners had ever attended. Among men reporting homosexual partners, more than half of those with five or more partners in the last year had attended a clinic in the same period. These may well be minimum estimates in view of the possible under-reporting of clinic attendance. Figure 9.9 demonstrates the very clear relationship between number of partners and STD clinic attendance when both heterosexual and homosexual partnerships are taken into account. The proportion of men who report STD clinic attendance but no heterosexual partners in Table 9.7 is largely accounted for by those with homosexual partners. The high proportion of individuals with multiple partnerships who attend STD clinics confirms the relationship between sexual lifestyle and probability of STD acquisition, but also underlines the importance of such clinics for assisting individuals to reduce their risk of acquiring further STD.

Multivariate analysis

A logistic model was constructed to assess the simultaneous effects of age, marital status, numbers of heterosexual and homosexual partners and non-prescribed drug injecting on the likelihood of attendance at an STD clinic in the last 5 years (Fig. 9.10).

After adjustments for other factors in the analysis, numbers of heterosexual partners in the last 5 years exerted the strongest effect in the model for both men and women. The adjusted odds ratio for STD attendance for women reporting five or more partners was in excess of 9 and for men more than 12. Homosexual partnerships exerted a strong effect in the model for men only (odds ratio 12.4), confirming the strong association between behaviour and clinic attendance. For women, injecting drug use was associated with a significantly increased likelihood of clinic attendance. The effects of age and marital status after controlling for other variables in the model were somewhat weaker. Men aged 25–44 were more likely to have been to an STD clinic in the last 5 years than older or younger men. For women, the age range was younger, those

Table 9.7. Proportions of respondents attending an STD clinic in relation to number of homosexual and heterosexual partners
[Source: booklet, questions 7a,b, 8a,b; 16]

Number of homosexual partners ever
Ever attended

STD clinic	*0*	*1*	*2*	*3–4*	*5–9*	*10+*
Men						
(%)	7.4	20.3	15.1	33.9	44.3	67.3
Base	7 325	148	37	48	12*	55
Women						
(%)	5.3	27.9	16.9	32.7	26.6	—
Base	9 409	120	32	13*	10*	3†

Number of heterosexual partners ever
Ever attended

STD clinic	*0*	*1*	*2*	*3–4*	*5–9*	*10+*
Men						
(%)	9.2	1.7	2.8	3.8	7.8	20.2
Base	184	1 628	841	1 447	1 549	1 943
Women						
(%)	0.5	1.3	2.4	6.1	12.2	26.7
Base	182	3 896	1 679	1 816	1 308	678

Number of homosexual partners in last 5 years
Attended STD clinic

last 5 years	*0*	*1*	*2*	*3–4*	*5+*
Men					
(%)	3.1	7.9	9.4	32.0	51.4
Base	7 505	49	11*	18*	41
Women					
(%)	2.6	8.1	5.2	—	—
Base	9 518	40	16*	3†	6†

Number of heterosexual partners in last 5 years
Attended STD clinic

last 5 years	*0*	*1*	*2*	*3–4*	*5+*
Men					
(%)	7.5	0.7	2.9	4.5	13.7
Base	357	4 490	798	958	1 017
Women					
(%)	0.3	1.2	4.1	8.0	15.7
Base	510	6 503	1 062	771	431

* Note small base.
† Base <10.

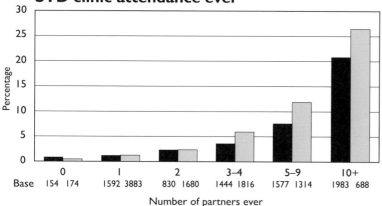

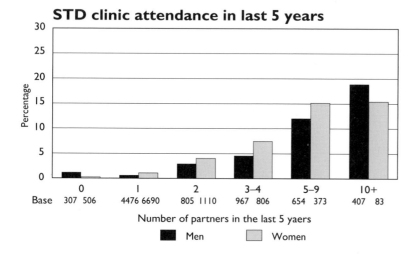

Fig. 9.9. STD clinic attendance by number of heterosexual and homosexual partners. [Source: booklet, questions 7a,b; 16]

aged 16–34 being most likely to attend. Marital status had a weaker effect among men than among women, with only single status being associated with a significantly raised odds of clinic attendance.

HIV antibody testing

HIV antibody testing has been widely available in STD clinics, hospitals and other settings since 1985. All donated blood is routinely screened for HIV antibody. HIV screening is sometimes undertaken in other circumstances, for example, for life insurance, for travel to certain countries and in connection with pregnancy. Understanding the proportion of the population who have undergone testing is important in assessing the likely extent of undiagnosed HIV infection and the degree to which those at high risk of infection have actively sought testing.

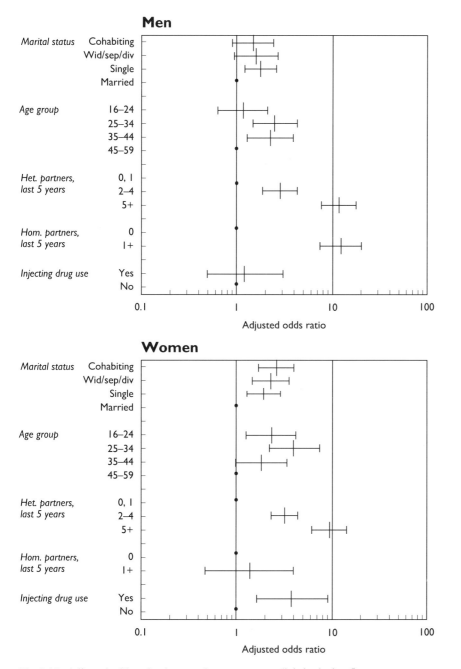

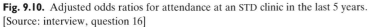

Fig. 9.10. Adjusted odds ratios for attendance at an STD clinic in the last 5 years.
[Source: interview, question 16]

Table 9.8. HIV testing by age group
[Source: booklet, question 20]

	Men					Women				
	16–24 (%)	25–34 (%)	35–44 (%)	45–59 (%)	All ages (%)	16–24 (%)	25–34 (%)	35–44 (%)	45–59 (%)	All ages (%)
Blood test										
Yes	12.7	15.5	14.9	8.9	13.1	15.9	18.9	12.8	7.0	13.7
No	81.9	79.5	80.6	87.1	82.2	77.2	74.2	81.1	89.7	80.6
Unsure	5.4	5.0	4.4	4.1	4.7	6.9	6.9	6.1	3.3	5.8
Reason for test										
Blood donor	7.4	8.9	9.1	4.4	7.5	6.1	7.5	6.8	4.0	6.2
Pregnancy	0.4	0.6	0.3	0.0	0.3	6.4	8.9	3.0	0.1	4.6
Insurance, mortgage, etc.	0.8	1.4	1.7	1.5	1.4	0.6	0.7	0.5	0.4	0.5
'Other'	4.5	5.5	4.2	2.7	4.2	3.6	3.3	2.7	2.1	2.9
Base	1648	2066	1919	1939	7572	1852	2731	2439	2435	9456

Respondents reported whether they had had an HIV test in the last 5 years and for what reason. Options given were 'being a blood donor (giving blood)', 'pregnancy' (for men 'a pregnancy of your wife/partner'), 'insurance, mortgage or travel' or 'other reason(s)'. This last category was of particular interest because it was likely to include respondents who had actively sought HIV testing because they perceived themselves to be at risk of infection. Unless data on reasons for testing were collected, incidence of testing might be overestimated because of confusion in the minds of respondents who had had blood tests in the last 5 years as to whether this included HIV testing. Overall, more than 13% of the sample reported that they had had an HIV test (Table 9.8). The commonest reason for testing was blood donation (7.5% of men, 6.2% of women) but 4.2% of men and 2.9% of women had an HIV test for reasons other than blood donation, or pregnancy, or insurance/travel. Testing rates declined in those aged 45 or more.

HIV testing and sexual behaviour

The relationship between reported behaviour and the likelihood of testing is shown in Table 9.9. More than one in five men and one in four women with five or more heterosexual partners in the last 5 years reported having an HIV test, and one in 10 had done so other than for blood donation, etc. Amongst men with homosexual partners in the last 5 years, the

Table 9.9. HIV testing and sexual behaviour
[Source: booklet, questions 7b; 8b; 17; 20]

	HIV test for any reason				HIV test for 'other' reason			
	Men		Women		Men		Women	
	(%)	Base	(%)	Base	(%)	Base	(%)	Base
Heterosexual partners in the last 5 years								
0,1	11.1	4791	11.2	7108	3.1	4777	1.9	7081
2–4	13.8	1752	19.7	1897	3.9	1747	5.1	1893
5+	21.0	1016	26.7	441	10.2	1016	8.9	441
Homosexual partners in the last 5 years								
0	12.6	7446	13.6	9391	3.9	7427	2.8	9360
1+	43.0	118	24.0	64	27.0	118	13.1	65
Injecting drug use								
Ever	41.5	58	62.7	35	31.4	58	48.6	35
Last 5 years	47.9	33	76.2	24	37.4	33	60.6	24
Never	12.8	7436	13.5	9344	4.1	7417	2.7	9310

proportion rose to over four out of 10, with more than one out of four seeking testing for an 'other' reason. For those injecting non-prescribed drugs, nearly half had been tested. All these rates are in excess of those of the population as a whole, suggesting that a considerable proportion of those with high-risk behaviours perceive their increased risk and have responded by undertaking HIV testing. The proportions of men who have sex with men and those with a history of injecting drug use who have undergone HIV testing are similar to those reported from drug users recruited through treatment and other agencies and volunteer samples of homosexual men (Dawson *et al.*, 1991; Hart *et al.*, 1991; Report of a Working Group, 1993).

Logistic regression models were constructed to examine the demographic and behavioural influence on HIV testing for any reason other than blood donation, pregnancy, insurance or travel (Fig. 9.11). For men and women, the dominant effects were numbers of heterosexual partners, any homosexual partners and injecting drug use. After controlling for other variables in the model, age and marital status were not significantly associated with an HIV test for 'other' reasons. This analysis confirms the strong relationship between behaviour and seeking testing, since the

ticular the routine religious practice of circumcision amongst Jews and Moslems. Analysis by ethnic group shows white males to be the least likely to be circumcised.

In our data there was no relationship in bivariate analysis between circumcision and rates of attendance at an STD clinic.

Infertility, adverse pregnancy outcomes and sexual behaviour

The relationships between sexual behaviour and a number of adverse outcomes with respect to fertility are explored here. These include infertility, loss of pregnancy through miscarriage or stillbirth and termination of an unwanted or abnormal pregnancy. In this section patterns of infertility, miscarriage and abortion are examined in relation to demographic and behavioural characteristics of the sampled population.

Infertility

The incidence of infertility was measured by two questions (booklet, questions 15a and 15b): 'Have you ever had a time lasting 6 months or longer when you (and your partner) were trying to get pregnant but it did not happen?' This measure was used as an indicator of delay in conception. Any time cut-off, however, has its drawbacks. Studies of couples of proven fertility indicate that a significant minority will conceive within 6 months and 1 year of first trying and a further minority will conceive after 1 year (Tietze, 1956, 1968). To assess action taken in response to infertility a second question was asked: 'Have you (or your partner) ever sought medical or professional help about infertility?' The reported incidence of both infertility for 6 months and professional help-seeking are shown in Table 9.11 and Fig. 9.12. Women were more likely than men to report both infertility for at least 6 months and seeking

Table 9.11. Infertility for at least 6 months and use of professional help by age group [Source: booklet, question 15]

	Men					Women				
	16–24 (%)	25–34 (%)	35–44 (%)	45–59 (%)	All ages (%)	16–24 (%)	25–34 (%)	35–44 (%)	45–59 (%)	All ages (%)
Infertility for at least 6 months	2.4	11.1	17.4	15.2	11.5	5.8	19.1	23.5	18.5	17.1
Professional help for infertility	0.9	5.3	10.4	8.9	6.4	2.0	8.9	12.3	9.5	8.3
Base	1887	2046	1847	1893	7673	2155	2730	2376	2390	9651

Table 9.12. Proportions of women reporting miscarriage or stillbirth and abortion by age group (women only)
[Source: booklet, questions 13; 14]

	Miscarriage or stillbirth					Abortion				
	16–24 (%)	25–34 (%)	35–44 (%)	45–59 (%)	All ages (%)	16–24 (%)	25–34 (%)	35–44 (%)	45–59 (%)	All ages (%)
In the last year	2.3	2.4	0.8	0.1	1.4	2.2	1.2	0.5	0.1	1.0
In the last 5 years	5.4	10.9	5.6	0.7	5.8	7.9	6.3	3.6	0.3	4.5
Ever	5.7	18.0	26.6	30.9	20.7	9.2	14.6	15.4	9.4	12.3
Base	2 184	2 772	2 450	2 477	9 882	2 161	2 752	2 424	2 480	9 818

professional help. This may reflect more accurate recall amongst women than men of the time taken to conceive, related to awareness of the menstrual cycle. What differences there are between male and female reporting of professional help-seeking are smaller, and may arise either from lack of awareness that their partner has been seeking advice or a tendency for respondents to consider that the majority of fertility problems lie with women.

Table 9.11 and Fig. 9.12 indicate marked variability in experience of infertility and use of professional help by age group, with the incidence peaking in men and women aged 35–44. The lower apparent incidence in the oldest age group may reflect either a genuine increase in infertility in younger cohorts or simply a changing awareness of infertility and the professional help available. Several studies have shown that the proportion of women seeking professional help for infertility has increased over recent decades (Aral & Cates, 1983; Johnson *et al.*, 1987). Johnson *et al.* estimated that 7% of women born in 1950 had consulted an infertility specialist by the time they were 35, a figure that is consistent with the 12.3% of 35- to 44-year-old and 9.5% of 45- to 59-year-old women seeking professional help in this sample. On the basis of general practice records, Johnson *et al.* estimated that there had been no significant increase in rates of primary infertility *per se*, although rates of voluntary childlessness had increased. Templeton *et al.* (1990), on the basis of a postal survey, estimated that 14% of women aged 46–50 in Aberdeen had experienced difficulty in becoming pregnant for more than 2 years, compared with 17% for more than 6 months for 45- to 59-year-olds in this sample. Since approximately one-fifth of couples who do not conceive within 6 months can be expected to conceive by 24 months,

A logistic regression model, exploring the relationship between age, marital status, a history of having one or more child and infertility, confirmed the findings of the bivariate analysis (Fig. 9.13). The likelihood of reporting and seeking help for infertility was greatest in women aged 35–44; the single were those least likely to have sought help, although cohabitees and the widowed, separated and divorced were less likely than the married to report infertility problems.

Stillbirth, miscarriage and abortion

Miscarriage and stillbirth are unwanted outcomes of pregnancy, while abortion (or therapeutic termination of pregnancy) is generally a response to unwanted pregnancy. Secular changes in rates of reported abortion must be expected following the legalization of termination of pregnancy the Abortion Act of 1967. Reporting of abortion is a sensitive matter and in her 1976 survey, Dunnell estimated that only half the abortions expected from official statistics were reported (Dunnell, 1979). Results from this survey indicate that although age-specific reporting rates of abortions consistently lay slightly below those expected from official statistics for 1990, the 95% confidence limits for the rates reported in the survey always included the recorded national rates (see Chapter 3, Table 3.10).

As Table 9.12 and Fig. 9.14 indicate, there are substantial variations in rates of reporting by age and the patterns for miscarriage and stillbirth differ substantially from those for abortion. Lifetime reporting of miscarriage is extremely common for women (20.7% of all respondents) and, as expected, increases with age as women accumulate experience of pregnancy. Nearly one-third of women aged 45–59 reported experience of miscarriage or stillbirth in their lifetime. Recent experience (in the last 5 years) was most common (10.9%) amongst women in the most active reproductive years (25–34).

In contrast, lifetime experience of abortion was highest at 15.4% amongst women aged 35–44, the majority of whom would have had therapeutic abortion potentially available to them throughout their sexually active careers. For those aged over 45, abortion would have become available after their most sexually experimental period and this is reflected in less frequent experience of abortion (9.4%). Recent abortion (last 5 years) was most common amongst those aged 16–24 (7.9%), possibly reflecting poor use of contraception, greater numbers of sexual partners and a higher prevalence of uncommitted relationships resulting in unwanted pregnancy in this group.

The pattern of miscarriages, stillbirth and abortion in relation to marital status is entirely consistent with known demographic patterns in

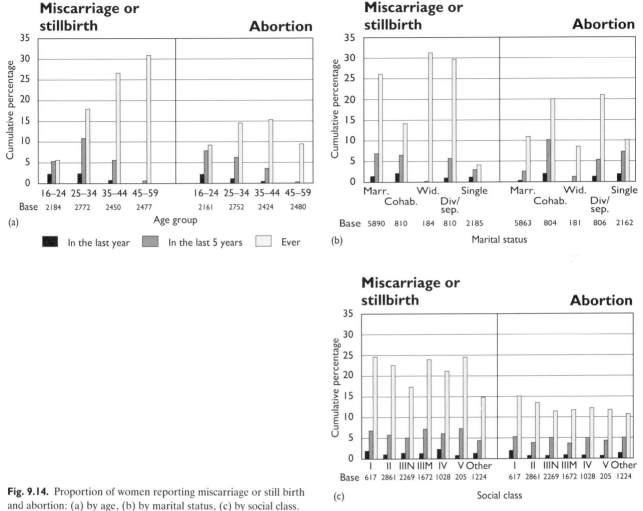

Fig. 9.14. Proportion of women reporting miscarriage or still birth and abortion: (a) by age, (b) by marital status, (c) by social class. [Source: booklet, questions 13; 14]

relation to childbirth (Botting, 1991; OPCS, 1993). Miscarriage, both in the last 5 years and ever, is least common amongst the single, although this relationship will also be affected by current age. Different patterns are seen for abortion in the last 5 years, which was least common amongst the widowed (1.3%) and married (2.6%). Single women reported higher rates (7.3% in the last 5 years), but the highest rates were amongst cohabiting women (10.2%). This last finding can be compared with data reported in Chapters 5 and 6 showing the less monogamous lifestyles of those cohabiting. Though making sufficient commitment to a relationship to live with a partner, they appear to have a less exclusive attitude to that relationship, and possibly also to the responsibilities of child care.

more than five times more likely to have an abortion than those who had only one partner (34.4% and 6.0%).

The various influences on miscarriage or stillbirth and abortion were examined in logistic regression, with age, marital status and numbers of heterosexual partners included. The 5-year models are shown in Fig. 9.16. After controlling for all other variables in the likelihood of miscarriage or stillbirth in the last 5 years was significantly increased among those aged 16–34, decreased among the unmarried and only weakly (and non-significantly) related to numbers of heterosexual partners in the last 5 years. By contrast, the dominant effect in the 5-year model for abortion was number of heterosexual partners in the same time period. The adjusted odds ratio for abortion among women with between five and nine partners in the last 5 years was close to 4 and for those with 10 or more in excess of 10. The effects of both age and marital status were attenuated, so that age effects were weak and non-significant, whilst only those cohabiting showed a significantly raised odds ratio for abortion. The strong effect of numbers of partners was also sustained in the model when lifetime data were considered (data not shown).

Thus, sexual lifestyle, as measured by numbers of partners, appears to exert a strong influence over the likelihood of an abortion. Such a relationship is not unexpected, in terms of both increased exposure to risk and less commitment to partners, and is supported by the increased rates of sexually acquired infections observed in women attending abortion clinics (Cohn & Stewart, 1992).

Summary

This chapter has explored physical health, health behaviour, health service use and aspects of reproductive health in relation to sexual behaviour.

Self-reported health behaviour was found to have only a very weak relationship with sexual behaviours as measured by frequency of heterosexual acts of sex and numbers of heterosexual partners.

Both alcohol consumption and smoking were found to be associated with patterns of sexual behaviour. After controlling for age, social class and marital status, reporting of multiple partnerships was significantly associated with smoking and with increasing levels of alcohol consumption.

A history of injecting non-prescribed drugs was reported by less than 1% of the sample. Reporting rates were however higher amongst those under 45 and those resident in London. More than half those injecting non-prescribed drugs had shared a needle at some time. Although these estimates should be regarded as minima, they are consistent with limited data from other sources.

A history of attendance at an STD clinic was strongly associated with number of heterosexual partners and with a history of homosexual partnership, even after controlling for age and marital status. Over one in seven of those with five or more heterosexual partners in the last 5 years had attended a clinic in that time. Among men reporting five or more homosexual partners in the last 5 years, more than half had attended. This finding indicates that a high proportion of those at risk of STD and HIV are attending STD clinics and emphasizes the importance of these health service settings for assisting individuals in risk reduction strategies.

Over 13% of respondents reported that they had had an HIV test, showing that a relatively high proportion of the population has already been tested. After excluding those tested for blood donation, pregnancy, insurance or travel, a history of HIV testing was strongly associated with patterns of HIV risk behaviour. In particular, a history of HIV testing was much more likely amongst those with five or more heterosexual partners in the last 5 years, any homosexual partners in the last 5 years or a history of injecting non-prescribed drugs. These findings suggest that those at increased risk of HIV infection have perceived their risk and chosen to undergo HIV testing.

Amongst men, 21.9% had been circumcised. The prevalence of circumcision increased markedly with age and was also related to religious affiliation and ethnic group. White men were least likely to be circumcised.

Experience of infertility and seeking help for it were not surprisingly related to age and marital status. No relationship was detected between numbers of heterosexual partners and experience of infertility.

A history of miscarriage or stillbirth was common, involving more than one in five women of all ages and nearly one in three women aged 45–59. While the likelihood of miscarriage or stillbirth was related to age and marital status, no relationship was found with numbers of heterosexual partners. In contrast, the likelihood of termination of pregnancy increased markedly with increasing numbers of heterosexual partners independent of age and marital status.

The findings in this chapter indicate close associations between a number of risk-taking behaviours. They confirm the strong relationship between sexual behaviour and the probability of STD clinic attendance, abortion and HIV testing. These findings indicate both general awareness of the risk of HIV infection and other adverse outcomes for sexual health, and also emphasize the importance of health service provision in the design and implementation of sexual health programmes.

Chapter 10
Risk Reduction Strategies

JANE WADSWORTH & KAYE WELLINGS

This chapter looks at aspects of sexual attitudes and behaviour in the context of prevention, describing evidence of strategies used to reduce the risk of adverse effects of sexual activity. In terms of sexual health, these adverse effects can be principally identified as unplanned pregnancy and STD, and the preventive practices as contraception and prophylaxis.

Safer-sex practices vary in the extent to which they confer protection, and strategies that may be effective in one context do not always transfer to another. Behaviour adopted to prevent infection will not necessarily serve to prevent pregnancy, and the reverse is also true. With the exception of the condom, methods of contraception do not normally protect against infection, and although condom use may be the best available strategy for reducing the risk of infection, there are more effective means of preventing conception. Reducing the number of partners may lower the probability of infection but not that of pregnancy. Avoiding penetrative sex reduces the risk of HIV transmission and pregnancy but not necessarily other sexually transmitted infections, such as herpes.

The preventive practices described here have relevance for many areas of sexual health, but the questions asked in this survey mostly concerned safer sex in the context of preventing pregnancy and HIV transmission. The first part of this chapter describes patterns of contraceptive use among different subgroups of the population. The second looks at knowledge of risk reduction strategies, awareness of risk of HIV and reported behaviour change in response to the threat of AIDS.

Contraceptive use

Two questions on contraception were asked in the face-to-face interview of all those with experience of sexual intercourse with someone of the opposite sex after reaching the age of 13. The questions were phrased similarly to those of the GHS (OPCS, 1991). Although the term 'contraception' does not feature in the question, all the response options are clearly contraceptive methods. Respondents were presented with a show-card listing contraceptive methods, including 'other' and 'no method' options, and asked which, if any, they had used with a partner ever, and which in the past year. (The method used on the occasion of first intercourse is described in Chapter 4.) In addition, the self-completion booklet contained questions on condom use in the past 4 weeks and on the last occasion of sex.

Contraceptive users and non-users

No method of contraception used was reported by 21.1% of women and 17.6% of men in the past year (Table 10.1). These data are based on responses from those with at least one heterosexual partner in the past year and therefore exclude the 13.9% of women and 13.1% of men who reported no partner during that period. It cannot be assumed that those who were not sexually active in that recent period were not using some method of contraception, but it can be assumed that they were not at risk of heterosexually acquired infection or pregnancy.

Among those using no method, it is not possible to distinguish between those who were sexually active and at risk of an unplanned pregnancy, and those who were pregnant, seeking pregnancy or sterile for non-contraceptive reasons, and therefore not at risk. Even on the most conservative estimate of these categories, the residual category of those sexually active and not protected against unplanned pregnancy is probably well under 10% of the total. Just how much progress has been made in contraceptive practice in Britain can be appreciated when we recall that at the turn of the century only 10% of women used any contraceptive method at all (Wellings, 1986a).

Contraceptive use decreases with age. More than nine out of 10 sexually active 16- to 24-year-old men and women reported the use of at least one method in the past year, compared with two-thirds of men and just over half of women in the oldest age group (many of whom will no longer be of childbearing age) (Table 10.1). Compared with those who were married, contraceptive use was higher among the single or cohabiting, lower among those who were divorced or separated and lowest among the widowed, reflecting varying levels of sexual activity and need for protection against pregnancy in these different groups (Table 10.2).

Contraceptive methods used

Respondents were asked to list *all* methods used in the past year, so that more than one method could have been reported and used concurrently or sequentially in this time period. Some methods – especially those conferring lower levels of protection against pregnancy – are more likely

Table 10.1. Contraception used in the last year by age group
[Source: interview, question 30b; booklet, question 7d]

	16–24 (%)	25–34 (%)	35–44 (%)	45–59 (%)	All ages (%)
Men					
Pill	53.1	49.4	18.7	4.9	30.4
IUD	2.2	5.0	7.8	3.8	4.9
Condom	60.8	44.4	28.1	19.6	36.9
Diaphragm	1.8	2.2	2.3	1.5	2.0
Pessaries	0.3	0.8	0.5	0.7	0.6
Sponge	0.3	0.2	0.0	0.0	0.1
Douche	0.5	0.2	0.1	0.1	0.2
Safe period	3.9	2.9	2.7	1.8	2.7
Withdrawal	9.4	8.2	5.4	4.7	6.8
Female sterilization	0.5	4.8	14.3	14.8	9.1
Vasectomy	0.1	4.7	22.1	21.6	12.8
Abstinence	2.6	1.6	1.1	1.0	1.5
Other method	0.4	0.2	0.3	0.2	0.3
None	9.0	11.2	14.7	33.7	17.6
Base*	1 439	1 955	1 875	1 886	7 154
Women					
Pill	64.1	43.6	11.3	2.5	28.8
IUD	3.1	8.9	9.3	3.8	6.6
Condom	41.9	31.0	20.7	12.8	25.9
Diaphragm	1.0	3.9	2.3	1.3	2.3
Pessaries	0.5	1.0	1.1	0.3	0.8
Sponge	0.1	0.2	0.1	0.0	0.1
Douche	0.2	0.1	0.1	0.2	0.1
Safe period	2.3	2.5	2.1	0.7	1.9
Withdrawal	6.6	4.3	3.6	3.0	4.2
Female sterilization	0.4	6.2	17.8	17.9	11.0
Vasectomy	1.1	7.4	24.3	15.0	12.6
Abstinence	1.7	1.6	0.6	0.1	1.0
Other method	0.9	0.9	0.5	0.5	0.7
None	9.5	12.7	16.2	45.3	21.1
Base*	1 692	2 667	2 344	2 208	8 911

Note: Percentages sum to more than 100% because more than one contraceptive method could be reported.
* Excludes respondents with no heterosexual partners in the last year.

Table 10.2. Contraception used in the last year by marital status
[Source: interview, question 30b; booklet, question 7d]

	Married (%)	Cohabit. opp. sex (%)	Widowed (%)	Divorced, separated (%)	Single (%)	All (%)
Men						
Pill	21.3	51.9	15.7	26.7	48.7	30.4
IUD	5.6	5.7	5.0	5.9	2.5	4.9
Condom	27.9	31.0	32.4	37.1	64.2	36.9
Diaphragm	1.8	2.9	0.0	1.6	2.1	2.0
Pessaries	0.7	1.3	0.0	0.2	0.3	0.6
Sponge	0.0	0.2	0.0	0.2	0.3	0.1
Douche	0.0	0.5	0.0	1.3	0.3	0.2
Safe period	2.1	3.8	7.7	3.2	3.9	2.7
Withdrawal	5.4	10.0	7.3	8.5	9.3	6.8
Female sterilization	11.9	7.8	0.0	12.6	1.1	9.1
Vasectomy	18.2	7.5	6.8	9.2	0.1	12.8
Abstinence	1.0	2.5	0.0	1.7	2.4	1.5
Other method	0.2	0.3	0.0	0.6	0.4	0.3
None	20.4	11.4	40.1	24.9	10.3	17.6
Base*	4584	597	21	307	1639	7149
Women						
Pill	19.7	48.7	4.6	24.5	59.0	28.8
IUD	7.1	5.7	4.4	12.0	3.2	6.6
Condom	21.8	26.2	2.2	19.1	46.7	25.9
Diaphragm	2.1	3.5	0.8	3.4	2.0	2.3
Pessaries	0.8	0.8	0.0	0.5	0.8	0.8
Sponge	0.1	0.1	0.0	0.2	0.2	0.1
Douche	0.1	0.0	0.0	0.3	0.2	0.1
Safe period	1.7	2.7	0.0	1.3	2.6	1.9
Withdrawal	3.5	4.5	0.0	3.7	7.5	4.2
Female sterilization	13.1	9.8	16.8	16.7	0.5	11.0
Vasectomy	17.1	4.9	3.5	5.7	0.6	12.6
Abstinence	0.6	1.8	0.7	0.8	2.4	1.0
Other method	0.5	1.3	0.0	1.4	0.9	0.7
None	23.9	12.4	67.7	26.7	9.9	21.1
Base*	6053	816	64	544	1429	8906

Note: percentages sum to more than 100% because more than one contraceptive method could be reported.
* Excludes respondents with no heterosexual partner in the last year.

to be used together, for example, barrier methods and natural family planning. Even those methods with higher effectiveness rates, such as sterilization and oral contraception, may be reported in addition to another – for example, by those with more than one sexual relationship in the last year, or those who seek prophylactic as well as contraceptive protection. Analysis of highly effective methods of contraception together with condom use in the past year is described below (see p. 319).

According to reports of use in the past year, the three contraceptive methods most commonly relied on are the pill (reported by 28.8% of women and 30.4% of men), the condom (25.9% of women and 36.9% of men) and male or female sterilization (23.3% of women and 21.4% of men) (Table 10.1). No other single method is reported by more than 10% of respondents.

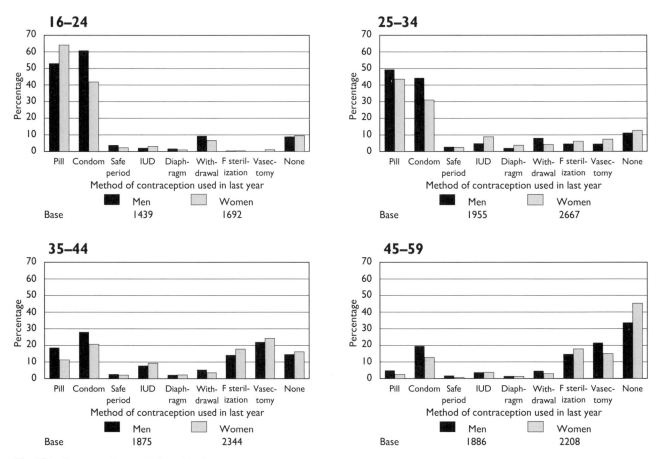

Fig. 10.1. Contraceptive method used in the last year by age group. [Source: interview, question 30b]

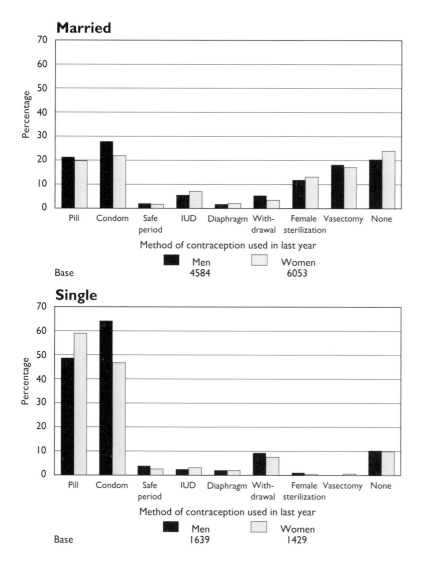

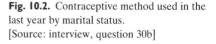

Fig. 10.2. Contraceptive method used in the last year by marital status.
[Source: interview, question 30b]

Oral contraception

Although the pill is the method of choice for a quarter of British women, reliance on this method varies markedly with age group and marital status (Tables 10.1 & 10.2). Oral contraceptive use declines steeply with age. Nearly two-thirds (64.1%) of women aged 16–24 reported the use of this method in the past year, but scarcely more than one in 10 of those aged 35–44 did so, and the proportion falls to one in 40 (2.5%) in the age group 45–59 (Table 10.1 & Fig. 10.1). Similarly, well over half of single women and nearly half of those cohabiting reported the use of oral contraceptives in the past year, compared with fewer than one in five of those who were married (Table 10.2 & Fig. 10.2).

The sharpest fall in the level of oral contraceptive use occurred between women in the 25–34 age group (43.6% of whom reported pill use in the past year) and those in the 35–44 age group (11.3% of whom did so). This may well concur with DHSS guidelines relating to use of the combined pill for those aged 40 and over (DHSS, 1979).

Although age and marital status are clearly related, each exerts a separate effect on method choice, as shown in Table 10.3. The decline in use of the pill with increasing age, however, is more marked at an earlier age for married women than it is for those who are single, reflecting a

Table 10.3. Contraceptive method* used in past year by age and marital status
[Source: interview, question 30b; booklet, question 7d]

	Pill (%)	Condom (%)	Female sterilization (%)	Vasectomy (%)	Total sterilization (%)	None (%)	Base†
Men							
16–24 years							
Married	57.7	38.9	1.8	0.6	2.4	13.5	163
Cohab. opp. sex	71.4	37.9	1.3	0.0	1.3	7.5	146
Widowed	—	—	—	—	—	—	0
Separated, divorced	57.9	20.0	0.0	0.0	0.0	2.0	16‡
Single	50.0	67.6	0.3	0.0	0.3	73.7	1114
Total	53.1	60.8	0.5	0.1	0.6	9.0	1439
25–34 years							
Married	45.5	40.2	5.7	7.2	12.8	11.8	1224
Cohab. opp. sex	66.5	37.0	1.7	0.4	2.1	8.7	240
Widowed	—	—	—	—	—	—	0
Separated, divorced	45.9	46.7	10.3	1.1	11.4	18.1	96
Single	52.0	61.3	2.6	0.1	2.7	9.0	396
Total	49.4	44.4	4.8	4.7	9.4	11.2	1955
35–44 years							
Married	17.0	26.5	14.8	24.2	38.6	13.8	1549
Cohab. opp. sex	27.7	20.1	16.1	20.8	32.9	12.9	130
Widowed	—	—	—	—	—	—	4‡
Separated, divorced	19.2	44.2	14.9	10.4	24.9	22.8	94
Single	31.5	47.7	3.1	0.9	4.0	24.3	96
Total	18.7	28.1	14.3	22.0	35.7	14.7	1873
45–59 years							
Married	3.8	18.9	14.7	22.5	36.5	33.7	1648
Cohab. opp. sex	12.8	18.7	24.3	20.2	39.2	25.4	82
Widowed	3.1	34.5	0.0	8.4	8.4	47.9	17‡
Separated, divorced	13.4	24.0	14.8	17.2	31.0	34.7	101
Single	15.2	36.5	4.6	1.3	6.0	42.9	33
Total	4.9	19.6	14.8	21.6	35.5	33.7	1882

continued

Table 10.3. *Continued*

	Pill (%)	Condom (%)	Female sterilization (%)	Vasectomy (%)	Total sterilization (%)	None (%)	Base†
Women							
16–24 years							
Married	61.3	29.1	0.5	1.5	2.0	17.6	353
Cohab. opp. sex	70.1	35.3	0.9	3.1	4.0	5.7	302
Widowed	—	—	—	—	—	—	1‡
Separated, divorced	48.7	31.5	0.0	0.0	0.0	21.0	33
Single	63.9	48.8	0.2	0.4	0.6	7.2	1 000
Total	64.1	41.9	0.4	1.1	1.5	9.4	1 689
25–34 years							
Married	40.2	30.2	6.9	9.8	16.6	12.7	1 822
Cohab. opp. sex	51.8	28.4	6.1	2.8	8.6	12.1	313
Widowed	—	—	—	—	—	—	2‡
Separated, divorced	39.8	22.3	9.6	3.6	12.9	17.3	185
Single	56.0	42.3	1.0	1.2	2.1	11.0	343
Total	43.6	31.0	6.2	7.4	13.5	12.7	2 666
35–44 years							
Married	10.1	20.9	17.0	27.5	44.5	15.6	1 935
Cohab. opp. sex	14.6	10.7	30.8	14.1	43.5	14.3	147
Widowed	9.1	0.0	34.7	0.0	34.7	52.0	11
Separated, divorced	19.7	19.8	19.7	9.0	28.7	18.7	187
Single	18.5	46.3	2.6	1.7	4.3	24.2	63
Total	11.3	20.7	17.8	24.3	41.6	16.2	2 344
45–59 years							
Married	2.4	13.4	17.5	16.5	33.5	43.8	1 942
Cohab. opp. sex	4.2	4.6	23.9	1.9	25.7	46.9	54
Widowed	0.0	1.8	13.8	4.5	18.3	74.2	50
Separated, divorced	4.7	10.7	26.1	5.4	30.1	51.6	138
Single	0.0	20.7	2.6	0.0	2.6	68.0	23
Total	2.5	12.8	17.9	15.0	32.4	45.3	2 207

* Three most commonly used methods.
† Excludes respondents with no heterosexual partners in the last year.
‡ Note small scale.

diminishing need amongst married women for reliable contraception in the peak childbearing years, and a continuing need amongst single women (Table 10.3).

Sterilization

While the pill is more commonly the method of choice amongst single women, and decreases in use with age, surgical methods of birth control find favour with married women and increase in popularity with age. The proportion of women relying on their own sterilization or that of their partner increased with age up to 44 years (Table 10.1 & Fig. 10.1). Reliance on female sterilization or vasectomy was reported by very small proportions of men and women aged 16–24. Use of these methods peaks in the age group 35–44, falling slightly in the oldest age group, 45–59.

As shown in Table 10.3, sterilization is far more common among married than single women, and vies with the pill as the method of choice for married women as a whole. There is, however, an abrupt reversal in the popularity of the two methods in the middle years of the lives of married women. While pill users outnumber those who rely on sterilization in the 25–34 age range, they are heavily outnumbered in the 35–44 age group. Reports of reliance on sterilization peaked among married women aged 35–44, 44.0% of whom are protected by their partner's or their own sterilization. The prevalence of sterilization in the 45–59 age group of women was lower than among those aged 35–44, but the proportion using no method was higher — 43.8% compared with 15.6 — so that sterilization accounted for more than half of all contraceptive use in the 45–59 age range.

The ratio of male to female sterilization also varies with age. For women, reliance on vasectomy is more common than reliance on female sterilization in all age groups save the oldest. For men, reliance on female sterilization is more common in those aged under 35 and vasectomy in those aged 35 and older. The trend towards greater reliance on male than female sterilization in recent decades documented elsewhere (Bone, 1985; Wellings, 1986b) is also demonstrated here.

Condoms

Condom use is described among contraceptive methods but it should be borne in mind that the question wording made no mention of contraception as such, so that respondents might be equally likely to be reporting prophylactic use of condoms. Condom use on the last occasion of heterosexual sex and in the last 4 weeks was also probed in the booklet, and these data are described below (see p. 334).

Until recently, the method of contraception that showed the most striking rise in popularity was sterilization, reflecting the decline of the pill, since for those looking for a highly effective methods free from side-effects, this is the only serious alternative (Wellings, 1986b). However, following the wide publicity given to the advantages of condom use in response to the HIV epidemic, the condom has increased in prominence as a contraceptive method.

Overall, 25.9% of women and 36.9% of men report having used a condom in the past year. Generally speaking, the popularity of condoms declines with age (Table 10.1). The proportion of young women aged 16–24 who reported condom use in the past year is twice that of 35- to 44-year-old women and more than three times that of those aged 45–59. Similar trends are evident for men, although a higher proportion of men than women in all age groups report condom use in the last year. Despite the pattern of decreasing use with increasing age, reports of condom use at least once in the past year outnumber reports of pill use in men and women aged 35 and over.

Other methods

Methods of contraception other than those described above are reported by far fewer respondents. The next most commonly reported method, the intrauterine device (IUD), is more popular among women in their middle

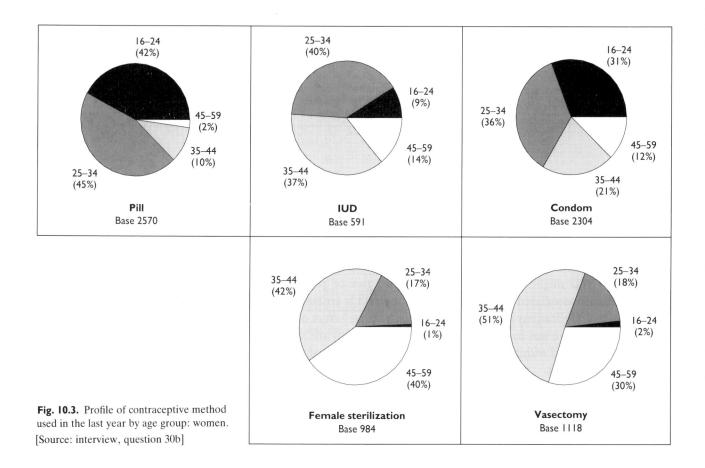

Fig. 10.3. Profile of contraceptive method used in the last year by age group: women. [Source: interview, question 30b]

Female barrier methods are used by very small proportions of respondents. The diaphragm is used by little more than 2% of women; its use is highest amongst cohabiting women and those women who are divorced and separated.

Contraceptive use by social class

Earlier surveys have shown some variation in contraceptive method use by social class. In 1970, Bone (1973) found significant variation in use between women in manual and non-manual social classes. In particular women in the lowest socioeconomic groups were most likely to report abstinence or the use of no method. Differences in contraceptive practice between social classes were still just perceptible in 1975 (the year in which contraceptive provision was made freely available to all under the NHS), but they had diminished (Bone, 1978). Dunnell's data (1979) showed that when only those who were currently sexually active were considered, there was little social class difference in contraceptive behaviour among single women.

In common with these findings, these data show the association with social class to be more marked for whether a method is used at all, than for specific choice of method. In bivariate analysis, the data show a social class gradient for use of any contraceptive method in the past year, particularly for men (Table 10.4). In social classes I and II, 14.2% of men reported the use of no method in this time period compared with 20.7% of those in social classes IV and V. For women, the comparable figures were 19.4% and 23.6%.

Social class variation is apparent for some but not all methods used. Use seems to be differentiated more in terms of intrusiveness. Those in non-manual groups, for example, seem to be more likely to use intercourse-related methods. Women in upper socioeconomic groups were more likely to have used female barrier methods in the past year – the diaphragm and pessaries – and also to have used the safe period.

The ratio of male to female sterilization also varies with social class. Women reporting reliance on male sterilization outnumber those reporting reliance on female sterilization in all social classes except IV and V, in which the reverse holds. This finding from bivariate analysis is consistent with that of Hunt & Annandale (1990), i.e. that women who were sterilized themselves were of lower social class than those with a sterilized partner. The difference may be partly explained by parity, women in manual groups being more likely to have a larger number of children (see p. 310). Bivariate analysis shows no consistent social class effect on pill use, though women in social class I seem less likely than those in other social class groups to report its use (Table 10.4).

Table 10.5. Contraceptive method used in the last year by religion
[Source: interview, question 30b; booklet, question 7d]

	No religion (%)	Christian C of E (%)	Christian RC (%)	Christian other (%)	Non-Christian (%)	Total (%)
Men						
Pill	36.0	23.3	28.5	23.9	23.1	30.4
IUD	4.5	5.0	5.5	5.0	6.8	4.9
Condom	40.0	31.2	35.4	35.3	42.8	36.9
Diaphragm	2.2	1.6	0.8	2.4	2.3	2.0
Pessaries	0.6	0.7	0.7	0.4	0.5	0.6
Sponge	0.1	0.1	0.1	0.1	0.4	0.1
Douche	0.2	0.2	0.5	0.0	0.0	0.2
Safe period	3.0	2.7	2.8	2.1	1.6	2.7
Withdrawal	7.4	5.6	8.3	5.5	6.1	6.8
Female sterilization	8.4	10.9	7.5	10.5	4.6	9.0
Vasectomy	10.8	18.6	9.0	14.4	4.5	12.8
Abstinence	1.8	0.9	1.6	1.9	0.4	1.5
Other method	0.2	0.2	0.6	0.4	0.4	0.3
None	15.1	18.7	22.6	19.8	26.5	17.6
Base*	3676	1823	639	736	274	7148
Women						
Pill	37.7	21.4	31.0	29.0	17.0	28.8
IUD	6.9	6.3	7.1	5.8	8.8	6.6
Condom	27.7	23.8	25.8	25.6	27.6	25.9
Diaphragm	2.6	2.0	1.9	2.3	3.2	2.3
Pessaries	0.8	0.6	0.5	1.0	1.2	0.8
Sponge	0.2	0.0	0.2	0.1	0.0	0.1
Douche	0.1	0.1	0.2	0.2	0.2	0.1
Safe period	2.1	1.2	2.9	2.1	2.6	1.9
Withdrawal	4.2	4.1	5.3	3.7	4.8	4.2
Female sterilization	9.4	13.4	7.0	13.7	8.6	11.1
Vasectomy	10.3	16.4	8.8	13.8	7.0	12.6
Abstinence	1.0	0.8	1.7	0.8	1.8	1.0
Other method	0.5	0.7	1.4	0.6	1.9	0.7
None	16.9	22.6	24.3	23.0	32.1	21.0
Base*	3339	2978	1004	1277	299	8897

Note: percentages sum to more than 100% because more than one contraceptive method could be reported.
* Excludes respondents with no heterosexual partners in the last year.

Table 10.6. *Continued*

Number of children	Pill (%)	Condom (%)	Female sterilization (%)	Vasectomy (%)	Total sterilization (%)	Base†
Women						
16–24 years						
0	66.8	47.8	0.2	0.9	1.1	1 253
1	58.4	24.2	0.2	0.5	0.7	295
2	53.5	27.4	0.9	3.4	4.3	109
3	45.2	18.8	10.9	6.1	17.0	28
4+	—	—	—	—	—	4‡
Total	64.1	41.8	0.4	1.1	1.5	1 690
25–34 years						
0	56.7	39.4	0.4	1.6	1.9	837
1	48.5	29.7	1.7	1.7	3.3	564
2	37.5	28.2	8.5	12.5	20.9	841
3	25.3	20.9	16.6	16.8	33.3	313
4+	19.3	23.4	26.2	15.7	41.9	111
Total	43.7	31.0	6.2	7.4	13.5	2 665
35–44 years						
0	19.5	24.7	6.1	9.4	15.5	224
1	16.7	22.7	10.1	14.7	24.8	303
2	8.0	21.8	17.7	30.7	47.7	1 086
3	11.4	18.1	24.7	25.8	49.8	487
4+	11.5	14.5	25.1	18.7	43.8	242
Total	11.3	20.7	17.8	24.4	41.7	2 341
45–59 years						
0	4.0	19.5	7.8	3.8	11.6	165
1	3.0	15.7	8.9	11.5	20.0	278
2	2.0	14.7	17.1	18.9	35.4	851
3	2.9	11.5	20.7	16.5	36.8	555
4+	2.1	5.0	27.3	11.4	37.7	358
Total	2.5	12.8	17.9	15.0	32.4	2 207

* Three most commonly used methods only.
† Excludes respondents with no heterosexual partners in the last year.
‡ Base <10.

Contraceptive method use and number of heterosexual partners

Data on risk and preventive practice can be used to explore whether risk reduction strategies are related to current or past patterns of behaviour. In this context those with multiple sexual partners are clearly of interest, and method use was examined in relation to partner numbers in the last year (Table 10.7). Those with more than one partner are less likely to have used no method than those who report having been monogamous

Table 10.7. Contraceptive method used in the last year by number of heterosexual partners in the last year
[Source: interview, question 30b; booklet, question 7d]

	1 (%)	2 (%)	3–4 (%)	5+ (%)
Men				
Pill	28.0	38.4	56.8	54.6
IUD	5.1	4.9	2.6	5.2
Condom	33.2	55.9	61.8	71.6
Diaphragm	1.9	1.9	4.2	3.2
Pessaries	0.6	0.5	0.9	0.5
Sponge	0.1	0.5	0.1	0.9
Douche	0.1	0.3	1.1	2.4
Safe period	2.3	5.1	7.4	1.7
Withdrawal	5.6	10.5	15.5	22.7
Female sterilization	10.0	5.3	4.6	4.6
Vasectomy	14.2	8.0	4.9	0.7
Abstinence	1.5	1.3	1.8	4.7
Other method	0.3	0.4	0.3	0.0
None	18.0	9.2	8.3	8.9
Base*	5 799	655	328	125
Women				
Pill	27.6	46.2	53.4	70.2
IUD	6.6	7.0	7.7	4.4
Condom	24.8	39.6	52.3	60.4
Diaphragm	2.3	3.8	1.3	2.7
Pessaries	0.7	1.2	1.8	1.4
Sponge	0.1	0.3	1.0	0.0
Douche	0.1	0.3	0.0	0.0
Safe period	2.0	1.3	5.9	1.4
Withdrawal	4.1	6.7	8.3	4.4
Female sterilization	11.5	9.2	4.2	0.0
Vasectomy	13.4	6.1	4.2	2.8
Abstinence	1.0	1.2	1.3	4.6
Other method	0.8	0.1	0.0	0.0
None	20.8	11.3	8.0	0.0
Base*	7 914	476	159	35

Note: percentages sum to more than 100% because more than one contraceptive method could be reported.
* Excludes respondents with no heterosexual partners last year.

in the past year. Pill use increases with numbers of partners. This is particularly marked for women. Oral contraception was used by 70.2% of women reporting five or more partners in the past year, compared with 27.6% of those reporting only one partner.

proportion of the small number of those with five or more partners, 39.6% of women and 28.4% of men, do not report any condom use in the past year. The use of almost all non-surgical methods – IUD, condom, diaphragm, safe period, withdrawal – seems to show little variation with increase in numbers of partners. Use of sterilization and vasectomy is highest amongst those with only one partner.

Multivariate analysis

Logistic regression models were used to explore the relationship between age, marital status, social class, parity and numbers of partners, and contraceptive method (Figs 10.5 & 10.6). Age exerts a strong effect on any use of contraception, increasing for both men and women after controlling for other factors (Fig. 10.5). The social class effect was sustained – men in manual social class groups were twice as likely as those in non-manual social class groups to report use of no method, though for women this effect was weaker. The effect of numbers of partners was more marked for men than for women, those with more than one sexual partner in the past year being four times less likely to report no method use than those with one. For both men and women, having children was significantly associated with using some method of contraception.

When looking at the pattern for the main methods used (Fig. 10.6), oral contraception is positively associated, for both men and women, with younger current age, with cohabiting, widowed, separated or divorced status and, for men, with having three or more sexual partners. Those with children are less likely to use oral contraception. The age effect is reflected in condom use, though it is less marked, and the effect of marital status is reversed for condom use for women. Those with two or more sexual partners are more likely to report condom use, but the effect is weaker than the effect of age. The most striking effects on sterilization are those of age, marital status and children. Women with children are nearly five times as likely, and men four times as likely, as those with none to rely on sterilization for contraceptive protection. Not surprisingly, those aged 16–24 and those who are single are very unlikely to rely on sterilization for contraception.

Gender differences in contraceptive reporting

Tables 10.1 & 10.2 show there that is some disparity between the sexes in their reporting of the use of any contraceptive methods. Several factors might account for gender differences. The age difference between partners is such that a proportion of men in each age range will report the method used by women 2 or 3 years younger, on average, than themselves. The lower proportion of men in the younger age group reporting partner's pill use may be explained by the fact that a proportion of these younger men will be having a sexual relationship with young women who have not yet started taking the pill. The higher proportion of men aged 35–44 reporting pill use in the last year may reflect the fact that a proportion of these men will have partners in the younger age range amongst whom the prevalence of pill use is higher. This effect is also apparent in the sterilization data.

Lack of familiarity with the partner's method might also explain some of the discrepancy, and so the difference could be expected to be more pronounced for the single than the married and for younger rather than older respondents.

Contraceptive trends

It is difficult to determine to what extent these cross-sectional patterns of contraceptive use should be interpreted in terms of lifestage effects and to what extent in terms of historical trends. Needs relating to ferility control vary throughout the lifecourse. At the start of the sexual career, before childbearing, the need is for a reliable and reversible method of contraception. During the period of starting and spacing a family, a concern for efficacy may take second place to a need for safety and acceptability. On completion of childbearing and possible resumption of a woman's employment the need for a reliable method returns, but this time the need for reversibility is less, and with advancing years the concern for side-effects greater.

Amongst older women, the decline in pill use no doubt reflects declining fertility and the decreasing need for a totally efficacious contraceptive method, together with increasing awareness of adverse side-effects with advancing years, and is therefore to some extent a function of lifestage. Similarly the increase in popularity of sterilization with parity and age reflects a continuing need for a high degree of efficacy, together with a greater tolerance for a method which is irreversible, on completion of family size.

Nevertheless, the notion of an orderly 'reproductive career' has not gone unchallenged. The concept of a linear lifecourse comprising three consecutive stages – a sexually active period before childbearing, a period of childbearing during which pregnancies are spaced, and the remaining fertile years when no further children are wanted – is oversimplified and ignores changes in marital status (Hunt, 1991). Age is the only reliably progressive variable; marital status and even family spacing do not dependably follow a sequential course.

At any one point in the life of an individual, a decision relating to

reported the use of condoms and at least one other method of contraception in the last year is clearly of interest in the context of sexual health. Whilst reporting of both cannot be taken to indicate that those reporting use of both another contraceptive method as well as a condom would have used them together on the same occasion of sex (Table 10.8), it is reasonable to assume that a proportion would have done so.

These data show sizeable proportions reporting both a reliable method of contraception and a condom, particularly amongst the young and those with between two and four partners, though clearly the variety of contraceptive methods encountered by both men and women will increase with the number of sexual partners.

Safer sex

The focus in this section of the chapter is on behaviour which tends to reduce the likelihood of sexually transmitted infection. Of interest in this context is awareness of personal risk and knowledge of the means by which to reduce it, whether people take preventive health action and what strategies are adopted. The exact relationship between these variables is unclear. It has long been accepted that information is insufficient to prompt behaviour change (Gatherer *et al.*, 1979) and others have noted an absence of any clear association between awareness of unsafe sexual practices and a change to safer sex (Joseph *et al.*, 1987; Becker & Joseph, 1988; Memon, 1991).

Questions asked in the survey relate to several of these variables. Respondents were asked, for example, to describe their understanding of safer sex, to assess their own risk status in relation to HIV transmission, and to report any behaviour change made because of the AIDS epidemic. Information provided elsewhere in the questionnaire enables the relationship between self-perceived risk and risky behaviour to be explored, together with the extent of adoption of risk reduction strategies. These data also afford an opportunity for exploring the relationship between reported behaviour change and actual practice.

Meaning of safer sex

The question relating to safer sex was included in the context of the AIDS epidemic. Respondents were asked, 'There has been a lot of publicity about AIDS in the last year or two. From what you have heard or read, what does the phrase "safer sex" mean to you?' Respondents' answers were recorded verbatim and interviewers were instructed to probe until no further responses were forthcoming. This was the only open-ended question in the schedule and responses were subsequently post-coded

Table 10.9. Meaning of phrase 'safer sex' by age group
[Source: interview, question 43]

	16–24 (%)	25–34 (%)	35–44 (%)	45–59 (%)	All ages (%)
Men					
Use of condom	75.6	79.0	74.5	72.1	75.3
Use of other contraception	14.5	7.2	6.5	4.9	8.2
Safer sex practices	6.8	9.6	9.2	4.7	7.7
Monogamy	19.3	25.9	32.3	33.9	27.9
Restrict number of partners	31.8	28.6	26.8	21.2	27.1
Know partner	21.5	22.8	22.0	14.8	20.4
Abstain from sex	2.2	3.9	4.1	4.9	3.8
Avoid drug use	5.8	4.8	7.3	4.4	5.6
Avoid STDs/pregnancy	5.8	5.9	3.5	6.0	5.3
Other	5.1	4.7	6.0	8.8	6.1
Base*	508	546	537	497	2088
Women					
Use of condom	80.5	84.8	79.2	79.0	81.0
Use of other contraception	13.5	5.0	4.6	3.5	6.3
Safer sex practices	2.8	4.9	4.4	3.5	4.0
Monogamy	21.2	27.8	33.4	33.8	29.4
Restrict number of partners	44.5	37.3	30.6	31.5	35.6
Know partner	28.4	26.1	20.7	18.8	23.3
Abstain from sex	4.2	5.8	6.9	7.8	6.3
Avoid drug use	6.8	4.2	4.3	3.0	4.4
Avoid STDs/pregnancy	4.0	4.9	4.4	4.3	4.4
Other	1.2	4.7	4.8	3.9	3.8
Base*	536	721	634	686	2577

* All respondents given long questionnaire.

according to the categories that emerged from respondents. These are summarized in Table 10.9.

The dominant messages of the British AIDS public education campaigns have been to remain within a sexually exclusive relationship or, where this is not feasible, to use a condom. Choosing a partner carefully has been implied rather than explicit in the messages to avoid casual sex, but there has been no real attempt to promote non-penetrative sex amongst heterosexuals except in a few advertisements in the women's press, and in campaigns mounted by voluntary agencies (Wellings, 1992). This has, however, been a prominent message for risk reduction amongst homosexual men.

Responses to the survey question tend to correspond fairly closely to official advice. What the data show most strikingly is the widespread equation of safer sex with condom use (Table 10.9). More than three-quarters of respondents saw safer sex in terms of condom use. No other single strategy was mentioned by more than 36% of respondents. The next most common (in order of frequency) were sexual exclusivity, reducing the number of partners and knowing a partner well, mentioned by approximately a quarter of respondents in each case. Restricting numbers of partners was mentioned more often by women than men; younger respondents were more likely to report restricting numbers of partners, while older respondents interpreted safer sex more in terms of monogamy.

Comparatively few references were made to sexual practices, including non-penetrative sex, which is perhaps not surprising given its relative rarity in the heterosexual repertoire (see Chapter 6). Nor is it surprising, since the question was asked within the context of the AIDS epidemic, that use of contraception (other than condoms) does not feature prominently among responses. It is mentioned by only 8.2% of men and 6.3% of women. This meaning was more likely to be given by younger respondents aged 16–24 (14.5% men and 13.5% of women) who were brought up in the era in which safer sex was almost synonymous with the prevention of transmission of HIV.

Perceived risk

An important question here is to what extent subjective ratings relate to actual behaviour. Respondents were asked for their assessment of whether they felt themselves to be at risk of HIV. Interviewers told them, 'Nobody yet knows for sure how many people are at risk of becoming infected with the AIDS virus, but we would like to know what you think about . . . (a) the risks to you personally with your present sexual life-style?'

The response options were: 'greatly at risk'; 'quite a lot'; 'not very much'; 'not at all at risk'. The respondents who chose any but the last of these were aggregated to form a category of those who saw themselves to be at any risk. The results are summarized in Table 10.10 in relation to number of heterosexual partners, homosexual partners and injecting drug use in the last 5 years.

Six out of 10 men and women with five or more partners in the past 5 years see their current lifestyle as presenting some risk — more than four times as many as those with only one partner. Men who report more than five heterosexual partners in the past 5 years are less likely to see themselves to be at risk for HIV than are those with five or more homosexual partners (Table 10.10). The numbers of women with homosexual

Table 10.10. Proportions of respondents who perceive themselves to be at some risk of AIDS
[Source: interview, question 45a]

	Men		Women	
	(%)	Base	(%)	Base
Heterosexual partners in the last 5 years				
0	25.7	689	12.4	910
1	14.1	4 536	15.0	6 750
2	33.9	802	31.5	1 104
3–4	46.0	964	44.3	808
5–9	58.2	630	61.9	362
10+	61.6	388	63.3	81
Homosexual partners in the last 5 years				
0	26.0	8 153	20.5	10 294
1	51.4	49	53.8	40
2	—	9†	52.5	16*
3–4	56.9	18*	—	3†
5–9	74.2	11*	—	5†
10+	82.0	30	—	1†
Injecting drug use in the last 5 years				
Yes	59.0	33	70.0	23
No	26.9	7 522	21.3	9 462
Total	26.5	8 318	20.7	10 419

* Note small base.
† Base <10.

partners are too small to make the same comparison. Fifty-nine per-cent of men and 70.0% of women reporting injecting non-prescribed drugs consider themselves to be at some risk. These data show that risk perception is higher among those reporting behaviours that carry a higher risk of HIV infection.

Prevalence and distribution of unsafe sex

Since an important aim of this survey was to identify the size and nature of the section of the population at higher risk of adverse outcomes, we sought to construct a variable measuring unsafe heterosexual sex. A broad measure of risk-taking behaviour is obtained by defining a group of

Table 10.11. Proportions reporting 'unsafe' sex (two or more heterosexual partners and no condom use) in the last year
[Source: interview, question 30b; booklet, question 7d]

	Men (%)	Base*	Women (%)	Base*
Age				
16–24	9.7	1534	9.2	1732
25–34	5.8	2029	3.8	2729
35–44	5.7	1929	3.1	2453
45–59	3.7	1983	1.6	2534
Marital status				
Married	3.0	4545	1.3	6003
Cohabiting	10.4	593	5.7	817
Widowed, separated, divorced	15.7	421	8.0	1013
Single	9.6	1914	10.6	1613
Social class				
I, II	5.5	2734	2.6	3455
III NM	5.0	1453	5.4	2164
III M	7.7	1838	1.7	1696
IV, V, other	5.9	1444	6.6	2126
Homosexual partners in the last year				
0	6.0	7404	4.0	9415
1+	7.4	64	11.0	32
All respondents	6.0	7476	4.0	9448

* All respondents who have had sexual intercourse.

people who have had 'unsafe' sex as those who have had two or more heterosexual partners in the last year but *never* used a condom in that time. This is not an all-inclusive definition of unsafe sexual behaviour. It excludes those who use a condom inconsistently, and those who have had only one partner but who may have been at risk as a result of their partner's behaviour, and so is likely to underestimate the prevalence of unsafe sex. These uncertainties are difficult to resolve in a large-scale quantitative survey and are better addressed by means of other investigative techniques. Nevertheless, defining a group in this way provides an indicator for the likely attributes of those who may be at increased risk.

From Table 10.11, it is clear that the likelihood of having 'unsafe' sex decreases with age. In all age groups, men were more likely to have had 'unsafe' sex than women (6.0% cf. 4.0%). More than 9% of men and women under 25 reported two or more partners and no condom use in the last year. These proportions decreased very noticeably with age for

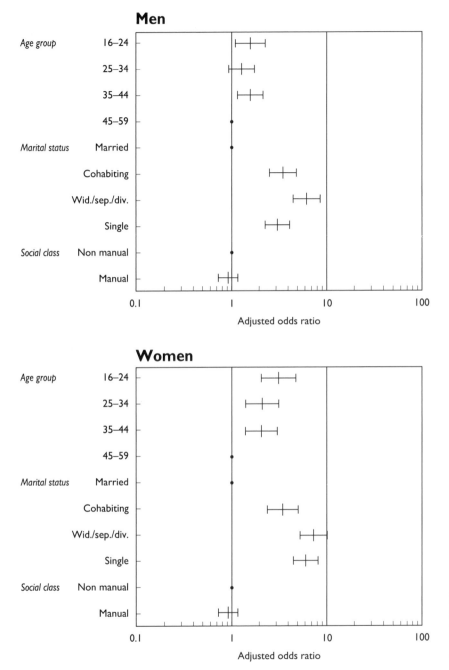

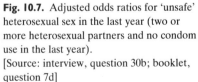

Fig. 10.7. Adjusted odds ratios for 'unsafe' heterosexual sex in the last year (two or more heterosexual partners and no condom use in the last year).
[Source: interview, question 30b; booklet, question 7d]

women; only 1.6% of those over 44 had 'unsafe' sex in the last year.

Marital status also has a strong effect, with only 3.0% of married men and 1.3% of married women reporting 'unsafe' sex in the last year. Men who were cohabiting were three times as likely to report 'unsafe' sex as were those who were married. 'Unsafe' sex was reported by 9.6% of single men and 10.6% of single women. However, the highest proportions of 'unsafe' practice were reported by men who were widowed, separated or divorced, 15.7% of whom fall into this category. There was little social class difference in reporting 'unsafe' sex.

Since some of these variables are interrelated, logistic regression models were used to explore the relationships between them and the likelihood of reporting 'unsafe' sex in the last year. The effects of age remained for men and women, but they were considerably attenuated by the inclusion of the other factors in the model (Fig. 10.7). The effects of marital status remained strong. The group apparently most likely to be exposed to risk are the widowed, separated and divorced, who are more than six times as likely to report 'unsafe' sex as those who are married, and so might form a neglected audience in terms of health education intervention.

Behaviour change because of AIDS

Change in sexual behaviour may result from a variety of factors, which are mostly not amenable to exploration in this type of study. However,

Table 10.12. Proportions who report sexual lifestyle change because of AIDS by age group [Source: interview, question 44b]

	Men					Women				
	16–24 (%)	25–34 (%)	35–44 (%)	45–59 (%)	All ages (%)	16–24 (%)	25–34 (%)	35–44 (%)	45–59 (%)	All ages (%)
Having fewer partners	12.0	8.0	4.1	1.8	6.4	9.1	4.6	2.0	0.8	3.9
Know partner before having sex	20.1	11.1	5.5	2.0	9.5	18.0	7.5	3.9	1.8	7.4
Using a condom	26.4	13.7	7.0	2.1	12.1	16.8	7.5	4.1	1.5	7.1
Not having sex	3.6	3.2	1.7	0.9	2.3	4.2	2.8	1.6	1.4	2.4
Sticking to one partner	15.6	11.2	6.5	3.0	9.0	16.3	9.2	4.7	1.7	7.6
Avoiding some sexual practices	5.0	3.6	2.4	0.8	2.9	3.2	1.3	1.1	0.6	1.5
Other change(s)	1.1	0.8	0.8	0.2	0.7	1.0	1.1	0.7	0.2	0.7
Base	1 983	2 153	2 042	2 172	8 350	2 233	2 889	2 572	2 754	10 448
Any change in sexual lifestyle	36.2	22.9	13.9	6.2	19.5	29.7	15.7	9.4	4.5	14.2
Base	1 983	2 154	2 042	2 173	8 352	2 236	2 892	2 572	2 758	10 458

Table 10.13. Proportions of respondents reporting lifestyle change because of AIDS
[Source: interview, question 44a; booklet, questions 7b; 8b; 17]

	Men		Women	
	(%)	Base	(%)	Base
Total	19.5	8 352	14.2	10 458
Heterosexual partners in the last 5 years				
0	25.0	696	19.1	914
1	7.8	4 539	6.2	6 768
2	27.2	804	28.1	1 106
3–4	36.7	967	40.8	810
5–9	50.5	635	49.0	364
10+	45.2	388	60.1	82
Homosexual partners in the last 5 years				
0	18.9	8 180	14.1	10 326
1	49.1	49	44.4	40
2	58.2	11*	26.9	16*
3–4	66.6	18	—	3†
5–9	73.1	11*	—	5†
10+	89.7	30	—	1†
Injecting drug use in the last 5 years				
Yes	38.4	33	64.6	24
No	19.8	7 336	14.2	9 487

* Note small base.
† Base <10.

responses to a series of questions probing behaviour change, and the type of changes made, provide some insight into the extent and nature of the response to HIV and AIDS.

Respondents were asked, in the face-to-face section of the questionnaire, 'Have you changed your own sexual lifestyle in any way or made any decisions about sex because of concern about catching AIDS or HIV virus'. If the answer was yes, the following response options were presented, on a show-card, to the respondent: 'having fewer partners'; 'finding out more about a person before having sex'; 'using a condom'; 'not having sex'; 'sticking to one partner'; 'avoiding some sexual practices'; 'other change(s)'.

Some behaviour change because of AIDS was reported by 19.5% of men and 14.2% of women. Not surprisingly, the proportions of people doing so decreased with increasing age (Table 10.12). There are marked differences in reporting with sexual lifestyle. Those at apparently greater risk are more likely to have adopted preventive strategies in the context of AIDS. Reporting of changes increases with numbers of partners for both men and women reporting heterosexual partners in the past 5 years, and also for men reporting homosexual partners in that time period (Table 10.13). Changes were reported to have been made by 48.5% of men with five or more heterosexual partners in the last 5 years, compared with 7.8% of those with only one, and for women the comparable proportions were 51.0% and 6.2%.

Men reporting homosexual partners were generally more likely to have made changes, nearly half of those with only one partner in the last 5 years having done so. Evidence of the most widespread behaviour modification was found among the small number of men reporting 10 or more homosexual partners in the last 5 years, nearly 90% of whom reported having made changes. Those who reported having injected non-prescribed drugs were much more likely to have made lifestyle changes than those who had never done so (Table 10.13).

Looking at preferred options for behaviour change for all respondents, there are clear gender differences in preferences for different strategies (Table 10.12). The lifestyle change most commonly reported by men was the use of condoms (12.1%) and by women, *'sticking to one partner'* (7.6%). *'Finding out more about a person before having sex'* was

Table 10.14. Reported behaviour change for those with any homosexual partners two or more heterosexual partners or injecting drug use in the last 5 years
[Source: interview, question 44; booklet, questions 7b; 8b; 17]

	Men			Women		
	Homosexual partner (%)	2+ heterosexual partners (%)	Injecting drug use (%)	Homosexual partner (%)	2+ heterosexual partners (%)	Injecting drug use (%)
Having fewer partners	29.2	15.1	28.1	8.8	13.9	32.4
Know partner before having sex	29.7	21.1	21.7	18.9	20.9	9.5
Using a condom	44.2	26.2	31.0	14.9	20.5	37.1
Not having sex	11.6	3.9	14.0	4.7	5.6	1.9
Sticking to one partner	17.8	15.8	18.9	22.6	20.3	23.4
Avoiding some sexual practices	40.2	5.5	23.9	7.5	3.5	3.6
Other change(s)	3.6	1.2	0.0	2.5	1.2	1.8
Any change in sexual lifestyle	65.0	38.3	38.4	37.3	36.8	64.6
Base	118	2 795	33	65	2 361	24

next most commonly cited by both men and women (9.5% and 7.4% respectively), followed by '*sticking to one partner*' for men (9.0%) and '*using a condom*' for women (7.1%). Having fewer partners was less commonly reported, possibly because the majority of respondents have not had more than one partner in the last 5 years. '*Not having sex*' and '*avoiding some sexual practices*' were rare behaviour changes reported by fewer than 3% of respondents. When these responses were stratified by age group, this overall pattern was reflected for each age group (Table 10.12).

Table 10.14 summarizes patterns of reported behaviour change made in response to AIDS by different behaviours. Selected strategies varied widely, according to whether respondents reported having homosexual partners, having more than one heterosexual partner or injecting drugs in the last 5 years. Men with homosexual partners are considerably more likely to report behaviour changes than are those with two or more heterosexual partners or who report injecting drug use, reflecting their

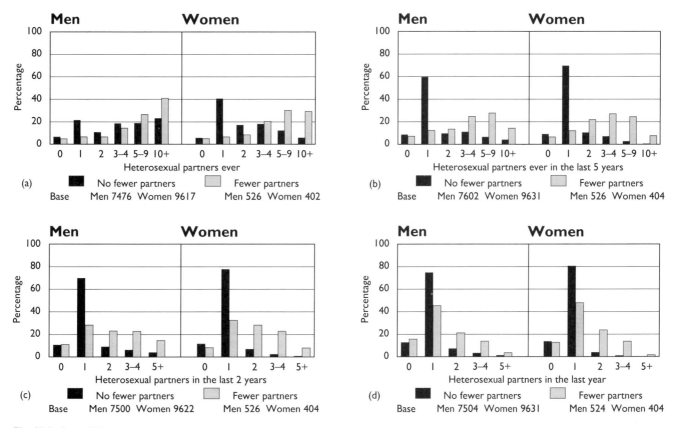

Fig. 10.8. Sexual lifestyle change in response to AIDS: fewer partners (a) ever, (b) in the last 5 years, (c) in the last 2 years, (d) in the last year.
[Source: interview, question 44b; booklet, question 7a–d]

who had never had a sexual partner, twice as many reported abstinence as a lifestyle change in response to AIDS as reported no such change. This ratio increased steadily over 5 years and 2 years, and in the last year 37.0% of men and 45.3% of women with no sexual partners reported a change to abstinence, compared with 12.5% of men and 13.0% women who did not report this change. In absolute terms, the numbers reporting abstinence as a risk reduction strategy is small, but it cannot be a useful consequence of AIDS public education to deter people from having sex altogether.

An encouraging pattern is seen for those who report 'sticking to one partner' as their preventive action and it is particularly clear for women. When lifetime partners are considered, those who have one partner are less likely to report such a change than are those with two or more. The same pattern is seen for partners in the last 5 years, but the proportions become steadily closer with more recent time periods. In the last year there is very little difference between those who report a change to monogamy and those who do not. It should be noted that the trend towards monogamy is also age-related, so that change over time could also be a consequence of lifestage. Nevertheless, these data are entirely consistent with claimed behaviour change.

Claims of adopted condom use in response to AIDS can also be compared with reports of recent use (Table 10.15): 49.7% of men and 41.3% of women who reported having adopted this risk reduction strategy used a condom on the last occasion of sex compared with 19.6% of men and 15.6% of women who reported no such change. Women who reported having taken up condom use as a preventive strategy were almost three times more likely to have reported using a condom on every occasion in the last 4 weeks than those reporting no such change. Nevertheless, 45.7% of men and 50.6% of women did not use a condom at all in the last 4 weeks despite claims of having adopted this preventive measure.

The data also allow a comparison of claims of avoiding certain (unspecified) sexual practices, with reports of experience of sexual practices over different time periods. Vaginal intercourse, for example, was reported less frequently by those who claimed to be avoiding certain practices (Fig. 10.10) than by those who did not, and this difference is more marked in recent time intervals for men. The numbers of those reporting anal sex are small, but there are noticeable changes in reporting of both ever experience and more recent experience, with claims of avoiding some sexual practices. Those reporting avoidance of some practices are markedly more likely to have reported experience of anal sex at some time in their life, compared to those making no such claim, but the excess diminishes steadily over decreasing time periods and for

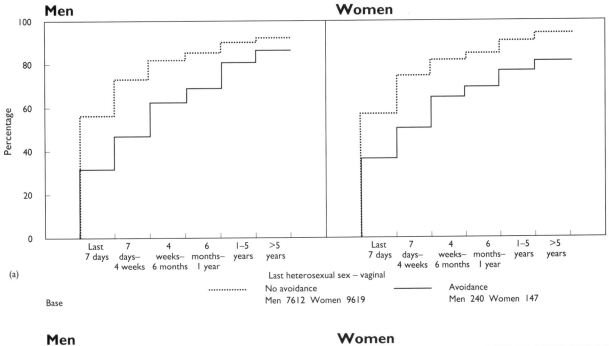

(a)

Base

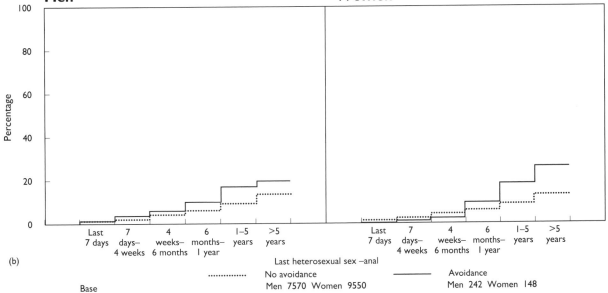

(b)

Base

Fig. 10.10. Relationship between sexual practices and reported avoidance of certain practices: (a) vaginal sex, (b) anal sex.
[Source: interview, question 44b; booklet, question 3a,d]

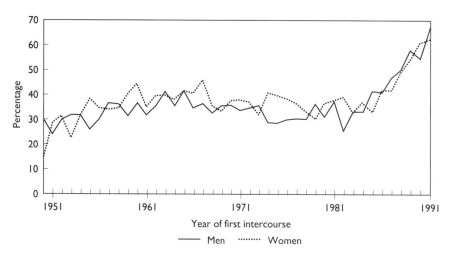

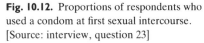

Fig. 10.12. Proportions of respondents who used a condom at first sexual intercourse. [Source: interview, question 23]

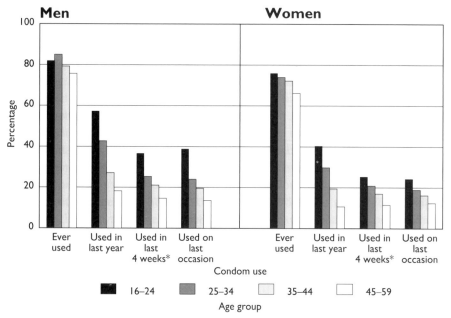

Fig. 10.13. Condom use by age. (*Respondents who were sexually active in the last 4 weeks.) [Source: interview, question 30a,b; booklet, questions 1c; 2d]

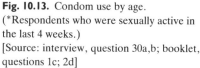

However, the important result of these models is the reduction in effect of number of heterosexual partners as the time interval decreases from ever to the last year. This is the expected pattern if those who report having changed their behaviour by reducing their numbers of partners have in fact done so.

Condom use

As stated above, a great deal of emphasis has been placed on the use of condoms in the context of the HIV/AIDS epidemic and this traditional barrier to infection and pregnancy has once again become one of the cornerstones of preventive practice. Correct and consistent use is not assessed in this survey, but estimates can be made of reported use at first intercourse, at the most recent sexual encounter, as well as consistency of use in the last 4 weeks.

These data provide ample evidence that the early health education campaigns that encouraged the use of condoms had a considerable effect on behaviour at first intercourse (see Chapter 4). The secular trend in Fig. 10.12 shows the increase in the proportions of men and women who reported using a condom at first intercourse since 1985. Although official Government public education campaigns did not start until early 1986, the print and broadcast media gave a good deal of publicity to the potential value of condoms in the fight against AIDS before that.

In general, condoms are more commonly used by young people, and this is clearly seen in Fig. 10.13. Condom use ever, in the last year, in the last 4 weeks and on the last occasion all show similar trends: a decrease in their use with increasing age. This pattern is not found for ever use in men aged under 25 and this is probably accounted for by the proportion of young men with no heterosexual experience. Given that older men, especially those aged 45–59, would have lived through an era in which condoms were one of the few contraceptive options available, these age-related differences are even more notable.

Condom use is of the greatest importance in preventing the occurrence of sexually transmitted infections in new and non-exclusive relationships. Looking in some detail at the last 4 weeks, reported use of condoms has been examined in relation to numbers of partners and numbers of new partners. Four weeks is a short interval in which to examine multiple or new partnerships, but it was the longest interval over which it was realistic

Table 10.16. Proportion of respondents with new partners in the last 4 weeks
[Source: booklet, question 2b,c]

Number of partners in the last 4 weeks	Men			Women		
	No new partners (%)	One or more new partner (%)	Base	No new partners (%)	One or more new partner (%)	Base
1	97.7	2.3	5 554	99.0	1.0	7 044
2	54.3	45.8	122	65.5	34.5	75
3+	38.1	61.9	20	—	—	5†

† Base <10.

of consistent condom use in the last 4 weeks with age group, multiple partners and new partners in the same time interval (Fig. 10.14). For men and women, those under 45 were significantly more likely to use a condom on every occasion of sex than older people, even after patterns of new partnerships had been taken into account. For men, those with a new partner were significantly more likely to have used a condom every time than those with no new partner, but those with two or more partners in the last 4 weeks were significantly less likely to use a condom than those with only one partner. For women the picture is slightly less clear-cut. They are significantly more likely to use condoms on every occasion if they have a new partner, but there is no significant effect of numbers of partners. This model needs to be interpreted with caution because of the small number of women with multiple or new partners in the last 4 weeks.

Decisions about condom use rest on a multitude of factors, not all of which bear rational examination after the event. Nevertheless, the demographic and behavioural characteristics of those who used a condom on the last occasion of sex can be compared with those who did not. Age and marital status are obvious variables to choose, given the expectation of greater risk among the young and the single. The selection of behavioural variables was guided by other considerations. Failure to use condoms has often been attributed to alcohol use (Leigh, 1990; Gillies, 1991; Gold et al., 1991). In addition, the suggestion in Chapter 9 of a consistent profile over different areas of risk-taking behaviour prompted the addition of smoking and drinking behaviour to the model. Smoking and alcohol consumption have been combined with the timing (more or less than 5 years ago) and status of partner (new or not new) on the last occasion of sex.

As shown in Fig. 10.15, men and women under 45 were significantly more likely to have used a condom on the last occasion than older people. Single people were more than twice as likely and cohabiting people significantly less likely to have used a condom on the last occasion. As far as behavioural characteristics are concerned, smoking is significantly associated with increased likelihood of using a condom, whereas alcohol consumption is associated with a decrease in likelihood of condom use on the last occasion. There is no significant difference in condom use at the last occasion of sex for men between those for whom this took place more than 5 years ago and those for whom it was more recent. For women there was a weak trend showing greater likelihood of condom use when the last occasion of sex took place more than 5 years ago. Both men and women were significantly more likely to use a condom with a new partner, but the size of the odds ratio (1.8 for men and 2.1 for women) indicates that this difference was not as great as might have been hoped for in the light of recent health education efforts.

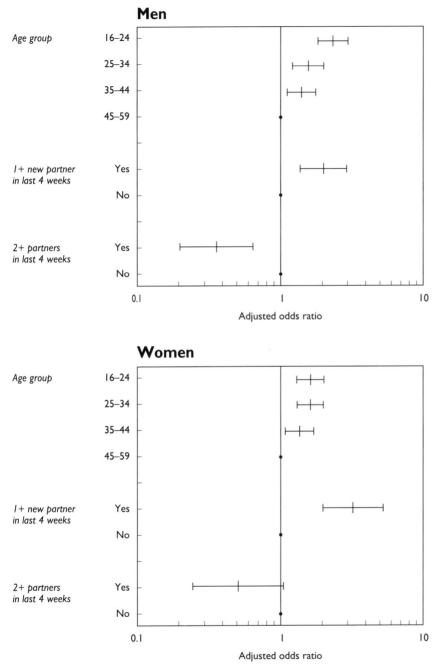

Fig. 10.15. Adjusted odds ratios for condom use on the last occasion of sex. [Source: booklet, question 1c]

Wellings, K. (1986a) Trends in contraceptive method usage since 1970. *British Journal of Family Planning*, **12**, 15–22.

Wellings, K. (1986b) Sterilisation trends. *British Medical Journal*, **292**, 1029.

Wellings, K. (1992) Assessing HIV/AIDS preventive strategies in the general population. In: Paccaud, F., Vader, J.P. & Gurtzwiller, F. (eds) *Assessing AIDS Prevention*. Birkhauser, Switzerland.

Appendix 1
Survey Questionnaires

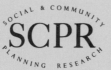

35 NORTHAMPTON SQUARE

LONDON EC1V 0AX

SOCIAL & COMMUNITY PLANNING RESEARCH

SCPR

TELEPHONE 071- 250 1866

FAX 071- 250 1524

CONFIDENTIAL

THE NATIONAL SURVEY OF SEXUAL ATTITUDES AND LIFESTYLES, 1990

Confidentiality

The questions in this booklet are mostly very personal. Your answers will be treated in strict confidence; the interviewer does not need to see them.

When you have finished, put the booklet in the envelope and seal it. Your name will not be on the booklet or envelope.

How to answer

Just put a tick in the box opposite the appropriate answer like this ✓ , OR write in a number on a line, like this 19 90

Not all the questions will apply to you; follow arrows and instructions.

Please ask for help or explanations if you are not sure.

Importance

It is very important to the whole study that you answer these questions completely honestly and as accurately as you can.

Some things may be hard to remember, so please take your time.

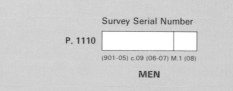

Survey Serial Number

P. 1110

(901-05) c.09 (06-07) M.1 (08)

MEN

Please read these notes before answering the questions.

They are just to make sure everyone applies the same meaning to certain terms we use.

Partners

> People who have had sex together — whether just once, or a few times, or as regular partners, or as married partners.

Genital area

> A man's penis or a woman's vagina — that is, the sex organs.

Vaginal sexual intercourse

> A man's penis entering a woman's vagina.

Oral sex (oral sexual intercourse)

> A man's or a woman's mouth on a partner's genital area.

Anal sex (anal sexual intercourse)

> A man's penis entering a partner's anus (rectum or back passage).

Genital contact NOT involving intercourse

> Forms of contact with the genital area NOT leading to intercourse (vaginal, oral or anal), but intended to achieve orgasm, for example, stimulating by hand.

Any sexual contact or experience

> This is a wider term and can include just kissing or cuddling, not necessarily leading to genital contact or intercourse.

QUESTION 1

a) When, if ever, was the last occasion you had
sex with a woman?
**This means vaginal intercourse,
oral sex, anal sex.**

(Tick one box)

Have never had sex with a woman ☐ 8 → GO TO QUESTION 4 (page 6)

909

Last occasion was:

In the last 7 days ☐ 1

Between 7 days and 4 weeks ago ☐ 2

Between 4 weeks and 3 months ago ☐ 3

Between 3 months and 6 months ago ☐ 4

Between 6 months and 1 year ago ☐ 5

Between 1 year and 5 years ago ☐ 6

Longer than 5 years ago ☐ 7

b) Was this the **first** occasion with that
partner, or not?

(Tick one box)

Yes, first occasion with that partner ☐ 1

No, not the first occasion ☐ 2

10

c) Did you use a condom (sheath) on that
occasion?

(Tick one box)

Yes ☐ 1

No ☐ 2

11

d) What was her age (at that time)?

WRITE IN AGE ....

12-13

NOW
PLEASE
ANSWER
QUESTION 2

QUESTION 2

OFFICE
USE
ONLY

a) On how many occasions in the last **4 WEEKS**
have you had sex with a woman?

TICK THIS BOX IF **NONE** [0] → [AND GO TO
QUESTION 3]

914-16

OR, IF **ANY**, WRITE IN THE NUMBER
OF OCCASIONS IN LAST **4 WEEKS**, ...

OR, GIVE YOUR BEST
ESTIMATE HERE ....

E/R(i)
17-19

R(ii)
20-22

b) With how many women have you had sex
in the last 4 weeks?

WRITE IN THE NUMBER ....

23-24

E/R(i)
25-26

R(ii)
27-28

c) How many of these were new partners with whom
you had not had sex before?

WRITE IN THE NUMBER ....

*(If none,
enter '0')*

29-30

E/R(i)
31-32

R(ii)
33-34

d) Did you use a condom (sheath) on any occasions
in the last 4 weeks?

(Tick one box)

Yes, on all the occasions [1]

Yes, on some occasions [2]

No, not in the last 4 weeks [3]

35

e) On how many occasions in the last **7 DAYS**
have you had sex with a woman?

WRITE IN THE NUMBER OF
OCCASIONS IN LAST **7 DAYS** ....

36-37

*(If none,
enter '0')*

E
38-39

QUESTION 3

This is about different kinds of sex with women. In case you are not sure of the meanings, they are defined in the front of this booklet.

a) When, if ever, was the last occasion you had **vaginal sexual intercourse** with a woman?

(Tick one box)

If never, tick the last box

In the last 7 days	1
Between 7 days and 4 weeks ago	2
Between 4 weeks and 6 months ago	3
Between 6 months and 1 year ago	4
Between 1 year and 5 years ago	5
Longer than 5 years ago	6
Never had vaginal intercourse	7

940

b) When, if ever, was the last occasion you had **oral sex** with a woman — **by you to a partner?**

(Tick one box)

If never, tick the last box

In the last 7 days	1
Between 7 days and 4 weeks ago	2
Between 4 weeks and 6 months ago	3
Between 6 months and 1 year ago	4
Between 1 year and 5 years ago	5
Longer than 5 years ago	6
Never had oral sex — by me to partner	7

41

c) When, if ever, was the last occasion you had **oral sex** with a woman — **by a partner to you?**

(Tick one box)

If never, tick the last box

In the last 7 days	1
Between 7 days and 4 weeks ago	2
Between 4 weeks and 6 months ago	3
Between 6 months and 1 year ago	4
Between 1 year and 5 years ago	5
Longer than 5 years ago	6
Never had oral sex — by partner to me	7

42

(Question 3 continued)

d) When, if ever, was the last occasion you
had **anal sex** with a woman?

*If never, tick
the last box*

(Tick one box)

943

In the last 7 days | 1

Between 7 days and 4 weeks ago | 2

Between 4 weeks and 6 months ago | 3

Between 6 months and 1 year ago | 4

Between 1 year and 5 years ago | 5

Longer than 5 years ago | 6

Never had anal sex | 7

e) When was the last occasion you had **genital
contact** with a woman **NOT involving intercourse?**
(For example, stimulating sex organs by hand but not
leading to vaginal, oral or anal intercourse)

*If never, tick
the last box*

(Tick one box)

44

In the last 7 days | 1

Between 7 days and 4 weeks ago | 2

Between 4 weeks and 6 months ago | 3

Between 6 months and 1 year ago | 4

Between 1 year and 5 years ago | 5

Longer than 5 years ago | 6

Never had genital contact without intercourse as well | 7

QUESTION 6

This question is about different kinds of sex with **male** partners, involving contact with the genital/penis area. In case you are not sure of the meanings, they are defined in the front of this booklet.

a) When, if ever, was the last occasion you had **oral sex** with a man — **by you to a partner?**

(Tick one box)

1012

If never, tick
the last box

- In the last 7 days ☐ 1
- Between 7 days and 4 weeks ago ☐ 2
- Between 4 weeks and 6 months ago ☐ 3
- Between 6 months and 1 year ago ☐ 4
- Between 1 year and 5 years ago ☐ 5
- Longer than 5 years ago ☐ 6
- Never had oral sex — by me to partner ☐ 7

b) When, if ever, was the last occasion you had **oral sex** with a man — **by a partner to you?**

(Tick one box)

13

If never, tick
the last box

- In the last 7 days ☐ 1
- Between 7 days and 4 weeks ago ☐ 2
- Between 4 weeks and 6 months ago ☐ 3
- Between 6 months and 1 year ago ☐ 4
- Between 1 year and 5 years ago ☐ 5
- Longer than 5 years ago ☐ 6
- Never had oral sex — by partner to me ☐ 7

c) When, if ever, was the last occasion you had **anal sex** with a man — **by you to a partner?**

(Tick one box)

14

If never, tick
the last box

- In the last 7 days ☐ 1
- Between 7 days and 4 weeks ago ☐ 2
- Between 4 weeks and 6 months ago ☐ 3
- Between 6 months and 1 year ago ☐ 4
- Between 1 year and 5 years ago ☐ 5
- Longer than 5 years ago ☐ 6
- Never had anal sex — by me to partner ☐ 7

(Question 6 continued)

d)   When, if ever, was the last occasion you
had **anal sex** with a man — **by a partner to you?**

(Tick one box)

1015

In the last 7 days	☐ 1

*If never, tick
the last box*

Between 7 days and 4 weeks ago	☐ 2
Between 4 weeks and 6 months ago	☐ 3
Between 6 months and 1 year ago	☐ 4
Between 1 year and 5 years ago	☐ 5
Longer than 5 years ago	☐ 6
Never had anal sex — by partner to me	☐ 7

e)   When was the last occasion you had any **other form of sex**
with a man that involved genital contact but NOT
also oral or anal sex?
(For example, stimulating sex organs by hand)

(Tick one box)

16

In the last 7 days	☐ 1

*If never, tick
the last box*

Between 7 days and 4 weeks ago	☐ 2
Between 4 weeks and 6 months ago	☐ 3
Between 6 months and 1 year ago	☐ 4
Between 1 year and 5 years ago	☐ 5
Longer than 5 years ago	☐ 6
Never had genital contact without oral/anal sex as well	☐ 7

QUESTION 9

Thinking now of female and/or male partners you have had sex with in the last 5 years (whether just once, a few times, a regular partner or wife) . . .

. . . if **one** partner or **no** partners in the last 5 years, tick here [ ]₁ → AND GO TO QUESTION 13 (page 14)

Or . . . if **two or more** partners in the last 5 years, tick here [ ]₂ → AND PLEASE ANSWER QUESTION 10 (below)

(1140)

(1141-53)

OFFICE USE ONLY		
(Q.10)	(Q.11)	(Q.12)
a. 1141-44	1154-57	1168-71
b. 45	58	72
c. 46-49	59-62	73-76
d. 50-51	63-64	77-78
e. 52	65	79
f. 53	66	80
g. –	67	–

QUESTION 10

These questions are about the partner you had sex with most recently.

a) When was the most recent occasion you had sex with that partner?

WRITE IN: Month .... Year 19 ....

b) Was this the first occasion with that partner, or not?

Yes, the first [ ]₁ → GO TO d)

No, not the first [ ]₂ → ANSWER c)

c) When was the first occasion with that partner?

WRITE IN: Month .... Year 19 ....

d) How old was that partner on the first occasion?

WRITE IN AGE ....

e) Is that partner . . . . . . female [ ]₁

or, male? [ ]₂

f) Are you (or were you ever) . . .

. . . married to each other [ ]₁

or, living together (but never married) [ ]₂

or, regular partners (but never lived together) [ ]₃

or, not regular partners (so far)? [ ]₄

NOW PLEASE ANSWER QUESTION 11 (opposite)

– 12 –

(1154-67)   (1168-80)

QUESTION 11

These questions are about your 2nd most recent partner in the last 5 years.

a) When was the most recent occasion you had sex with that partner?

WRITE IN: Month .... Year 19 ....

b) Was this the first occasion with that partner, or not?

Yes, the first [1] → [GO TO d)]

No, not the first [2] → [ANSWER c)]

c) When was the first occasion with that partner?

WRITE IN: Month .... Year 19 ....

d) How old was that partner on the first occasion?

WRITE IN AGE ....

e) Is that partner . . .   . . . female [1]

or, male? [2]

f) Are you (or were you ever) . . .

. . . married to each other [1]

or, living together (but never married) [2]

or, regular partners (but never lived together) [3]

or, not regular partners (so far)? [4]

g) In the last 5 years have you had sex with anyone else in addition to the two most recent partners?

Yes [1] → [Please Answer Question 12]

No [2] → [Go to Question 13 (overleaf)]

QUESTION 12

These questions are about your 3rd most recent partner in the last 5 years.

a) When was the most recent occasion you had sex with that partner?

WRITE IN: Month .... Year 19 ....

b) Was this the first occasion with that partner, or not?

Yes, the first [1] → [GO TO d)]

No, not the first [2] → [ANSWER c)]

c) When was the first occasion with that partner?

WRITE IN: Month .... Year 19 ....

d) How old was that partner on the first occasion?

WRITE IN AGE ....

e) Is that partner . . .   . . . female [1]

or, male? [2]

f) Are you (or were you ever) . . .

. . . married to each other [1]

or, living together (but never married) [2]

or, regular partners (but never lived together) [3]

or, not regular partners (so far)? [4]

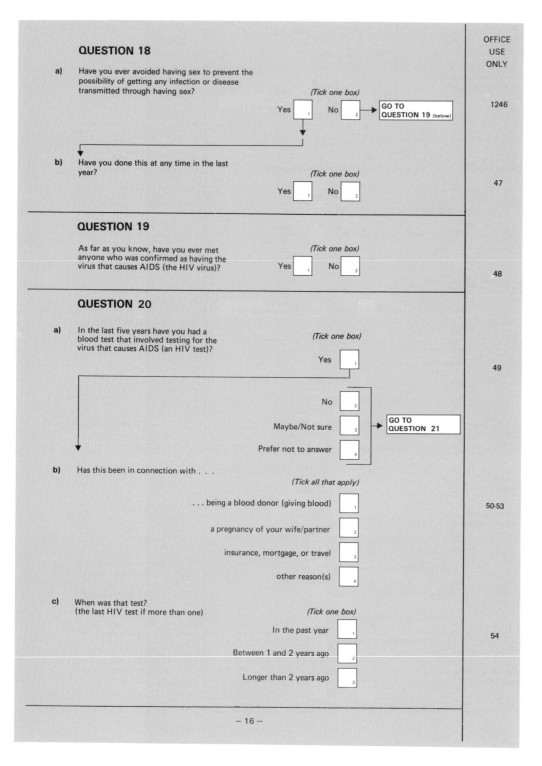

QUESTION 18

a) Have you ever avoided having sex to prevent the possibility of getting any infection or disease transmitted through having sex?

(Tick one box)

Yes ☐₁   No ☐₂ → GO TO QUESTION 19 (below)

1246

b) Have you done this at any time in the last year?

(Tick one box)

Yes ☐₁   No ☐₂

47

QUESTION 19

As far as you know, have you ever met anyone who was confirmed as having the virus that causes AIDS (the HIV virus)?

(Tick one box)

Yes ☐₁   No ☐₂

48

QUESTION 20

a) In the last five years have you had a blood test that involved testing for the virus that causes AIDS (an HIV test)?

(Tick one box)

Yes ☐₁

No ☐₂
Maybe/Not sure ☐₃   → GO TO QUESTION 21
Prefer not to answer ☐₄

49

b) Has this been in connection with . . .

(Tick all that apply)

. . . being a blood donor (giving blood) ☐₁

a pregnancy of your wife/partner ☐₂

insurance, mortgage, or travel ☐₃

other reason(s) ☐₄

50-53

c) When was that test?
(the last HIV test if more than one)

(Tick one box)

In the past year ☐₁

Between 1 and 2 years ago ☐₂

Longer than 2 years ago ☐₃

54

QUESTION 21

Are you circumcised?   *(Tick one box)*

Yes ☐₁   No ☐₂

55

(W. 56-57)

THANK YOU VERY MUCH FOR YOUR HELP IN ANSWERING THESE QUESTIONS.

We greatly appreciate your help and hope you have felt able to answer the questions without too much trouble.

If there is anything you would like to add, or comments that you would like to make about the survey or the questions, please write them below.

58-67

NOW PUT THIS QUESTIONNAIRE IN THE ENVELOPE PROVIDED, SEAL IT, AND HAND IT TO THE INTERVIEWER.

THANK YOU.

Please read these notes before answering the questions.

They are just to make sure everyone applies the same meaning to certain terms we use.

Partners

> People who have had sex together — whether just once, or a few times, or as regular partners, or as married partners.

Genital area

> A man's penis or a woman's vagina — that is, the sex organs.

Vaginal sexual intercourse

> A man's penis entering a woman's vagina.

Oral sex (oral sexual intercourse)

> A man's or a woman's mouth on a partner's genital area.

Anal sex (anal sexual intercourse)

> A man's penis entering a partner's anus (rectum or back passage).

Genital contact NOT involving intercourse

> Forms of contact with the genital area NOT leading to intercourse (vaginal, oral or anal), but intended to achieve orgasm, for example, stimulating by hand.

Any sexual contact or experience

> This is a wider term and can include just kissing or cuddling, not necessarily leading to genital contact or intercourse.

370   APPENDIX 1

QUESTION 1

a) When, if ever, was the last occasion you had sex with a man?

This means vaginal intercourse, oral sex, anal sex.

(Tick one box)

Have never had sex with a man [8] → GO TO QUESTION 4 (page 6)

Last occasion was:

In the last 7 days [1]

Between 7 days and 4 weeks ago [2]

Between 4 weeks and 3 months ago [3]

Between 3 months and 6 months ago [4]

Between 6 months and 1 year ago [5]

Between 1 year and 5 years ago [6]

Longer than 5 years ago [7]

b) Was this the **first** occasion with that partner, or not?

(Tick one box)

Yes, first occasion with that partner [1]

No, not the first occasion [2]

c) Was a condom (sheath) used on that occasion?

(Tick one box)

Yes [1]

No [2]

d) What was his age (at that time)?

WRITE IN AGE ....

NOW PLEASE ANSWER QUESTION 2

OFFICE USE ONLY

909

10

11

12-13

– 2 –

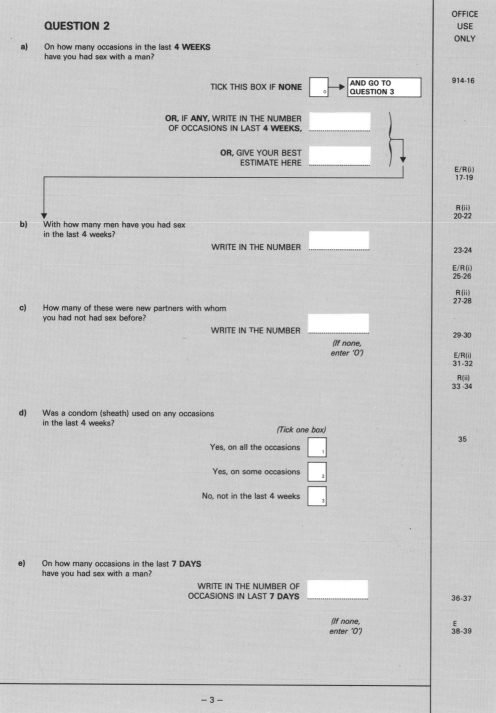

QUESTION 2

a) On how many occasions in the last **4 WEEKS** have you had sex with a man?

TICK THIS BOX IF **NONE** [0] → AND GO TO QUESTION 3

OR, IF **ANY,** WRITE IN THE NUMBER OF OCCASIONS IN LAST **4 WEEKS,** ....

OR, GIVE YOUR BEST ESTIMATE HERE ....

b) With how many men have you had sex in the last 4 weeks?

WRITE IN THE NUMBER ....

c) How many of these were new partners with whom you had not had sex before?

WRITE IN THE NUMBER ....

(If none, enter '0')

d) Was a condom (sheath) used on any occasions in the last 4 weeks?

(Tick one box)

Yes, on all the occasions [1]

Yes, on some occasions [2]

No, not in the last 4 weeks [3]

e) On how many occasions in the last **7 DAYS** have you had sex with a man?

WRITE IN THE NUMBER OF OCCASIONS IN LAST **7 DAYS** ....

(If none, enter '0')

OFFICE USE ONLY

914-16

E/R(i) 17-19

R(ii) 20-22

23-24

E/R(i) 25-26

R(ii) 27-28

29-30

E/R(i) 31-32

R(ii) 33-34

35

36-37

E 38-39

QUESTION 3

This is about different kinds of sex with men. In case you are not sure of the meanings, they are defined in the front of this booklet.

a) When, if ever, was the last occasion you
    had **vaginal sexual intercourse** with a man?   *(Tick one box)*

940

In the last 7 days	1
Between 7 days and 4 weeks ago	2
Between 4 weeks and 6 months ago	3
Between 6 months and 1 year ago	4
Between 1 year and 5 years ago	5
Longer than 5 years ago	6
Never had vaginal intercourse	7

*If never, tick
the last box*

b) When, if ever, was the last occasion you had
    oral sex with a man — **by you to a partner?**   *(Tick one box)*

41

In the last 7 days	1
Between 7 days and 4 weeks ago	2
Between 4 weeks and 6 months ago	3
Between 6 months and 1 year ago	4
Between 1 year and 5 years ago	5
Longer than 5 years ago	6
Never had oral sex — by me to partner	7

*If never, tick
the last box*

c) When, if ever, was the last occasion you had
    oral sex with a man — **by a partner to you?**   *(Tick one box)*

42

In the last 7 days	1
Between 7 days and 4 weeks ago	2
Between 4 weeks and 6 months ago	3
Between 6 months and 1 year ago	4
Between 1 year and 5 years ago	5
Longer than 5 years ago	6
Never had oral sex — by partner to me	7

*If never, tick
the last box*

(Question 3 continued)

d)   When, if ever, was the last occasion you
     had **anal sex** with a man?

(Tick one box)

943

In the last 7 days | 1 |

*If never, tick
the last box*

Between 7 days and 4 weeks ago | 2 |

Between 4 weeks and 6 months ago | 3 |

Between 6 months and 1 year ago | 4 |

Between 1 year and 5 years ago | 5 |

Longer than 5 years ago | 6 |

Never had anal sex | 7 |

e)   When was the last occasion you had **genital
     contact** with a man **NOT involving intercourse?**
     (For example, stimulating sex organs by hand but not
     leading to vaginal, oral or anal intercourse)

(Tick one box)

44

In the last 7 days | 1 |

*If never, tick
the last box*

Between 7 days and 4 weeks ago | 2 |

Between 4 weeks and 6 months ago | 3 |

Between 6 months and 1 year ago | 4 |

Between 1 year and 5 years ago | 5 |

Longer than 5 years ago | 6 |

Never had genital contact without intercourse as well | 7 |

QUESTION 4

a)   Have you ever had ANY kind of sexual experience or sexual contact with a **female**?

*Please tick 'yes' here, even if it was a long time ago or did **not** involve contact with the genital area/vagina.*

Yes ☐₁   No ☐₂ → GO TO QUESTION 7 (page 10)

945

b)   How old were you the first time that ever happened?

WRITE IN AGE ....

46-47

E
48-49

c)   Have you ever had sex with a woman involving genital area/vaginal contact?

Yes ☐₁   No ☐₂ → GO TO QUESTION 7 (page 10)

50

d)   When was the last occasion?   *(Tick one box)*

In the last 7 days ☐₁

Between 7 days and 4 weeks ago ☐₂

Between 4 weeks and 3 months ago ☐₃

Between 3 months and 6 months ago ☐₄

Between 6 months and 1 year ago ☐₅

Between 1 year and 5 years ago ☐₆

Longer than 5 years ago ☐₇

51

e)   Was this the **first** occasion with that partner, or not?   *(Tick one box)*

Yes, first occasion with that partner ☐₁

No, not first occasion ☐₂

52

(M.53)

f)   What was her age (at that time)?

WRITE IN AGE ....

54-55

NOW
PLEASE
ANSWER
QUESTION 5

QUESTION 5

a) On how many occasions in the last **4 WEEKS** have you had sex with a woman?

TICK THIS BOX IF **NONE** [0] → AND GO TO QUESTION 6   956-58

OR, IF **ANY,** WRITE IN THE NUMBER OF OCCASIONS IN LAST **4 WEEKS,** ....

OR, GIVE YOUR BEST ESTIMATE HERE ....   E/R(i) 59-61

R(ii) 62-64

b) With how many women have you had sex in the last 4 weeks?

WRITE IN THE NUMBER   65-66

E/R(i) 67-68

R(ii) 69-70

c) How many of these were new partners with whom you had not had sex before?

WRITE IN THE NUMBER   71-72

(If none, enter '0')

E/R(i) 73-74

R(ii) 75-76

(M.77)

d) On how many occasions in the last **7 DAYS** have you had sex with a woman?

WRITE IN THE NUMBER OF OCCASIONS IN LAST **7 DAYS**   78-79

(If none, enter '0')

980
1006-07
C.10
E/R(i)
08-09
R(ii)
10-11

QUESTION 6

This question is about different kinds of sex with **women** partners, involving contact with the genital/vaginal area. In case you are not sure of the meanings, they are defined in the front of this booklet.

a)   When, if ever, was the last occasion you had
oral sex with a woman — **by you to a partner?**

(Tick one box)

1012

In the last 7 days ☐ 1

*If never, tick
the last box*

Between 7 days and 4 weeks ago ☐ 2

Between 4 weeks and 6 months ago ☐ 3

Between 6 months and 1 year ago ☐ 4

Between 1 year and 5 years ago ☐ 5

Longer than 5 years ago ☐ 6

Never had oral sex — by me to partner ☐ 7

b)   When, if ever, was the last occasion you had
oral sex with a woman — **by a partner to you?**

(Tick one box)

13

In the last 7 days ☐ 1

*If never, tick
the last box*

Between 7 days and 4 weeks ago ☐ 2

Between 4 weeks and 6 months ago ☐ 3

Between 6 months and 1 year ago ☐ 4

Between 1 year and 5 years ago ☐ 5

Longer than 5 years ago ☐ 6

Never had oral sex — by partner to me ☐ 7

(M.14-15)

(Question 6 continued)

c)   When was the last occasion you had any **other form of sex**
with a woman that involved genital contact but NOT
also oral sex?
(For example, stimulating sex organs by hand)   *(Tick one box)*

*If never, tick
the last box*

In the last 7 days	1
Between 7 days and 4 weeks ago	2
Between 4 weeks and 6 months ago	3
Between 6 months and 1 year ago	4
Between 1 year and 5 years ago	5
Longer than 5 years ago	6
Never had genital contact without oral sex as well	7

1016

QUESTION 9

Thinking now of male and/or female partners you have had sex with in the last 5 years (whether just once, a few times, a regular partner or husband) . . .

. . . if **one** partner or **no** partners in the last 5 years, tick here ☐₁ → AND GO TO QUESTION 13 (page 14)

Or . . . if **two or more** partners in the last 5 years, tick here ☐₂ → AND PLEASE ANSWER QUESTION 10 (below)

(1140)

(1141-53)

OFFICE USE ONLY		
(Q.10)	(Q.11)	(Q.12)
a. 1141-44	1154-57	1168-71
b. 45	58	72
c. 46-49	59-62	73-76
d. 50-51	63-64	77-78
e. 52	65	79
f. 53	66	80
g. —	67	—

QUESTION 10

These questions are about the partner you had sex with most recently.

a) When was the most recent occasion you had sex with that partner?

WRITE IN: Month .... Year 19 ....

b) Was this the first occasion with that partner, or not?

Yes, the first ☐₁ → GO TO d)

No, not the first ☐₂ → ANSWER c)

c) When was the first occasion with that partner?

WRITE IN: Month .... Year 19 ....

d) How old was that partner on the first occasion?

WRITE IN AGE ....

e) Is that partner . . .   . . . male ☐₁

or, female? ☐₂

f) Are you (or were you ever) . . .

. . . married to each other ☐₁

or, living together (but never married) ☐₂

or, regular partners (but never lived together) ☐₃

or, not regular partners (so far)? ☐₄

→ NOW PLEASE ANSWER QUESTION 11 (opposite)

(1154-67)   (1168-80)

QUESTION 11

These questions are about your 2nd most recent partner in the last 5 years.

a)   When was the most recent occasion you had sex with that partner?

WRITE IN: Month .... Year 19 ....

b)   Was this the first occasion with that partner, or not?

Yes, the first [1] → GO TO d)

No, not the first [2] → ANSWER c)

c)   When was the first occasion with that partner?

WRITE IN: Month .... Year 19 ....

d)   How old was that partner on the first occasion?

WRITE IN AGE ....

e)   Is that partner . . .

. . . male [1]

or, female? [2]

f)   Are you (or were you ever) . . .

. . . married to each other [1]

or, living together (but never married) [2]

or, regular partners (but never lived together) [3]

or, not regular partners (so far)? [4]

g)   In the last 5 years have you had sex with anyone else in addition to the two most recent partners?

Yes [1] → **Please Answer Question 12**

No [2] → **Go to Question 13** (overleaf)

QUESTION 12

These questions are about your 3rd most recent partner in the last 5 years.

a)   When was the most recent occasion you had sex with that partner?

WRITE IN: Month .... Year 19 ....

b)   Was this the first occasion with that partner, or not?

Yes, the first [1] → GO TO d)

No, not the first [2] → ANSWER c)

c)   When was the first occasion with that partner?

WRITE IN: Month .... Year 19 ....

d)   How old was that partner on the first occasion?

WRITE IN AGE ....

e)   Is that partner . . .

. . . male [1]

or, female? [2]

f)   Are you (or were you ever) . . .

. . . married to each other [1]

or, living together (but never married) [2]

or, regular partners (but never lived together) [3]

or, not regular partners (so far)? [4]

QUESTION 18

a) Have you ever avoided having sex to prevent the possibility of getting any infection or disease transmitted through having sex?

(Tick one box)

Yes ☐₁   No ☐₂   → GO TO QUESTION 19 (below)

1246

b) Have you done this at any time in the last year?

(Tick one box)

Yes ☐₁   No ☐₂

47

QUESTION 19

As far as you know, have you ever met anyone who was confirmed as having the virus that causes AIDS (the HIV virus)?

(Tick one box)

Yes ☐₁   No ☐₂

48

QUESTION 20

a) In the last five years have you had a blood test that involved testing for the virus that causes AIDS (an HIV test)?

(Tick one box)

Yes ☐₁

No ☐₂

Maybe/Not sure ☐₃

Prefer not to answer ☐₄

→ GO TO QUESTION 21

49

b) Has this been in connection with . . .

(Tick all that apply)

. . . being a blood donor (giving blood) ☐₁

being pregnant ☐₂

insurance, mortgage, or travel ☐₃

other reason(s) ☐₄

50-53

c) When was that test?
(the last HIV test if more than one)

(Tick one box)

In the past year ☐₁

Between 1 and 2 years ago ☐₂

Longer than 2 years ago ☐₃

54

QUESTION 21

How old were you when you started
menstruating (having periods)?

(M.55)

WRITE IN AGE ....

56-57

THANK YOU VERY MUCH FOR YOUR HELP IN ANSWERING THESE QUESTIONS.

We greatly appreciate your help and hope you have felt able to answer the questions
without too much trouble.

If there is anything you would like to add, or comments that you would like to make
about the survey or the questions, please write them below.

58-67

NOW PUT THIS QUESTIONNAIRE IN THE ENVELOPE PROVIDED, SEAL IT, AND HAND
IT TO THE INTERVIEWER.

THANK YOU.

- 2 -

ASK ALL

3.a) I am going to read out two statements; please say which one
comes closest to how you feel about things, ... **READ OUT**

... there is a lot that people can do to keep themselves
in good health, ... 1   (220)

or, when it comes down to it, good health is mostly a
matter of luck? ... 2

(Can't choose/Don't know) ... 8

b) Now which of these two comes closest to how you
feel, ... **READ OUT**

... on the whole I am happy with the way I am ... 1   (221)

or, I often wish I could be a different sort of person? ... 2

(Can't choose/Don't know) ... 8

c) And which of these two comes closest to how you
feel, ... **READ OUT**

... I mostly find that things just happen in my life ... 1   (222)

or, I usually feel that I control what happens to me in life? ... 2

(Can't choose/Don't know) ... 8

d) What about this statement: 'To have good health
is the most important thing in life! Do you ... READ OUT   (223)

... strongly agree, ... 1

agree, ... 2

disagree, ... 4

or, strongly disagree? ... 5

(All depends/Don't know) ... 3

4.a) On average, how often do you
drink alcohol, is it ... **READ OUT**

... every day or nearly every day	1	
several days a week	2	**ASK b)**
at least once a week	3	
less than once a week	4	
or, never?	5	**GO TO Q.5**
(Varies a great deal)	6	**ASK b)**

(224)

b) About how many drinks do you usually have on the
days when you have any, apart from parties or
special occasions?

(PROBE BY READING OUT
IF NECESSARY)

One or two ... 1   (225)

Three or four ... 2

More than four ... 3

Other answer, AFTER PROBE (STATE) ... 7

ONE DRINK IS:-
½ pint of beer/lager
1 glass of wine
1 tot of spirits (gin/whisky)

- 3 -

ASK ALL

5.a) Do you ever smoke cigarettes?

	Yes	1	**ASK b)**	(226)
	No	2	**GO TO c)**	

b) About how many do you smoke a day?

ENTER NUMBER PER DAY ☐☐   **GO**   (227-28)

Doesn't smoke every day   96   **TO**

Varies (STATE RANGE) _____   97   **Q.6**

	OFFICE USE	(229-30)
	_____	(231-32)

c) Have you ever smoked as much as a
cigarette a day for as long as a year?

Yes ... 1   (233)

No ... 2

ASK ALL

6.a) About how much do you weigh?

	(st.)	(lbs)		
ENTER WEIGHT AS:- Stones/pounds	☐☐	☐☐	**ASK b)**	(234-37)
OR AS:- Pounds	☐☐☐	(lbs)	**ASK b)**	(238-40)
OR AS:- Kilograms	☐☐☐	(kg)	**ASK b)**	(241-43)
OR:- Weight not known	998		**GO TO c)**	

b) Are you fairly sure of your weight or
is that an estimate?

Fairly sure ... 1   (244)

Estimate ... 2

c) And how tall are you?

ENTER HEIGHT AS:- Feet/inches ☐(ft) ☐☐(in's)   (245-47)

OR AS:- Centimetres ☐☐☐(cms)   (248-50)

Height not known   998

- 6 -

ASK ALL WHO LIVED WITH ONE OR BOTH PARENTS TO 16

10.a) When you were about 14, comparing your (parents/mother/father) with the parents of your friends, would you say that your (parents/mother/father) (were/was) <u>more strict</u> or <u>more easy going</u> about allowing you to go out at night, to parties, social events, and so on?
IF <u>MORE</u> STRICT/EASY GOING, PROBE: Much more or a little more (strict/easy going)?

Much more strict ... 1	(270)
A little more strict ... 2	
About the same as others ... 3	
A little more easy going ... 4	
Much more easy going ... 5	
Didn't apply (eg. I didn't want to go out) ... 6	
Can't say/Can't remember ... 8	

b) Also when you were about 14, did you find it easy or difficult to talk to your (parents/mother/father) about sexual matters, or didn't you discuss sexual matters with (them/her/him) at that age?

Easy (with one or both) ... 1	(271)
Difficult ... 2	
Didn't discuss (with either) ... 3	
Varied/depended on topic ... 4	
Can't remember ... 8	

11.a) {**IF AGED 16/17 NOW:** Can you tell me what are ...
{**IF AGED 18+:** Now think of when you were about 16, can you remember what were ...

... the views of your (parents/mother/father) on young people having sex before marriage; could you say whether, in general, (they/she/he) approve(d) or disapprove(d) or (have/had) mixed feelings?

IF MIXED, PROBE: Would you say (they/she/he) were more inclined to approve or to disapprove, or were (they/she/he) equally balanced?

b) What about your own views {**IF AGED 16/17:** now,..................}
{**IF AGED 18+ :** when you were about 16,}
on young people having sex before marriage. In general (do/did) you approve or disapprove, or have mixed feelings?

IF MIXED, PROBE: (Are/were) you more inclined to approve or to disapprove or (are/were) you equally balanced?

	(a) Parents	(b) Self at 16	
Approve(d) ...	1	1	(272)(273)
Mixed feelings (PROBE) → { Inclined to approve ...	2	2	
Equally balanced ...	3	3	
Inclined to disapprove ...	4	4	
Disapprove(d) ...	5	5	
Other answers: Disapprove(d) for girls ...	6	6	
Disapprove(d) for me ...	7	7	
Parents had different views ...	8	-	
Don't know/Can't remember ...	9	9	

- 7 -

ASK ALL WHO LIVED WITH ONE OR BOTH PARENTS TO 16

<u>**CARD A**</u>

12.a) IF AGED 16/17: Now, ... } how important
IF AGED 18+ : When you were about 16, }
would you say religion and religions beliefs
(are/were) to your (parents/mother/father)?

Very important ...	1
Fairly important ...	2
Not very important ...	3
Not important at all ...	4
Important to one parent, not the other ...	5
Don't know/Can't remember ...	8

(274)

12.b) INTERVIEWER CHECK CODE: Respondent is aged 16/17 | 1 **GO TO d)**
FOR <u>**ALL RESPONDENTS**</u>   Respondent is aged 18+ | 2 **ASK c)**

(275)

<u>**CARD A**</u>

c) When you were about 16, how important
were religion and religious beliefs to <u>you</u>?

Very important ...	1
Fairly important ...	2
Not very important ...	3
Not important at all ...	4
Don't know/Can't remember ...	8

(276)

ASK ALL

<u>**CARD A**</u>

d) How important are religion and religious
beliefs to you, now?

Very important ...	1
Fairly important ...	2
Not very important ...	3
Not at all important ...	4

(277)

- 8 -

ASK ALL

13.a) Do you regard yourself as belonging
to any particular religion?

Yes	A	**ASK b)**
No, none	00	**GO TO Q.14**

(278-79)

b) Which one?

Christian - no denomination ...	01
Roman Catholic ...	02
Church of England/Anglican ...	03
United Reform Church (URC) ...	04
Congregational ...	05
Baptist ...	06
Methodist ...	07
Presbyterian/Church of Scotland ...	08

CHRISTIAN DENOMINATIONS

Other Christian (SPECIFY) _____ ...	09
Hindu ...	10
Jew ...	11
Islam/Muslim ...	12
Sikh ...	13
Buddhist ...	14

OTHER RELIGIONS

Other non-Christian (SPECIFY) _____ ... 15

c) Apart from such special occasions as weddings, funerals and
baptisms, how often nowadays do you attend services or
meetings connected with your religion?

Once a week or more ...	1
Less often but at least once in two weeks ...	2
Less often but at least once a month ...	3
Less often but at least twice a year ...	4
Less often but at least once a year ...	5
Less often ...	6
Never or practically never ...	7
Varies ...	8

(280)

- 9 -

ASK ALL

14.a) Do you have, or have you had any children of your
own, that you are the natural { **MEN:**   father of; } please
{ **WOMEN:** mother of; }
include any who don't now, or never did live
with you as part of your household?   (306-07)

      C.03

(IF MENTIONED, EXCLUDE   Yes | 1   **ASK b)**
MISCARRIAGE/ABORTION/ADOPTED)   No | 2   **GO TO Q.15**   (308)

b) How old were <u>you</u> when your first child was born?
(INCLUDE STILLBIRTH/DIED)   ENTER AGE [   ]   (309-10)

c) How many children have you had?   One only | 01 **GO TO Q.15** (311-12)

                    More than one:-
                  ENTER NUMBER [   ] **ASK d)**

d) How old is the youngest now?   ENTER AGE [   ]   (313-14)

e) Do (both/all) your children have
the same { **MEN:**   mother?   Yes; both/all the same ... 1   (315)
       { **WOMEN:** father?   No;   different ... 2

ASK ALL

15.a) Do you have any adopted or   Yes - adopted | 1
step-children?   - step | 2   **ASK b)**   (316)
                    - both | 3
                No, - none | 4 **GO TO Q.16**

b) How many (adopted/step) children
do you have?   ENTER NUMBER [   ]   (317-18)

16.a) **ALL:** INTERVIEWER CHECK CODE: <u>TOTAL</u> NUMBER OF
NATURAL AND ADOPTED/STEP CHILDREN IS:
             None ('No' at Q14a <u>and</u> Q15a) | 1 **GO TO Q.17** (319)
             One ('01' at Q14c <u>or</u> Q15b) | 2
             Two (at Q14c and/or Q15b) | 3 **ASK b)**
      Three or more (at Q14c and/or Q15b) | 4

b) May I check, is (the child/either/any of the children)
(including your own and adopted or stepchildren)
aged 14 or over now?
        Yes: one or more aged 14+ | 1 **ASK c)** (320)
        No: none aged 14+ | 2 **GO TO Q.17**

c) When your child(ren) were about 14, comparing yourself with
other parents, would you say you were more <u>strict</u> or more <u>easy going</u>
about allowing your child(ren) to go out at night, to parties, social
events, and so on?
IF <u>MORE</u> STRICT/EASY GOING, PROBE:
Much more or a little more   Much more strict ... 1
(scrict/easy going)?   A little more strict ... 2
                   About the same as others ... 3 (321)
              A little more easy going ... 4
                Much more easy going ... 5
    Doesn't apply (eg. child(ren) don't want to go out yet/
      none living with me when aged 14/not responsible for
                step-children, etc.) ... 6

- 10 -

CARD B (M OR W)

17.a) When you were growing up, in which of
the ways listed on this card did you
learn about sexual matters?
(EXPLAIN: You can just tell me the code letters.)
PROBE: What other ways? (UNTIL 'NO OTHERS')

CODE ALL
THAT APPLY

Mother (P)	01	(322-45)
Father (Z)	02	
Brother(s) (X)	03	**IF TWO OR**
Sister(s) (L)	04	**MORE CODES,**
Other relative(s) (N)	05	**ASK b)**
Lessons at school (D)	06	**IF ONE CODE**
Friends of about my own age (J)	07	**ONLY, GO TO**
{ MEN: First girlfriend or sexual partner } (S)	08	**Q.18**
{ WOMEN: First boyfriend or sexual partner }		
A doctor, nurse or clinic (A)	09	
Television (K)	10	
Radio (E)	11	
Books (G)	12	
Magazines or newspapers (V)	13	
Other (SPECIFY) _____ (Q)	14	
Can't remember at all (PROBE BEFORE CODING)	98	**GO TO Q.18**

(CARD B)

b) From which <u>one</u> of those did you
learn most?

ONE CODE
ONLY

Mother (P) ... 01		(346-47)
Father (Z) ... 02		
Brother(s) (X) ... 03		
Sister(s) (L) ... 04		
Other relative(s) (N) ... 05		
Lessons at school (D) ... 06		
Friends of about my own age (J) ... 07		
{ MEN: First girlfriend or sexual partner } (S) ... 08		
{ WOMEN: First boyfriend or sexual partner }		
A doctor, nurse or clinic (A) ... 09		
Television (K) ... 10		
Radio (E) ... 11		
Books (G) ... 12		
Magazines or Newspapers (V) ... 13		
Other (SPECIFY) _____ (Q) ... 14		
Can't choose just one (STATE MAIN ONES) _____ ... 96		
Don't know/Can't remember at all ... 98		

OFFICE USE	(348-49)
	(350-51)

11

ASK ALL

CARD C

18.a) Looking back to the time when you first felt ready to have some sexual experience yourself, is there anything on this list that you <u>now</u> feel you ought to have known more about?

Yes (ought to have known more)	1	**ASK b)**
No /none - felt I knew enough at the time	2	**GO TO Q.19**
No/None not ready for sexual experience yet	3	

(352)

b) Which ones?

PROBE: What others?

CODE ALL THAT APPLY

(353-72)

How girls' bodies develop	(A) ...	01
How boys' bodies develop	(Q) ...	02
How a baby is born	(B) ...	03
Sexual intercourse	(H) ...	04
Contraception, birth control	(R) ...	05
Homosexuality, lesbianism	(L) ...	06
Masturbation	(T) ...	07
How to make sex more satisfying	(K) ...	08
How to be able to say 'No'	(S) ...	09
Sexual feelings, emotions and relationships	(M) ...	10
Sexually transmitted diseases(eg.VD/AIDS/HIV infection)	(D) ...	11
All of them	...	97
Would have liked to know more but can't specify which	...	98

CARD B (AGAIN)

c) Looking at this list again, in which <u>one</u> or <u>two</u> of these ways would you have liked to learn more, at the time (you felt ready for some sexual experience) about the sexual matters you've just mentioned?

CODE <u>ONE</u> OR <u>TWO</u> ONLY

(373-76)

Mother	(P) ...	01
Father	(Z) ...	02
Brother(s)	(X) ...	03
Sister(s)	(L) ...	04
Other relative(s)	(N) ...	05
Lessons at school	(D) ...	06
Friends of about my own age	(J) ...	07
MEN: First girlfriend or sexual partner / **WOMEN**· First boyfriend or sexual partner	(S) ...	08
A doctor, nurse or clinic	(A) ...	09
Television	(K) ...	10
Radio	(E) ...	11
Books	(G) ...	12
Magazines or Newspapers	(V) ...	13
Other (SPECIFY) _____	(Q) ···	14
Don't know	...	98

OFFICE USE

(377-80)

- 12 -

SECTION TWO: FIRST EXPERIENCES

ASK ALL

CARD D

19. On this card are two questions about your own experience. For each question would you tell me your age at the time, or just say, 'this hasn't ever happened'. PAUSE, TO GIVE RESPONDENT TIME TO READ CARD. DO NOT READ OUT THE QUESTIONS IN ITALICS (WHICH ARE ON THE CARD) UNLESS THE RESPONDENT NEEDS HELP.

> A. *How old were you when you first had sexual intercourse with someone of the opposite sex, or hasn't this happened?*
>
> *B. *How old were you when you first had any type of experience of a sexual kind - for example, kissing, cuddling, petting - with someone of the opposite sex (or hasn't this happened either)?*

* IF RESPONDENT QUERIES MEANING OF 'B', EXPLAIN: <u>Any</u> kind of experience that <u>you</u> feel is sexual.

(406-07)
C.04
a(408-09)
a(410-11)
b(412-13)
b(414-15)

a) **ASK:** How about question 'A'?
RECORD ANSWER <u>AND</u> RING LETTER CODE

RING LETTER

ENTER EXACT AGE, IF **13+** ⟶ A

Not sure of age - PROBE: About how old?
WRITE IN ESTIMATE/RANGE IF 13+ _____ ⟶ A

Age **12** or under: ENTER ⟶ X

Hasn't ever happened ...96... ⟶ C

Refused to answer ...97... ⟶ D

(416-17)

b) **ASK:** And how about question 'B'?
RECORD ANSWER   ENTER EXACT AGE

Not sure of age - PROBE: About how old?
WRITE IN ESTIMATE/RANGE _____

Hasn't ever happened ...96

Refused to answer ...97

(418-19)

INTERVIEWER CHECK:

c) **LETTER CODE AT a) is ...**

A	1	**GO TO Q.20**
X	2	**ASK d)**
C or D	3	**GO TO Q.31; RING 'C' OR 'D' AT Q.31c) BEFORE ASKING Q.31a)**

(420)

d) Looking at question 'A' again, has this happened with anybody <u>else</u> since you were 13?

RECORD ANSWER <u>AND</u> RING LETTER CODE

<u>Yes</u> - ENTER EXACT AGE, IF 13+ ⟶ A   **ASK Q.20**

<u>Yes</u>, not sure of age - PROBE About how old?
WRITE IN
ESTIMATE/RANGE IF **13+** _____ ⟶ A

No, not with anybody else since
age 13 (RING 96 AND 'B') ... 96 ⟶ B   **GO TO Q.31; RING 'B' OR 'D' AT Q.31c) BEFORE asking Q.31a)**

Refused to answer (RING 97 AND 'D') ... 97 ⟶ D

(421-22)

OFFICE	_____	(423-24)
USE	_____	(425-26)

- 13 -

ALL WHO HAD (FIRST) intercourse at age 13+

20.a) **INTERVIEWER CODE YOUR ASSESSMENT OF INTERVIEW CIRCUMSTANCES:**

Private enough to <u>ask</u> Q.21-29	1 **GO TO Q.21**	(427)
Definitely <u>not</u> private enough to ask Q.21-29 ONLY RING CODE 2 IF ABSOLUTELY NECESSARY	2 **ASK b)**	

b) **HAND SELF-COMPLETION 'FIRST EXPERIENCES' SHEET-MEN'S/WOMEN'S VERSION**

You may prefer to answer the next few questions yourself,
on this sheet. You just need to tick boxes opposite the
answers that apply to you.

CODE: Sheet accepted	1 **ANSWER c)**	
Prefers to be <u>asked</u> the questions	2 **ASK Q.21-29**	(428)

c) **WHILE RESPONDENT COMPLETING, WRITE IN YOUR REASON
FOR DECIDING ON USE OF SELF-COMPLETION** (429-30)

_____

d) **WHEN COMPLETED, TAKE SHEET BACK AND SAY:**

Thank you. Was there anything you weren't sure about
that you'd like to check with me? EXPLAIN IF NECESSARY.

CODE: Sheet completed and attached - no queries	1 **NOW GO**	
Sheet completed and attached - after query	2 **TO Q.30**	(431)
Sheet not completed/Refused (STATE WHY)	3	

_____

21. The next few questions are about the first time you had sexual intercourse
with someone of the opposite sex (ADD IF Q.19d) WAS ASKED: that is, the
first new partner you had sex with after you were 13):

a) How old was your partner at that time?

ENTER AGE [ ][ ]   (432-33)

Not sure of age - PROBE: About how old?
WRITE IN ESTIMATE/RANGE _____

Never knew partner's age ... 97

Can't remember partner's age ... 98

b) As far as you <u>now</u> know, was it (also) your
partner's first time ever, or not?

OFFICE	(434-35)
USE	(436-37)

IF DON'T KNOW, PROBE:

Do you <u>think</u> it was { **MEN** : her / **WOMEN** : his } first time, or not?

Yes, first time ... 1   (438)

Think it was first time ... 2

Think it was <u>not</u> first time ... 3

No, not first time ... 4

Don't know ... 8

ALL WHO HAD (FIRST) INTERCOURSE AT AGE 13+

22.a) Would you say that you were both equally willing to
have intercourse that first time, or was one of you
more willing than the other?

IF ONE MORE WILLING: Who was more willing?

Both equally willing	1	**GO TO Q.23**
Respondent more	2	
Partner more	3	**ASK b)**
Can't remember	8	**GO TO Q.23**

(439)

b) Would you say ... **READ OUT**

... that you were also willing ...	1
or, that you had to be persuaded ...	2
or, that you were forced? ...	3

(440)

CARD E (M OR W)

23. Did you or your partner use any form
of contraception or take any precautions
that first time, or not?

Condom (Sheath/Durex) (1) ...	1
Other contraception (2) ...	2
MEN: I withdrew / WOMEN: Partner withdrew (3) ...	3
Made sure it was a 'safe period' (4) ...	4
No precautions by me, don't know about partner (5) ...	5
No precautions by either of us (6) ...	6
Can't remember ...	8

(441)

24. **CARD F (M OR W)**

Which one of these descriptions applies best to
you and your partner at the time you first had
intercourse?

(MEN ONLY) She was a prostitute (N)	01	
We had just met for the first time (T)	02	
We had met recently (X)	03	**ASK Q.25**
We had known each other for a while, but didn't have a steady relationship at the time (D)	04	
We had a steady relationship at the time (Q)	05	
We were living together (but not married or engaged) (J)	06	
We were engaged to be married (B)	07	
We were married (H)	08	**GO TO Q.27**
Other (SPECIFY) _____ (S)	97	**ASK Q.25**

(442-43)

- 15 -

ALL WHO WERE <u>NOT</u> MARRIED AT FIRST INTERCOURSE

<u>CARD G</u>

25. Which of these statements is closest to how that
first time of having intercourse came about?

It just happened on the spur of the moment	(A) ... 1	(444)
I expected it would happen soon, but wasn't sure when	(B) ... 2	
I expected it to happen at that time	(C) ... 3	
I planned it to happen at that time	(D) ... 4	
We planned it together beforehand	(E) ... 5	
Can't remember	... 8	

<u>CARD H</u>

26.a) Which, if any, of these things applied to you
<u>at the time</u>? Please choose <u>all</u> that applied.

CODE ALL THAT
APPLY

I was curious about what it would be like	(M)	01	
I got carried away by my feelings	(C)	02	**ASK b) IF**
Most people in my age group seemed to be doing it	(F)	03	**TWO+ CODES.**
It seemed like a natural 'follow on' in the relationship	(L)	04	**GO TO Q.27**
I was a bit drunk at the time	(R)	05	**IF ONE CODE ONLY.**
I wanted to lose my virginity	(H)	06	
I was in love	(D)	07	
Other particular factor (SPECIFY) _____	(S)	08	

(445-60)

None of these applied	97	**GO TO Q.27**
Can't remember	98	

b) Which <u>one</u> was the main one that
applied at the time?

CODE ONE ONLY

(461-62)

I was curious about what it would be like	(M) ... 01	
I got carried away by my feelings	(C) ... 02	
Most people in my age group seemed to be doing it	(F) ... 03	
It seemed like a natural 'follow on' in the relationship	(L) ... 04	
I was a bit drunk at the time	(R) ... 05	
I wanted to lose my virginity	(H) ... 06	
I was in love	(D) ... 07	
Other particular factor (SPECIFY) _____	(S) ... 08	
	...	
Can't choose/more than one main factor	... 97	
Can't remember	... 98	

NB. CODE HERE MUST
BE SAME AS ONE OF
THOSE RINGED AT a)

- 16 -

ALL WHO HAD (1ST) INTERCOURSE AT 13+

27. How long did the <u>sexual</u> relationship with your (first) partner
continue after the first time you had sex, or is it still
continuing now, or did it not continue at all?

            Still continuing now ... 01   (463-64)

            Did not continue at all
    (i.e. once only with 1st partner) ... 02

    Continued, but ended after:-

            1 month or less ... 03
            Over 1 to 3 months ... 04
            Over 3 to 6 months ... 05
            Over 6 to 12 months ... 06
            Over 1 to 5 years ... 07
            Over 5 to 10 years ... 08
    Over 10 years (STATE) _____ ... 09
            Can't remember how long ... 98

28. Looking back <u>now</u> to the <u>first</u> time you had sexual intercourse,
do you think ... **READ OUT**   (465)

      ... you should have waited longer
      before having sex with anyone ... 1

    or, that you should not have waited so long ... 2

      or, was it at about the right time? ... 3

        (Don't know/No opinion) ... 8

29.a) About how long was it after the <u>first</u> time you had intercourse
with your <u>(first)</u> partner till you had intercourse with a second
partner, that is, with a different

  { **MEN:** woman }
  { **WOMEN:** man } , or hasn't that happened?

Hasn't happened	02	**GO TO Q.30**	(466-67)
Happened after:-		
1 month or less	03	
Over 1 to 3 months	04	
Over 3 to 6 months	05	
Over 6 to 12 months	06	**ASK b)**
Over 1 to 5 years	07	
Over 5 to 10 years	08	
Over 10 years (STATE) _____	09	
Can't remember how long after	98	

b) And for how long did the relationship with that (second)
person continue, or is it still continuing now, or did it
not continue at all?

            Still continuing now ... 01   (468-69)

            Did not continue at all
    (i.e. once only with 2nd partner) ... 02

    Continued, but ended after:-
            1 month or less   03
            Over 1 to 3 months 04
            Over 3 to 6 months 05
            Over 6 to 12 months 06
            Over 1 to 5 years 07
            Over 5 to 10 years 08
    Over 10 years (STATE) _____ 09
            Can't remember how long 98

                    (470-480)

- 17 -

SECTION THREE: LIFESTYLE

ALL WHO HAD (FIRST) INTERCOURSE AT AGE 13+

30. Now I'd like to ask you a few more general
questions about things affecting sex.

CARD J (M OR W)

a) First, from this list, could you tell me which you or a partner
have <u>ever</u> used, together? Just tell me the code letters.
PROBE: Any others?

CODE ALL THAT APPLY UNDER a).   (506-07)
C.05

b) And which have you used at all with a partner in the past year?
PROBE: Any others?   a)
(508-27)

CODE ALL THAT APPLY UNDER b)

	a) <u>Ever</u>	b) <u>Past year</u>	b) (528-43)
The pill (J)	01	(J) 01	
The coil/IUD/Intra-uterine device (R)	02	(R) 02	
Condom/sheath/Durex (D)	03	(D) 03	
Cap/diaphragm/Dutch cap (Q)	04	(Q) 04	
Foam tablets/jellies/creams/ suppositories/pessaries/ (L) aerosal foam	05	(L) 05	
Sponge (U)	06	(U) 06	
Douching,washing (T)	07	(T) 07	
Safe period/rhythm method (K)	08	(K) 08	
MEN: I have } withdrawn/been **WOMEN:** partner has } careful (S)	09 ASK b)	(S) 09	
MEN: Partner } **WOMEN:** I am } sterilized (C)	10	(C) 10	
MEN: I am } sterilized (had **WOMEN:** Partner is } vasectomy) (M)	11	(M) 11	
Going without sexual intercourse to avoid pregnancy (B)	12	(B) 12	
Other method of protection (W)	13	(W) 13	
None of these - ever (F)	14	- -	
None of these - past year (F)	-	(F) 14	

GO TO Q.31, BUT FIRST RING
CODE 'A' AT Q.31c) BEFORE
ASKING Q.31a)

- 18 -

THIS PAGE IS FOR INTERVIEWER REFERENCE ONLY

IF RESPONDENT NEEDS HELP WITH Q.31, SHOW CARDS K AND/OR L, YOU MAY READ
OUT FROM HERE, USING MEN'S OR WOMEN'S VERSIONS AS APPROPRIATE.

MEN

CARD K (M) (Q.31a)

I have felt sexually attracted ...

... only to females, never to males	(K)
... more often to females, and at least once to a male	(C)
... about equally often to females and to males	(F)
... more often to males, and at least once to a female	(L)
... only ever to males, never to females	(D)

I have never felt sexually attracted to anyone at all   (N)

CARD L (M) (Q.31b)

*Sexual experience is any kind of contact with another person
that you felt was sexual (it could be just kissing or touching,
or intercourse, or any other form of sex).*

I have had some sexual experience ...

... only with females (or a female), never with a male	(R)
... more often with females, and at least once with a male	(Q)
... about equally often with females and with males	(T)
... more often with males, and at least once with a female	(O)
... only with males (or a male), never with a female	(Z)

I have never had any sexual experience with anyone at all   (W)

WOMEN

CARD K (W) (Q.31a)

I have felt sexually attracted ...

... only to males, never to females	(K)
... more often to males, and at least once to a female	(C)
... about equally often to males and to females	(F)
... more often to females, and at least once to a male	(L)
... only ever to females, never to males	(D)

I have never felt sexually attracted to anyone at all   (N)

CARD L (W) (Q.31b)

*Sexual experience   is any kind of contact with another person
that you felt was sexual (it could be just kissing or touching,
or intercourse, or any other form of sex).*

I have had some sexual experience ...

... only with males (or a male), never with a female	(R)
... more often with males, and at least once with a female	(Q)
... about equally often with males and with females	(T)
... more often with females, and at least once with a male	(O)
... only with females (or a female), never with a male	(Z)

I have never had any sexual experience with anyone at all   (W)

- 19 -

ASK ALL

CARD K (M) - MEN   [DO NOT READ OUT CARD UNLESS
                        RESPONDENT NEEDS HELP]

CARD K (W) - WOMEN

31.a) Now please read this card carefully as it is important that
       you understand it and are as honest as you can be in
       your answer.

       PAUSE TILL RESPONDENT HAS READ CARD, THEN ASK:

       Which letter represents your answer?

	K	C	F	L	D	N	Refused	
RING ONE CODE FOR a) ⟶	1	2	3	4	5	6	7	(544)

CARD L (M) - MEN   [DO NOT READ OUT CARD UNLESS
                        RESPONDENT NEEDS HELP]

CARD L (W) - WOMEN

b) As before, please read this card carefully and be as honest
    as you can be in your answer.

    PAUSE TILL RESPONDENT HAS READ CARD, THEN ASK:

    Which letter represents your answer?

	R	Q	T	O	Z	W	Refused	
RING ONE CODE FOR b) ⟶	1	2	3	4	5	6	7	(545)

	c) RING ONE							
c) ⟶ **TRANSFER LETTER CODE FROM Q.19 (BEFORE ASKING Q.31a)**	A	01	05	09	13	17	21	25
	B	02	06	10	14	18	22	26
	C	03	07	11	15	19	23	27	(546-47)
	D	04	08	12	16	20	24	28

d) **NOW**, IN GRID ABOVE, FOLLOW THE LINE FROM THE RINGED LETTER CODE AT c) TO THE
    POINT BELOW THE RINGED b) CODE: RING THE GRID CODE AT THAT POINT.

e) IF THE GRID CODE IS:-

    • 22, 23, 24   (RESPONDENT ANY AGE) .... 1 ⎫ BOOKLET IS <u>NOT TO BE</u> GIVEN,

    • 02, 03, 04 or 26, 27, 28 <u>AND</u> RESPONDENT IS AGED <u>16/17</u> ..... 2 ⎬ GO TO Q.33

    • 02, 03, 04 or 26, 27, 28 <u>AND</u> RESPONDENT IS AGED <u>18+</u> .... 3 ⎫ BOOKLET IS TO BE GIVEN,   (548)

    • 01, 05-20, 21, 25   (RESPONDENT ANY AGE) .... 4 ⎬ GO TO Q.32

- 20 -

ALL WHO ARE TO COMPLETE BOOKLET

32. **HAVE READY TO HAND TO RESPONDENT DURING INTRODUCTION:-**
    * GREY BOOKLET (MEN) OR TURQUOISE BOOKLET (WOMEN) - ENTER SERIAL NUMBER
    * ENVELOPE - ENTER SERIAL NUMBER
    * PEN OR PENCIL
    * SCRIBBLE PAPER.

    KEEP ANOTHER COPY OF BOOKLET BY YOU, TO REFER TO IF RESPONDENT ASKS FOR HELP.

    INTRODUCE BOOKLET:

a) The next set of questions, which are in this booklet, will probably be easier if you read and answer them yourself. Some questions may not apply to you at all, so it shouldn't take long to do. When you have finished, <u>put the booklet in the envelope and seal it.</u>

ADD IF 'FIRST EXPERIENCES' SELF-COMPLETION SHEET USED (OTHERWISE ADD IF NECESSARY)	• The questions are quite personal and this way your answers will be <u>completely confidential and I won't see them</u>. • We need to have a number on it in case it gets separated from the questionnaire. Our office can then check that all documents for one person are completed, but names are never attached to answers.

It is very important to the study that you answer honestly and accurately, so please take your time. There is a piece of scribble paper in case you find it useful for jotting things down to help you remember.

Most questions can be answered by ticking a box, or by entering a number;
SHOW Q.2a IN BOOKLET AND DEMONSTRATE BY POINTING - here, for example, if you were to answer 'none' you'd tick this box and go on to Question 3. Or you'd write in a number here, or here, and follow the arrow to b). **CLOSE BOOKLET AND HAND TO RESPONDENT.**

I should add that the booklet contains certain terms, like oral sex, anal sex and vaginal intercourse. So that everyone attaches the same meaning to these terms, they are defined in the front of the booklet. I'd like you to read them first.

If you need any help or explanations, do please ask. I will just be doing some paper work while you do the booklet.

(549)

(550-51)

WHEN RESPONDENT HAS FINISHED, BUT BEFORE ENVELOPE IS SEALED, ASK:

b) May I just ask you whether you understood how to answer all the questions, or is there anything you would like me to explain, just to be sure?

(552-53)

Booklet <u>not</u> completed (STATE WHY) _____ _____	1	ASK Q.33 - a) **MEN** b) **WOMEN**

Booklet completed and attached:
            - all understood/no help given
    - help given <u>during</u> completion (STATE BELOW)
    - help given <u>after</u> completion (STATE BELOW)
       (Q.No.'s) _____
	2
	3
	4
		TAKE BACK SEALED ENVELOPE; CHECK THAT SERIAL NO. IS ENTERED; GO TO Q.34

(554)

33.a) **MEN:**	Now may I just ask, are you circumcised?	Yes No Question not understood	1 2 ASK Q.34 3

(555)

b) **WOMEN:**	Now may I just ask, at what age did you start menstruating (having periods)?	ENTER AGE	☐☐ ASK Q.34

(556-57)

- 21 -

SECTION FOUR: ATTITUDES

ASK ALL

34. Now I would like to ask you some questions on your <u>views</u> about sexual relationships.

In general, is there an age below which you think young people nowadays ought not to start having sexual intercourse ...

a) ... first, for <u>boys</u>? ENTER AGE [ ] [ ] ASK b) AND c) (558-59)

Depends on individual, not age	95
Not before marriage	96
Other (SPECIFY) _____	97 ASK b)
No view/don't know	98

b) ... and for <u>girls</u>? ENTER AGE [ ] [ ] ASK c) (560-61)

Depends on individual, not age	95 IF 95-98
Not before marriage	96 AT a) AND b)
Other (SPECIFY) _____	97 GO TO Q.35
No view/Don't know	98

OFFICE	(562)
USE	(563)
	(564)

CARD M

c) What is the <u>main</u> reason you say (that/those) ages?

Before that age:-

- young people are not <u>physically</u> mature enough ... 1	(565)
- young people are not <u>emotionally</u> mature enough ... 2	
- young people have not <u>learnt</u> enough about sex ... 3	
- it is <u>morally</u> wrong ... 4	
- the risks to <u>health</u> are increased ... 5	
2(+) of the above equally/different ones for boys and girls (SPECIFY) ... 6	

_____

<u>Other</u> reason (SPECIFY) _____ ... 7	

_____

Don't know ... 8

35. Would you tell me whether you think each of these things is legal or illegal under the law ...

READ OUT

	LEGAL	ILLEGAL	DON'T KNOW	
a) ... For a woman aged <u>under</u> 16 to have sex?	1	2	8	(566)
b) For a man aged <u>under</u> 16 to have sex?	1	2	8	(567)
c) For a man to have sex with a woman of <u>under</u> 16?	1	2	8	(568)
d) For a woman to have sex with a man of <u>under</u> 16?	1	2	8	(569)
e) For two men aged over 16 but under 21 to have sex together?	1	2	8	(570)
f) For two women aged over 16 but under 21 to have sex together?	1	2	8	(571)

- 22 -

ASK ALL

IF INTERVIEWING IN ENGLAND OR WALES, ASK ABOUT "BRITAIN"
IF INTERVIEWING IN SCOTLAND, ASK ABOUT "SCOTLAND"

36. Do you think that divorce in (Britain/Scotland)
should be ... **READ OUT**

... easier to obtain than it is now, ... 1   (572)

or, more difficult, ... 2

or, should things remain as they are? ... 3

(Don't know) ... 8

37. **CARD N**

As I read from this list, please look at the card and tell me
how important you think each one is to a successful marriage
... **READ OUT**

		VERY IMPORTANT	QUITE IMPORTANT	NOT VERY IMPORTANT	NOT AT ALL IMPORTANT	(DON'T KNOW)	
a)	... Faithfulness?	1	2	3	4	8	(573)
b)	An adequate income?	1	2	3	4	8	(574)
c)	Mutual respect and appreciation?	1	2	3	4	8	(575)
d)	Shared religious beliefs?	1	2	3	4	8	(576)
e)	A happy sexual relationship?	1	2	3	4	8	(577)
f)	Sharing household chores?	1	2	3	4	8	(578)
g)	Having children?	1	2	3	4	8	(579)
h)	Tastes and interests in common?	1	2	3	4	8	(580)

38.a) In general, what age do you think is a good
age for a man to get married?   (606-07) C.06

ENTER AGE [ ][ ]   (608-09)

Varies/Depends/no particular age ... 96

Other answer including age range (STATE BELOW) ... 97

_____

Don't know ... 98

OFFICE USE   (610-11) (612-13)

b) And for a woman to get married?

ENTER AGE [ ][ ]   (614-15)

Varies/Depends/no particular age ... 96

Other answer including age range (STATE BELOW) ... 97

_____

Don't know ... 98

OFFICE USE   (616-17) (618-19)

- 23 -

ASK ALL

CARD O

39.   From this card, what are your opinions about the
following sexual relationships ... **READ OUT**

		ALWAYS WRONG	MOSTLY WRONG	SOME-TIMES WRONG	RARELY WRONG	NOT WRONG AT ALL	DEPENDS/ DON'T KNOW	
a)	... If a man and a woman have sexual relations before marriage, what would your general opinion be?	1	2	3	4	5	8	(620)
b)	What about a married person having sexual relations with someone other than his or her partner?	1	2	3	4	5	8	(621)
c)	What about a person who is living with a partner, not married, having sexual relations with someone other than his or her partner?	1	2	3	4	5	8	(622)
d)	And a person who has a regular partner they don't live with, having sexual relations with someone else?	1	2	3	4	5	8	(623)
e)	What about a person having one night stands?	1	2	3	4	5	8	(624)
	What is your general opinion about ...							
f)	Sexual relations between two adult men?	1	2	3	4	5	8	(625)
g)	And sexual relations between two adult women?	1	2	3	4	5	8	(626)
h)	Lastly, what is your general opinion about abortion?	1	2	3	4	5	8	(627)

- 24 -

ASK ALL

CARD P

40. Now please would you say how far you agree or disagree with each of these things ... **READ OUT**

	AGREE STRONGLY	AGREE	NEITHER AGREE NOR DISAGREE	DIS-AGREE	DIS-AGREE STRONGLY	DON'T KNOW	
a) ... It is natural for people to want sex less often as they get older?	1	2	3	4	5	8	(628)
b) Having a sexual relationship outside a regular one doesn't necessarily harm that relationship?	1	2	3	4	5	8	(629)
c) Companionship and affection are more important than sex in a marriage or relationship?	1	2	3	4	5	8	(630)
d) Sex without orgasm, or climax, cannot be really satisfying for a man?	1	2	3	4	5	8	(631)
e) Sex without orgasm, or climax, cannot be really satisfying for a woman?	1	2	3	4	5	8	(632)
f) A person who sticks with one partner is likely to have a more satisfying sex life than someone who has many partners?	1	2	3	4	5	8	(633)
g) Sex is the most important part of any marriage or relationship.	1	2	3	4	5	8	(634)
h) Sex tends to get better the longer you know someone?	1	2	3	4	5	8	(635)

ASK ALL

CARD Q

41.a) In general, do you think it is _easy_ or _difficult_ for two people who have sex together to talk openly about it, for example, to tell each other what they like and dislike in sex?

b) What about you, how easy or difficult would it be for you?

	(a) General	(b) You	
Easy with a husband, wife or regular partner, but difficult with a new partner (C)	...1	(C)...1	a(636)
Easy with a new partner, but difficult with a husband, wife or regular partner (L)	...2	(L)...2	b(637)
Easy with _any_ partner (B)	...3	(B)...3	
Difficult with _any_ partner (K)	...4	(K)...4	
Depends/Would vary/Can't say/Don't know	...8	...8	

- 25 -

CARD R

42.a) Which of these lifestyles would you regard as the ideal one for you at this stage of your life?

b) What about the future, say in five years time, which one do you think will be your ideal then?

	(a) Now	(b) Future
Prefer to have no sex activity (T)	...01	(T)...01
No regular partners but casual partners when I feel like it (Q)	...02	(Q)...02
A few regular partners (B)	...03	(B)...03
One regular partner but not living together (S)	...04	(S)...04
Living with a partner (not married) with some sex activity outside the partnership (L)	...05	(L)...05
Living with a partner (not married) and no other sex partners (Z)	...06	(Z)...06
Married, with some sex activity outside the marriage (O)	...07	(O)...07
Married, with no other sex partners (H)	...08	(H)...08
Have no ideal/None of these/Don't know	...98	...98

a(638-39)
b(640-41)

43. There has been a lot of publicity about AIDS in the last year or two. From what you have heard or read, what does the phrase 'safer sex' mean to you? What else? (UNTIL 'NOTHING').
PROBE: What else? (UNTIL 'NOTHING').   DO NOT PROMPT; RECORD VERBATIM

(642-55)

- 26 -

ASK ALL

44.a) Have you changed your own sexual lifestyle in
any way, or made any decisions about sex,
because of concern about catching AIDS or
HIV virus?

Yes	1	**ASK b)**	(656)
No	2	**GO TO**	
Lifestyle has changed but		**Q.45**	
not because of AIDS	3		

IF YES AT a)

CARD S

b) In which of these ways have you changed?
Please tell me the letters of all those
that apply to you.

Having fewer partners	(D)	... 1	(657-63)
Finding out more about a person before having sex	(L)	... 2	
Using a condom	(K)	... 3	
Not having sex	(C)	... 4	
Sticking to one partner	(X)	... 5	
Avoiding some sexual practices	(Q)	... 6	
Other change(s)	(N)	... 7	

ASK ALL

CARD T

45. Nobody yet knows for sure how many people are
at risk of becoming infected with the AIDS
virus, but we would like to know what you
think about ... **READ OUT**

	GREATLY AT RISK (A)	QUITE A LOT (B)	NOT VERY MUCH (C)	NOT AT ALL AT RISK (D)	DON'T KNOW	
a) ... the risks to you, personally, with your present sexual lifestyle?	1	2	3	4	8	(664)

Now please choose a phrase from
the card to tell me how much at
risk you think each of these
groups is from AIDS ... **READ OUT**

	(A)	(B)	(C)	(D)	Don't know	
b) ... People who have many different partners of the opposite sex?	1	2	3	4	8	(665)
c) Married couples who only have sex with each other?	1	2	3	4	8	(666)
d) Married couples who occasionally have sex with someone other than their regular partner?	1	2	3	4	8	(667)
e) Male homosexuals - that is gay men?	1	2	3	4	8	(668)
f) Female homosexuals - that is lesbians?	1	2	3	4	8	(669)

- C1 -

SECTION FIVE: CLASSIFICATION

ASK ALL

1.   Finally, a few questions about you and your household.   706-07
    a)   At present are you ... READ OUT AS FAR AS NECESSARY   C.07
       TO CODE

... married (and living with spouse)	1		708
living with a partner { of opposite sex	2	**ASK b)**	
of same sex	3		
widowed	4		
divorced	5	**GO TO Q.3**	
separated	6		
or, single?	7	**GO TO Q.2**	

    b)   What was your (husband's/wife's/partner's) age last birthday?   ENTER AGE [ ][ ]   709-10

    c)   For how long have you been married/living with your partner?   711-12

         Less than 6 months ... 95
         6 months, but less than 1 year ... 96
         1 year or longer : ENTER NUMBER OF YEARS [ ][ ]

    d)   And may I check, is this

       (EITHER) your first marriage ...
       (OR)   the first partner you have lived with ...

       ... or have you been married or lived with another partner before?   713

         This is <u>first</u> marriage/partner ... 1
       <u>Not the first</u>:   - been married before ... 2
         - lived with (another) partner before ... 3
         - married before <u>and</u> lived with a partner before (i.e. different people) ... 4

    e)   How old were you when you (got married/or/started living with a partner) (ADD IF NOT FIRST: the <u>first</u> time)?   ENTER AGE [ ][ ] **GO TO Q4**   714-15

ASK ALL WHO ARE SINGLE

2.a)   Have you ever lived with a partner* (as married)?
       IF YES, PROBE: Just once or more than once?

         Yes, once   1
         Yes, more than once: ENTER NUMBER [ ]   **Ask b)**   716
         No   0   **GO TO Q4**

    b)   How old were you when you first started to live with a partner?*   ENTER AGE [ ][ ] **GO TO Q.4**   717-18

       * Partner may be opposite sex <u>or</u> same sex.

- C2 -

3.a) How long ago were you widowed/separated?*

*NOTE: IF DIVORCED, CODE HOW LONG AGO SEPARATION HAPPENED; ACTUAL SEPARATION (RATHER THAN LEGAL)	Less than 6 months ago ... 95	719-20
	6 months, but less than 1 year ago ... 96	
	1 year or longer ago : ENTER NUMBER OF YEARS [ ]	

b) And for how long were you married?
(LAST MARRIAGE)

Less than 6 months ... 95	721-22
6 months, but less than 1 year ... 96	
1 year or longer : ENTER NUMBER OF YEARS [ ]	

c) And may I check, was that your first marriage or had you been married or lived with another partner before?

First marriage and not lived with any other partner ... 1	723
Not the first: - been married before ... 2	
- lived with a partner before ... 3	
- married before and lived with a partner before (i.e. different people) ... 4	

d) How old were you when you got married (or lived with a partner) (ADD IF NOT THE FIRST: the first time)?

ENTER AGE [ ]	724-25

ASK ALL

4.a) Including yourself, how many people live here regularly as members of this household?

ENTER TOTAL [ ]	726-27

b) How many are ... READ OUT

... children aged under 2? [ ]	728
- aged 2 to 5? [ ]	729
- aged 6 to 15? [ ]	730
Men aged 16 to 24? [ ]	731
Women aged 16 to 24? [ ]	732
Men aged 25 to 59? [ ]	733
Women aged 25 to 59? [ ]	734
Men aged 60 or older? [ ]	735
Women aged 60 or older? [ ]	736

- C3 -

ASK ALL

5.   Do you (or your household) own or rent this
(house/flat/accommodation)?

Own - outright or with mortgage/loan ... 1   737

Rent, from: - Council ... 2

- Housing Assoc. ... 3

- Private landlord ... 4

Tied to job (inc. rent free) ... 5

Squat ... 6

Other (STATE) _____ ... 7

6.a)   For how long have you lived in this
(city/town/village)?

Always (i.e. since birth and never lived else where)	1	**GO TO Q.7**
1 year or less	2	
Over 1-5 years	3	**ASK b)**
Over 5-10 years	4	
Over 10-20 years	5	
Over 20 years (but not always)	6	

738

b)   Were you born in ... READ OUT
AS FAR AS NECESSARY

... England	1	
Wales	2	**GO TO Q.7**
Scotland	3	
Northern Ireland/Eire	4	**ASK c)**
or, another country? (STATE)	7	

739

c)   How old were you when you (first)
came to live in Britain?

ENTER AGE ☐☐   740-41

- C4 -

ASK ALL

CARD C1

7. Which of these descriptions applies to what you were doing last week, that is, in the seven days ending last Sunday?
PROBE: Any others? RING ALL LETTER CODES THAT APPLY

IF ONLY ONE LETTER CODE, TRANSFER IT TO NUMBER CODE

IF MORE THAN ONE, TRANSFER HIGHEST ON LIST TO NUMBER CODE

In full-time education (not paid for by employer, including on vacation) ... A	01	
On government training/employment scheme (e.g. Employment Training, Youth Training Scheme, etc.) ... B	02	**ASK Q.8**
In paid work (or away temporarily) for at least 10 hours in the week ... C	03	
Waiting to take up paid work already accepted ... D	04	**GO TO Q.9**
Unemployed and registered for benefit ... E	05	
Unemployed, not registered, but actively looking for a job ... F	06	
Unemployed, wanting a job (of at least 10 hrs per week), but not actively looking for a job ... G	07	**ASK Q.8**
Permanently sick or disabled ... H	08	
Wholly retired from work ... J	09	
Looking after the home ... K	10	
Doing something else (SPECIFY) _____ ... L	11	

742-43

ASK ALL NOT IN PAID WORK

8. When did you last have a paid job of at least 10 hours a week (or have you never had a paid job since leaving full-time education/other than the government scheme you mentioned)?

Never had a paid job	1	**GO TO Q.11**
Within past 3 months	2	
Over 3-6 months ago	3	**ASK Q.10**
Over 6 months - 1 year ago	4	
Over 1-5 years ago	5	
Over 5-10 years ago	6	
Over 10-20 years ago	7	**GO TO Q.11**
Over 20 years ago	8	

744

ASK ALL IN PAID WORK OR WAITING TO TAKE UP PAID WORK

9.a) How many hours a week do you normally (expect to) work in your (main) job, including any paid overtime?   (10+ ONLY) ENTER NUMBER OF HOURS [ ][ ]   745-46

IF VARIES, TAKE LAST WEEK

b) Do (will) you do any shift work or night work in your (main) job?   Yes ... 1   No ... 2   747

c) Does (will) your job ever take you away from home for more than one night at a time?
IF YES: Is this often or just occasionally?   Yes, often ... 1   Yes, occasionally ... 2   No ... 3   748

(NOW ASK Q.10)

- C5 -

ASK ALL EXCEPT THOSE WHO HAVE NEVER HAD A PAID JOB OR WHOSE LAST JOB WAS OVER 10 YEARS AGO (ie. ALL EXCEPT Q.8 CODE 1, 7, 8)

- IF IN PAID WORK NOW, ASK ABOUT PRESENT (MAIN) JOB
- IF WAITING TO TAKE UP A JOB OFFERED, ASK ABOUT FUTURE JOB
- OTHERS, ASK ABOUT LAST (MAIN) JOB

Now I want to ask you about your (present/future/last) job. CHANGE TENSES FOR (BRACKETED) WORDS AS APPROPRIATE

OFFICE USE

O.C. 749-53

E.S. 754-55

S.E.G. 756-57

SC/NM.M 758-59

SIC 760-61

H-G 762-63

10.a) What (is) your job? <u>PROBE AS NECESSARY:</u>

What (is) the name or title of the job? _____

b) What kind of work (do) you do most of the time? <u>IF RELEVANT:</u> What materials/machinery (do) you use? _____

c) What training or qualifications do you have that (are) needed for that job? _____

d) (Do) you supervise or (are) you responsible for the work of any other people? <u>IF YES:</u> How many?

Yes: <u>WRITE IN NO.:</u> [   ]

No: (<u>RING</u>):   00

e) Can I just check: (are) you ... <u>READ OUT</u> ...

... an employee, ... 1

or - self-employed? ... 2

764

f) What (does) your employer (IF SELF-EMPLOYED: you) make or do a the place where you usually work? <u>IF FARM, GIVE NO. OF ACRES</u>

_____

g) Including yourself, how many people (are) employed at the place you usually (work) from? <u>IF SELF-EMPLOYED:</u> (Do) you have any employees? <u>IF YES:</u> How many?

(No employees) ... 0

Under 10 ... 1

10-24 ... 2

25-99 ... 3

100-499 ... 4

500 or more ... 5

765

- C6 -

IF RESPONDENT IS MARRIED OR LIVING WITH A PARTNER (Q.1a CODE 1-3),
ASK Q.11 ABOUT HUSBAND/WIFE/PARTNER. OTHERS GO TO Q.15 (on page 8)

CARD C1

11. Which of these descriptions applied to what your (husband/wife/
partner) was doing last week, that is in the seven days ending
last Sunday? PROBE: Any others? RING ALL LETTER CODES THAT APPLY

IF ONLY ONE LETTER CODE, TRANSFER IT TO NUMBER CODE
IF MORE THAN ONE, TRANSFER HIGHEST ON LIST TO NUMBER CODE

In full-time education (not paid for by employer, including on vacation) ... A	01	ASK Q.12	
On government training/employment scheme (eg. Employment Training, Youth Training Scheme etc.) ... B	02		766-67
In paid work (or away temporarily) for at least 10 hours in the week ... C	03	GO TO Q.13	
Waiting to take up paid work already accepted ... D	04		
Unemployed and registered for benefit ... E	05		
Unemployed not registered, but actively looking for a job ... F	06		
Unemployed, wanting a job (of at least 10 hrs per week), but not actively looking for a job ... G	07	ASK Q.12	
Permanently sick or disabled ... H	08		
Wholly retired from work ... J	09		
Looking after the home ... K	10		
Doing something else (SPECIFY) _____ ... L	11		

IF SPOUSE/PARTNER NOT IN PAID WORK

12. How long ago did your (husband/wife/partner) last have a
paid job of at least 10 hours a week (or has he/she never
had a paid job since leaving full-time education/other
than the government scheme you mentioned)?

Never had a paid job	1	GO TO Q.15	768
Within past 3 months	2		
Over 3-6 months ago	3	GO TO Q.14	
Over 6 months - 1 year ago	4		
Over 1-5 years ago	5		
Over 5-10 years ago	6		
Over 10-20 years ago	7		
Over 20 years ago	8	GO TO Q.15	

IF SPOUSE/PARTNER IN PAID WORK OR WAITING TO TAKE UP PAID WORK

13.a) How many hours a week does (he/she) normally
(expect to) work in (his/her) (main) job,
including any paid overtime?

ENTER NUMBER OF HOURS (10+ ONLY) [ ]   769-70

IF VARIES, TAKE LAST WEEK

b) Does (will) (he/she) do any shift work or
night work in his/her (main) job?

Yes ... 1   771
No ... 2

c) Does (will) (his/her) job ever take him/her away
from home for more than one night at a time?
IF YES: Is this often or just occasionally?

Yes, often ... 1   772
Yes, occasionally ... 2
No ... 3

(NOW ASK Q.14)

- C7 -

ASK IF SPOUSE/PARTNER:-

- IS IN A PAID JOB (Q.11 CODE 03) - ASK ABOUT PRESENT MAIN JOB

- IS WAITING TO TAKE UP A PAID JOB (Q.11 CODE 04) - ASK ABOUT FUTURE JOB

- HAD A PAID JOB IN PAST 10 YEARS (Q.12 CODES 2-6) - ASK ABOUT LAST MAIN PAID JOB

14.a) Now I want to ask you about your (husband's/wife's/partner's) job. CHANGE TENSES FOR (BRACKETED) WORDS AS APPROPRIATE

What (is) the name or title of that job? _____

_____

_____

b) What kind of work (does) he/she do most of the time? IF RELEVANT: What materials/machinery (does) he/she use? _____

_____

c) What training or qualifications does he/she have that (are) needed for the job? _____

_____

d) (Does) he/she supervise or (is) he/she responsible for the work of any other people? IF YES: How many?

Yes: WRITE IN NO.: [   ]

No: (RING):   00

e) (Is) he/she ... READ OUT ...

... an employee, ... 1

or - self-employed? ... 2   816

f) What (does) the employer (IF SELF-EMPLOYED: he/she) make or do at the place where he/she usually works? IF FARM GIVE NO. OF ACRES

_____

_____

g) Including him/herself, roughly how many people (are) employed at the place where he/she usually (works) (from)? IF SELF-EMPLOYED: (Does) he/she have any employees? IF YES: How many?

(No employees) ... 0   817

Under 10 ... 1

10-24 ... 2

25-99 ... 3

100-499 ... 4

500 or more ... 5

- C8 -

ASK ALL

CARD C2

15.a) Have you passed any exams or got any of
the qualifications on this card?

Yes	1	**ASK b)**
No, none	2	**GO TO Q.16**

818

b) Which ones? Any others?
CODE ALL THAT APPLY

GCSE Grades D-G	... 01
CSE Grades 2-5	
GCSE Grades A-C	
CSE Grade 1	
GCE 'O' level	... 02
School certificate	
Scottish (SCE) Ordinary	
GCE 'A' level/'S' level	
Higher certificate	... 03
Matriculation	
Scottish (SCE) Higher	
Overseas School Leaving Exam/Certificate	... 04
Recognised trade apprenticeship completed	... 05
RSA/other clerical, commercial qualification	... 06
City & Guilds Certificate - Craft/Intermediate/Ordinary/Part I	... 07
City & Guilds Certificate - Advanced/Final/Part II or Part III	... 08
City & Guilds Certificate - Full technological	... 09
BEC/TEC General/Ordinary National Certificate (ONC) or Diploma (OND)	... 10
BEC/TEC Higher/Higher National Certificate (HNC) or Diploma (HND)	... 11
Teachers training qualification	... 12
Nursing qualification	... 13
Other technical or business qualification/certificate	... 14
University or CNAA degree or diploma	... 15
Other (SPECIFY) _____	... 16

819-34

ASK ALL

16. Was the last school you attended a mixed school
or for boys/girls only? (EXCLUDE 6TH FORM COLLEGE;
INCLUDE 6TH FORM AT A SCHOOL IF RESPONDENT WAS IN
6TH FORM).

Mixed school	... 1
Single sex school	... 2
Single sex up to 6th form but mixed 6th form	... 3

835

- C9 -

ASK ALL

CARD C3

17. To which of the groups on this card do you consider you belong?

BLACK	... 01
WHITE	... 02
Indian	... 03
Pakistani	... 04
Bangladeshi	... 05
Chinese	... 06
Other Asian (STATE) ... 07	
ANY OTHER RACE OR ETHNIC GROUP (STATE) ... 08	
Refused	... 98

ASIAN (origin/descent)

836-37

18.a) Is there a telephone in (your part of) this accommodation?

| Yes | 1 | **GO TO c)** |
| No | 2 | **ASK b)** |

838

b) Do you have easy access to a 'phone where you can receive incoming calls? IF YES, ASK: Is this a home or a work number? IF BOTH, CODE HOME ONLY

Yes - home	1	**ASK c)**
No - work	2	
No	3	**GO TO Q.19**

839

c) A few interviews on any survey are checked by a supervisor to make sure that people are satisfied with the way the interview was carried out. In case my supervisor needs to contact you, it would be helpful if we could have your telephone number.

| Number given* | ... 1 |
| Number refused | ... 2 |

840

*RECORD HOME OR WORK NUMBER ON 'ARF'
ADDRESS SLIP ONLY - NOT HERE

ASK ALL

19. We may be doing surveys on similar subjects in future and we may wish to include you again. Would this be all right?

| Yes | ... 1 |
| No | ... 2 |

841

TIME INTERVIEW COMPLETED _____

TOTAL DURATION OF INTERVIEW (MINUTES)   842-44

DATE OF INTERVIEW   Day   Month   845-48

Interviewer's Name _____   NUMBER   849-52

THANK RESPONDENT FOR HIS/HER HELP

- C10 -

INTERVIEWER TO COMPLETE

20.a) Were any other people <u>in</u> the home at all during the interview?

Yes	1	**ANSWER b)**	853
No	2	**GO TO Q.21**	
Interview conducted outside (e.g. in garden, car)	3		

b) Was anyone else present in the room, <u>or</u> passing through, <u>or</u> nearby during any part of the interview and (possibly) able to overhear?

Yes	1	**ANSWER c)**	854
No	2	**GO TO Q.21**	

c) Who was present/passing through etc?
RING ONE CODE BELOW EACH CATEGORY OF PERSON

	Spouse/ partner	Parent(s)	Child(ren) (approx. age)		Young adult(s) 16-21	Other adult(s)		
			0-5	6-15				
Present throughout	1	1	1	1	1	1	**ANSWER d)**	855-60
Present some of time	2	2	2	2	2	2	**IF ANY 1-2**	
May have overhead all/part*	3	3	3	3	3	3	**GO TO Q.21**	
Passing through only	4	4	4	4	4	4	**(IF NONE**	
<u>Not</u> present (inc. not applicable)	5	5	5	5	5		**CODED 1-2)**	

* NOT IN ROOM BUT PASSING THROUGH OFTEN, OR NEARBY, SO
MAY HAVE LISTENED/OVERHEARD ALL/PART

d) Did anyone else look at or discuss any part of the self-completion booklet during completion?

Yes - looked at/read/ filled in together ... 1		861
Yes - discussed only ... 2		
No ... 3		
Booklet not given ... 4		

21.a) In your view, did the respondent have any difficulty during the interview because of ...

	Yes, severe	Yes, some	NO problem	
Language problems?	1	2	3	862
Literacy problems?	1	2	3	863
Other problems in understanding?	1	2	3	864

b) Did you need to read out any of the show cards?

Yes, all/most ... 1		865
Yes, some ... 2		
No ... 3		

c) In your view was the respondent ...

... very embarrassed/ill at ease ... 1		866
somewhat embarrassed/ill at ease ... 2		
only slightly embarrassed/ill at ease ... 3		
or, not at all embarrassed/ill at ease ... 4		

867-80

Appendix 2
Technical Details of the Survey

Stratification for selection of wards

1 The list of wards was ordered according to the Registrar General's Standard Regions, in this order: Scotland, Northern, Yorkshire and Humberside, North West, East Midlands, West Midlands, East Anglia, London and South East, South West, Wales.

2 Where there were fewer than 1500 delivery points in a ward, it was grouped with the next one (or two) so that no group of delivery points would be smaller than 1500 if selected.

3 Within each region, with the exception of Scotland, nine strata were created by listing actual wards in decreasing order of population density, based on OPCS mid-year estimates for 1988, then drawing cut-off points one-third and two-thirds of the way down the list to create three density bands. Within each density band, wards were listed in increasing order of percentage of population of pensionable age (1981 census) and cut-off points here again drawn one-third and two-thirds of the way down to create three pensionable age strata.

In Scotland four bands were created on the basis of types of regions:

(A) cities of Glasgow, Edinburgh, Aberdeen, Dundee;

(B) Strathclyde (excluding Glasgow);

(C) Central, Lothian, Fife;

(D) Borders, Dumfries and Galloway, Grampian (excluding Aberdeen), Highland (south of the Caledonian Canal), Tayside (excluding Dundee).

Then, as before, three pensionable age strata were created within each of the four bands, giving a total of 12 strata in Scotland.

There were a total of 93 stratification cells: nine regions of nine cells each and one region of 12 cells. These were numbered 01 to 93.

4 Within each of the 93 strata, the wards were ordered in ascending order of percentage of economically active males who were unemployed (achieved by using 1981 census Small Area Statistics, dividing cell 860 by cell 720; that is, unemployed males by economically active males).

5 From the fully stratified list, a random sample of 750 wards was drawn, with probability of selection proportional to the (weighted) number of delivery points. M was the total number of delivery points in all wards, a random start number was selected between 1 and $M/750$, and then every following ($M/750$th) delivery point was selected. The wards selected were the ones in which each selected delivery point fell. A three-digit ward code was assigned in the order that the wards appeared on the list (001–750).

6 If a selected ward was combined at stage **2** above with another ward (or wards), that group from then on formed a single Primary Sample Unit.

7 The selected wards were assigned to the two groups, A and B, by simply repeating the pattern of allocation ABBBABBBA until all 750 were assigned.

8 Within each ward, addresses remained ordered by postcode within Enumeration District (as in the standard PAF file).

Then followed the selection of clusters of addresses, the number of clusters per ward being dependent on the allocation to group A or B.

Group A. The ward was split into two equal-sized segments; a separate random start number was chosen for each segment (between 1 and the total number of delivery points, divided by 2) to give the first selected address, and then every following 14th address was selected until there were 50 in each cluster. Cluster numbers 1 and 2 were assigned.

Group B. A random start number between 1 and the total number of delivery points in the ward was selected to provide the first selected address. Every following 14th address was then selected until a total of 50 were drawn. Each resulting ward cluster was assigned a cluster code of 3.

Note: Following the delayed start to the survey, caused by the funding problems, the sample design was reassessed and it was decided that the design effects on sampling error might be very slightly reduced if the addresses in all the Group A sample clusters were allocated alternately for 'long' and 'short' interviews instead of whole clusters being so allocated. This improvement was at the cost of some administrative inconvenience to interviewers, who had to carry all the materials for both types of interview when working in any one of these areas.

For each sampled address the following information was provided:
(a) the full address, including the postcode;
(b) the Standard Region code;
(c) the ward code (assigned for the survey);
(d) the cluster code;
(e) the stratification cell number;
(f) an address serial number to provide a unique identifier for every address;
(g) the OPCS census ward identifier (which allows linkage to ward characteristics as portrayed by the census data);

(h) the ACORN code (this is a categorization, developed primarily for commercial purposes, which describes the ward in terms of the type of housing and resident);

(i) a Regional Health Authority code.

After the sample was delivered, a series of inspections and checks was run to establish that there were no errors in the design and selection. The final stage of sample selection, that of selecting a random adult for interview at each address, was carried out by the interviewers in the field according to a strict procedure.

Selection of respondent

All eligible individuals were listed on a grid in descending order of age and identified only by age and gender. Use was then made of the 'selection digits' that formed part of the individual address label. These are computer-generated, rotating random numbers, unique to each address, identifying which individual on the numbered listing should be selected depending on the number eligible, an improved variant of the standard Kish Grid (Kish, 1949). In the following example, 'Persons' refers to the number of eligible people in the household.

Persons	2	3	4	5	6	7	8	9	10	11	12
Select	1	2	4	3	6	5	3	8	7	3	9

Thus, if there were five persons in the household in the eligible age range, then the selected individual would be the third listed; that is, the third oldest of the five.

Interviewer training and briefing

On initial recruitment to the SCPR panel, all interviewers receive a basic training, which involves classroom tuition, home study and practice interviewing, irrespective of any previous experience of interviewing. Before starting work on any survey, the new interviewer attends a project briefing conference and is subsequently accompanied in the field for at least the first day of working by an experienced field supervisor.

All interviewers are briefed personally before undertaking any particular assignments. The dilemma for this survey was whether standard training and briefing procedures would be sufficient, given the sensitive nature of the subject and the general lack of experience in researching it. Early pilot work had suggested that an embarrassed interviewer was likely to result in an embarrassed and reluctant respondent. Interviewers had to be familiar with the terminology employed for the interview and willing to explain terms that might have been unfamiliar to the respondent. They needed to be as matter-of-fact about this subject as any other; they had to be professional enough not to allow any personal reactions of surprise, disgust, prejudice or admiration to surface, while at the same time listening to and recording the answers given to each question.

Various approaches to induction were explored during the early pilot work, including desensitizing exercises similar to those used in the initial training of marital counsellors. As work proceeded through the feasibility stage, the research team came to the view, endorsed by experienced interviewers, that, in the field, the survey operated in much the same way as any other. It was decided that no special training was needed, beyond normal interviewer training and careful project briefing. Administratively, the questionnaire was easy to work with and the effort that had been put into refining question content and wording had led to the minimizing of possible causes for embarrassment or offence. The most difficult part of the interviewer's task, again not unusually, would prove to be explaining, on the doorstep, the need for a survey on this subject, and obtaining the agreement for the interview to take place.

Each briefing conference was led by one of the four authors. Conference proceedings were divided into three main parts. During the first part, the researcher explained the background, history and purposes of the survey in some detail, taking the opportunity to introduce, as naturally as possible, a large number of sexual terms and phrases, so that interviewers could become used to hearing them said aloud and start to use them themselves without embarrassment. Discussion was encouraged, and topics such as interviewer safety, appropriate dress and methods of dealing with difficult situations, either of sexual advances to the interviewer or of respondents' distress about some aspect of their own lives, were addressed. Interviewers were instructed not to attempt to take on the role of counsellor, but to offer one or more of the help-line telephone numbers and addresses with which they had been supplied.

The second part of the conference consisted of instruction about technical and sampling aspects of the fieldwork task. The final part was devoted to familiarizing interviewers with the questionnaire by carrying out a dummy interview in which the researcher acted as respondent, answering the questions to a ready prepared script.

Reference

Kish, L. (1949) A procedure for objective respondent selection within the household. *Journal of the American Statistical Association*, **44**, 380–7.

Appendix 3
Appendix Tables

Table A3.1. Response rates quoted in different surveys on sexual behaviour

Country	Author/s†	Response rate (%)	Date of survey	Sample size	Age of population	Method
Great Britain	Gorer (1971)	65.6	1969	1 831	16–45	Interview
Great Britain	Schofield* (1968, 1973)	47.6	1972	1 873	25	Interview (follow-up from 1965 study)
Great Britain	Farrell* (1978)	74	1974	1 556	16–19	Interview (after postal sift)
Great Britain	Dunnell* (1979)	85	1976	6 589	16–49 (women only)	Interview (after postal sift)
Australia	Ross (1988)	60.2	1986	1 566 (postal returns)	16+	Interview and postal questionnaire
Norway	Kraft et al. (1989)	59.6	1987	665	19–24	Postal questionnaire
Norway	Sundet et al. (1988)	63	1987	6 300	18–60	Postal questionnaire
Sweden	Gothberg et al.* (1990)	68	1988	778	16–31	Postal request and self-completion questionnaire in a community hall
Great Britain	Wellings et al. (1990)	65	1988	977	16–65	Interview
Great Britain	McQueen et al. (1991)	65.2–77.5	Jan. 1989–Dec. 1990	Approx. 800 per month	18–60	Telephone
The Netherlands	Van Zessen & Sandfort (1991)	53.4	1989	1 001	18–50	Interview
Denmark	Melbye and Biggar (1992)	67.9	1989	4 680	18–59	Postal questionnaire
Great Britain	Johnson et al. (1992)	64.7	1990	18 876	16–59	Interview
France	Spira et al.* (1993)	77 (acceptance rate)	1991	20 055	18–69	Telephone

* Different basis for response rate calculation compared with NATSAL.
† For references, see Chapter 3.

Table A3.2. Weighted and unweighted bases

	Unweighted		Weighted	
	Men	Women	Men	Women
Age				
16–24	1 489	1 888	1 984	2 246
25–34	2 368	3 273	2 167	2 899
35–44	2 143	2 604	2 051	2 577
45–59	2 118	2 993	2 182	2 771
Social class				
I	586	616	575	648
II	2 332	3 059	2 331	2 997
III non-manual	1 485	2 402	1 555	2 382
III manual	1 969	1 831	2 011	1 842
IV	898	1 135	917	1 087
V	241	241	245	216
Other	589	1 452	733	1 300
Missing	18	22	16	20
Region				
North	486	679	454	590
North West	867	1 267	886	1 201
Yorkshire and Humberside	704	962	679	911
West Midlands	806	984	822	986
East Midlands	623	769	618	694
East Anglia	319	398	319	362
South West	638	884	634	810
South East	1 621	2 027	1 766	2 048
Greater London	906	1 100	1 128	1 319
Wales	414	613	369	542
Scotland	734	1 075	708	1 030
Ethnic group				
White	7 676	10 188	7 868	9 885
Black	149	239	161	223
Asian	155	156	198	203
Other	104	132	125	139
Missing	34	43	31	42

continued on p.430

Table A3.2. *Continued*

	Unweighted		Weighted	
	Men	Women	Men	Women
Religious affiliation				
None	4 121	3 957	4 299	3 875
Church of England	2 091	3 637	2 078	3 448
Roman Catholic	715	1 206	744	1 198
Other Christian	899	1 599	896	1 556
Non-Christian	280	341	358	397
Missing	12	18	8	19
Education				
Degree	1 034	863	1 012	839
A level or other non-degree	2 652	2 443	2 747	2 413
O level/CSE	2 341	4 031	2 495	3 984
Other	173	148	194	161
Missing	1 886	3 248	1 903	3 072
	32	25	32	24
Marital status				
Married	4 452	6 113	4 798	6 347
Cohabiting (opposite-sex partner)	579	801	606	834
Cohabiting (same-sex partner)	21	11	20	11
Widowed	71	310	49	201
Divorced, separated	628	1 361	396	860
Single	2 559	2 152	2 509	2 229
Missing	8	10	6	10
Smoking				
Non-smoker	3 164	4 733	3 295	4 792
Ex-smoker	1 803	1 795	1 828	1 699
Smokes <15 per day	1 172	1 741	1 258	1 701
Smokes 15+ per day	1 901	2 365	1 924	2 180
Missing	78	124	78	121
Alcohol				
None	696	1 510	741	1 475
Low intake	6 009	8 224	6 191	8 029
Moderate intake	1 113	961	1 154	925
High intake	285	43	284	44
Missing	15	20	13	20

Table A3.3. Complex standard errors and design factors (DEFT) for demographic variables

	Men				Women			
	% p	Complex SE (p)	DEFT	Weighted base	% p	Complex SE (p)	DEFT	Weighted base
Age								
16–24	23.7	0.6	1.278	8 384	21.4	0.5	1.252	10 492
25–34	25.8	0.6	1.177		27.6	0.5	1.166	
35–44	24.5	0.5	1.088		24.6	0.5	1.149	
45–59	26.0	0.6	1.231		26.4	0.5	1.236	
Married	57.3	0.7	1.250	8 378	60.6	0.6	1.343	10 483
Cohabiting	7.5	0.3	1.151		8.1	0.3	1.167	
Widowed, separated, divorced	5.3	0.3	1.105		10.1	0.3	1.065	
Single	29.9	0.7	1.384		21.3	0.5	1.304	
Social class of household								
I	6.9	0.3	1.196	8 368	6.2	0.3	1.380	10 472
II	27.9	0.6	1.290		28.6	0.6	1.361	
III NM	18.6	0.5	1.153		22.7	0.5	1.219	
III M	24.0	0.6	1.201		17.6	0.5	1.245	
IV	11.0	0.4	1.149		10.4	0.4	1.223	
V	2.9	0.2	1.296		2.1	0.1	1.079	
Other	8.8	0.4	1.388		12.4	0.4	1.353	
Census social class								
I	6.5	0.3	1.178	8 364	1.5	0.1	1.259	10 460
II	22.9	0.6	1.296		17.8	0.4	1.188	
III NM	11.1	0.4	1.156		25.7	0.5	1.286	
III M	32.6	0.6	1.200		5.3	0.2	1.096	
IV	13.3	0.4	1.137		12.8	0.4	1.148	
V	3.8	0.3	1.271		3.5	0.2	1.172	
Other	9.8	0.5	1.404		33.3	0.6	1.252	

continued on p. 432

Table A3.3. *Continued*

	Men				Women			
	% p	Complex SE (p)	DEFT	Weighted base	% p	Complex SE (p)	DEFT	Weighted base
Unemployed	8.4	0.4	1.362	8 369	4.7	0.3	1.341	10 469
In paid work	79.5	0.6	1.284		60.4	0.6	1.267	
Looking after home	1.9	0.4	1.034		27.2	0.7	1.193	
In full-time education	7.2	0.4	1.426		6.1	0.3	1.455	
Ethnic group								
Black	1.9	0.2	1.381	8 353	2.1	0.2	1.536	10 450
White	94.2	0.4	1.641		94.6	0.4	1.920	
Asian	3.2	0.4	1.793		2.5	0.3	1.955	
Indian/Pakistani	2.4	0.3	1.906		1.9	0.3	1.951	
Bangladeshi/other	1.5	0.2	1.155		1.3	0.1	1.249	
Religion								
None	51.3	0.7	1.296	8 375	37.0	0.6	1.333	10 474
Church of England	24.8	0.6	1.230		32.9	0.6	1.280	
Roman Catholic	8.9	0.4	1.133		11.4	0.4	1.308	
Other Christian	10.7	0.4	1.210		14.9	0.4	1.206	
Non-Christian	4.3	0.4	1.810		3.8	0.3	1.727	
Use of telephone	87.2	0.5	1.434	8 353	88.1	0.5	1.497	10 455

Table A3.4. Complex standard errors and design factors (DEFT) for sexual behaviour variables

	Men				Women			
	% p	Complex SE (p)	DEFT	Weighted base	% p	Complex SE (p)	DEFT	Weighted base
Age at 1st heterosexual sex								
<16	18.7	0.5	1.232	8 240	7.9	0.3	1.201	10 347
Contraception at 1st heterosexual sex								
Condom	37.3	0.6	1.142	7 577	40.4	0.6	1.255	9 570
Other	22.9	0.6	1.182		26.8	0.5	1.183	
None	39.8	0.7	1.233		32.8	0.6	1.349	
Heterosexual partners ever								
0	6.6	0.4	1.280	8 021	5.7	0.3	1.323	10 043
1	20.6	0.5	1.156		39.3	0.6	1.245	
2	10.6	0.4	1.141		16.9	0.4	1.106	
3–4	18.4	0.5	1.077		18.2	0.4	1.064	
5+	43.9	0.7	1.165		19.8	0.5	1.247	
Heterosexual partners in the last 5 years								
0	8.7	0.4	1.250	8 047	9.1	0.3	1.186	10 056
1	56.5	0.7	1.199		67.4	0.6	1.223	
2	10.0	0.4	1.129		11.0	0.4	1.217	
3–4	12.0	0.4	1.146		8.1	0.3	1.169	
5+	12.7	0.5	1.274		4.4	0.2	1.224	
Heterosexual partners in the last 2 years								
0	10.8	0.4	1.266	8 044	11.6	0.4	1.147	10 049
1	67.1	0.7	1.272		76.0	0.5	1.271	
2	10.0	0.4	1.162		7.9	0.3	1.251	
3+	12.2	0.4	1.216		4.4	0.3	1.335	
Heterosexual partners in the last year								
0	13.1	0.5	1.264	8 046	13.9	0.4	1.201	10 058
1	73.0	0.7	1.309		79.4	0.5	1.235	
2+	13.9	0.5	1.200		6.7	0.3	1.221	
Fellatio								
Never	29.3	0.6	1.137	7 759	35.7	0.6	1.148	9 645
In the last 5 years	65.1	0.7	1.185		58.6	0.6	1.128	
In the last year	56.2	0.7	1.166		50.5	0.6	1.121	
Cunnilingus								
Never	27.3	0.6	1.207	7 820	33.4	0.6	1.181	9 586
In the last 5 years	67.9	0.6	1.194		61.0	0.6	1.176	
In the last year	59.9	0.7	1.189		53.1	0.6	1.135	
Anal sex								
Never	86.1	0.4	1.119	7 828	87.1	0.4	1.223	9 721
In the last 5 years	9.9	0.4	1.124		8.9	0.3	1.186	
In the last year	6.5	0.3	1.092		5.9	0.3	1.114	

continued on p. 434

Table A3.4. *Continued*

	Men				Women			
	% p	Complex SE (p)	DEFT	Weighted base	% p	Complex SE (p)	DEFT	Weighted base
Non-penetrative sex								
Never	19.9	0.5	1.169	7 490	25.0	0.5	1.150	9 257
In the last 5 years	73.2	0.6	1.206		68.2	0.5	1.105	
In the last year	65.5	0.7	1.189		60.2	0.5	1.076	
Any homosexual experience	6.1	0.3	1.288	8 337	3.4	0.2	1.253	10 421
At least one homosexual partner								
Ever	3.6	0.3	1.259	8 321	1.7	0.2	1.279	10 411
In the last 5 years	1.4	0.2	1.260	8 323				
STD clinic attendance								
Never	91.6	0.4	1.129	7 636	94.3	0.3	1.174	9 590
In the last year	0.9	0.1	1.085					
Paid for sex with a woman								
Never	93.2	0.4	1.226	7 941				
In the last 5 years	1.8	0.2	1.228	7 938				
Abortion								
Never					87.5	0.4	1.088	9 842
In the last 5 years					4.5	0.2	1.154	

Table A4.1. Age at first heterosexual intercourse
[Source: interview, question 19]

	25th centile	50th centile	75th centile	Never had intercourse	Base‡	Missing‡	Under 16 years (%)	Base	Missing
Men									
Total	16	18	20	462	7 980	138	18.7	8 240	144
Age									
16–24	15	17	18	272	1 475	14	25.4	1 964	20
25–34	16	17	19	74	2 340	28	23.5	2 138	28
35–44	16	18	20	67	2 111	32	16.4	2 023	28
45–59	17	19	22	49	2 054	64	10.0	2 114	67
Social class									
I	17	19	23	24	581	5	5.9	571	5
II	16	18	20	54	2 295	37	15.0	2 292	39
III NM	16	18	20	58	1 460	25	17.0	1 526	29
III M	16	17	19	64	1 934	35	25.3	1 979	33
IV	16	17	†9	60	878	20	24.2	897	21
V	15	16	19	19	237	4	27.7	242	4
Other	16	18	20	181	579	10	16.8	721	12
Missing	16	19.5	23	2	16*	2	12.3	13*	2
Region									
North	16	17	19	34	473	13	23.0	441	14
North West	16	17	20	46	853	14	20.7	874	12
Yorkshire/Humberside	16	17	20	37	692	12	19.5	669	11
West Midlands	16	18	20	55	790	16	16.8	802	21
East Midlands	16	18	20	33	616	7	20.6	613	5
East Anglia	16	18	20	20	316	3	16.1	316	3
South West	16	17	20	32	630	8	18.4	623	11
South East	16	18	20	86	1 587	34	18.1	1 732	33
Greater London	16	18	20	54	892	14	17.5	1 113	14
Wales	16	17	20	19	407	7	19.6	362	7
Scotland	16	17	20	46	724	10	18.6	695	12
Ethnic group									
White	16	18	20	420	7 558	118	18.9	7 749	119
Black	15	17	18	10	142	7	26.3	157	4
Asian	17	20	25	16	148	7	10.7	186	12
Other	16	18	22	13	101	3	14.0	120	6
Missing	17	19	23	3	31	3	11.0	28	3
Religious affiliation									
None	16	17	19	230	4 061	60	22.7	4 240	59
Church of England	16	18	21	79	2 053	38	13.4	2 039	39
Roman Catholic	16	17	20	47	701	14	19.5	731	14
Other Christian	17	18	22	76	886	13	14.6	882	14
Non-Christian	17	20	24	30	270	10	10.8	342	16
Missing	—	—	—	0	9†	3	—	6†	2

continued on p. 436

Table A4.1. *Continued*

	25th centile	50th centile	75th centile	Never had intercourse	Base‡	Missing‡	Under 16 years (%)	Base	Missing
Education									
Degree	17	19	22	45	1 016	18	7.0	993	20
A level or other non-degree	16	18	20	124	2 622	30	15.8	2 716	31
O level/CSE	16	17	19	167	2 301	40	22.5	2 452	42
Other	16	18	20	5	169	4	16.9	187	7
None	16	17	20	117	1 842	44	24.5	1 861	42
Missing	16	19	21	4	29	2	18.3	30	2
Marital status									
Married	16	18	20	2	4 368	84	16.3	4 703	95
Cohabiting									
Opposite-sex partner	15	16	18	2	575	4	29.2	603	4
Same-sex partner	16	21	—	10	21	0	4.6	20	0
Widowed	17	18	20	0	70	1	9.6	48	1
Divorced, separated	16	17	19	1	616	12	21.9	387	8
Single	16	17	20	447	2 323	36	20.7	2 474	35
Missing	—	—	—	0	7†	1	—	5†	1
Smoking									
Non-smoker	17	18	21	343	3 104	60	10.5	3 237	59
Ex-smoker	16	18	20	29	1 769	34	15.5	1 792	36
Smokes <15 per day	15	17	18	35	1 150	22	27.7	1 234	24
Smokes 15+ per day	15	17	18	48	1 880	21	30.3	1 900	24
Missing	17	18	21	7	77	1	11.3	78	1
Alcohol									
None	16	18	23	107	674	22	15.7	718	23
Low intake	16	18	20	325	5 909	100	17.4	6 084	106
Moderate intake	16	17	19	22	1 099	14	24.0	1 141	13
High intake	15	16	18	7	284	1	32.0	284	1
Missing	15	18	19	1	14*	1	49.8	13*	1

continued

Table A4.1. *Continued*

	25th centile	50th centile	75th centile	Never had intercourse	Base‡	Missing‡	Under 16 years (%)	Base	Missing
Women									
Total	17	18	20	487	10 609	149	7.9	10 347	145
Age									
16–24	16	17	18	309	1 867	21	16.4	2 222	24
25–34	16	18	19	69	3 236	37	9.3	2 868	32
35–44	17	18	20	36	2 569	35	5.0	2 538	39
45–59	18	20	22	73	2 937	56	2.0	2 720	51
Social class									
I	18	20	22	7	608	8	1.6	638	10
II	17	19	21	63	3 026	33	5.3	2 965	32
III NM	17	18	20	116	2 364	38	8.1	2 347	35
III M	16	18	20	29	1 802	29	8.2	1 811	32
IV	16	18	20	48	1 122	13	11.8	1 075	12
V	17	18	20	8	238	3	9.3	214	2
Other	16	18	20	215	1 431	21	12.8	1 279	21
Missing	17	18	20	1	18*	4	2.8	18*	2
Region									
North	17	18	21	28	669	10	5.1	579	10
North West	17	18	20	54	1 250	17	7.7	1 186	15
Yorkshire/Humberside	16	18	20	35	948	14	9.1	896	15
West Midlands	17	18	20	53	955	29	9.5	955	31
East Midlands	17	18	20	26	767	2	9.7	692	2
East Anglia	17	19	21	21	396	2	8.6	361	2
South West	17	18	20	27	875	9	8.9	801	9
South East	17	18	20	89	1 993	34	8.7	2 017	31
Greater London	17	18	21	73	1 084	16	7.4	1 300	19
Wales	17	18	20	22	608	5	6.4	539	3
Scotland	17	19	21	59	1 064	11	4.6	1 021	9
Ethnic group									
White	17	18	20	435	10 057	131	8.0	9 760	125
Black	16	18	20	20	232	7	9.6	219	4
Asian	18	21	23	21	148	8	1.1	189	13
Other	18	19	23	9	132	0	5.0	139	0
Missing	17	18	20	2	40	3	11.2	40	2
Religious affiliation									
None	16	17	19	180	3 912	45	12.3	3 834	41
Church of England	17	19	21	108	3 591	46	5.1	3 403	45
Roman Catholic	17	19	21	54	1 180	26	5.1	1 171	27
Other Christian	17	19	21	104	1 576	23	5.7	1 538	18
Non-Christian	18	20	22	39	332	9	4.6	383	14
Missing	17	18	19	2	18*	0	30.4	19*	0

continued on p. 438

Table A4.1. *Continued*

	25th centile	50th centile	75th centile	Never had intercourse	Base‡	Missing‡	Under 16 years (%)	Base	Missing
Education									
Degree	18	19	22	30	855	8	5.7	832	7
A level or other non-degree	17	19	21	118	2 412	31	6.3	2 384	28
O level/CSE	16	18	20	237	3 982	49	8.6	3 937	47
Other	17	18	21	3	146	2	8.6	157	4
None	17	18	20	98	3 192	56	8.8	3 015	56
Missing	17	18	22	1	19*	3	0.0	20	2
Marital status									
Married	17	18	21	1	6 022	91	5.4	6 248	100
Cohabiting									
Opposite-sex partner	16	17	18	2	794	7	14.1	827	7
Same-sex partner	17	20	—	4	11*	0	8.4	11*	0
Widowed	18	20	22	0	307	3	2.9	200	1
Divorced, separated	16	18	20	2	1 342	19	9.9	844	16
Single	16	18	21	478	2 125	27	12.4	2 209	20
Missing	—	—	—	0	8†	2	—	8*	1
Smoking									
Non-smoker	17	19	21	393	4 657	76	4.7	4 716	75
Ex-smoker	17	18	20	15	1 768	27	7.0	1 674	25
Smokes <15 per day	16	17	19	45	1 722	19	11.8	1 685	17
Smokes 15+ per day	16	17	19	22	2 341	24	12.8	2 156	24
Missing	18	19	21	12	121	3	2.9	116	5
Alcohol									
None	17	19	21	140	1 480	30	7.7	1 440	35
Low intake	17	18	20	324	8 114	110	7.2	7 925	104
Moderate intake	16	17	19	20	952	9	13.5	918	7
High intake	16	17	19	1	43	0	11.8	44	0
Missing	17	18	19	2	20	0	9.9	20	0

* Note small base.
† Base <10.
‡ Unweighted data.

Table A5.1A. Numbers of female partners ever reported by men
[Source: booklet, question 7a]

	0 (%)	1 (%)	2 (%)	3–4 (%)	5–9 (%)	10+ (%)	99th centile	Median	Mean‡	Variance‡	Base	Missing
Total	6.6	20.6	10.6	18.4	19.4	24.4	75	4	9.9	6 575.1	8 021	363
Not asked											0	
Age												
16–24	20.4	16.3	9.8	19.4	17.9	16.2	45	3	5.3	98.1	1 936	48
25–34	3.1	15.0	9.2	18.2	23.1	31.4	100	5	10.3	720.5	2 098	68
35–44	1.9	20.5	10.7	17.1	20.9	28.9	75	5	10.2	2 838.5	1 966	85
45–59	1.5	30.5	12.6	18.9	15.8	20.8	100	3	13.6	22 093.0	2 021	161
Social class												
I	3.9	25.6	11.3	18.8	19.0	21.4	60	4			558	17
II	1.6	22.3	10.3	18.1	20.3	27.5	100	4			2 246	86
III NM	3.5	22.4	13.5	17.9	18.9	23.8	53	4			1 507	48
III M	3.4	20.2	10.0	18.6	21.3	26.5	75	5			1 913	98
IV	7.9	17.9	10.5	19.4	19.7	24.6	100	4			866	52
V	8.5	10.3	10.3	23.4	20.9	26.5	40	4			219	26
Other	37.0	14.7	7.0	16.7	12.3	12.3	60	2			705	27
Missing	—	—	—	—	—	—	—	—			7†	8
Region												
North	7.0	21.8	9.0	23.6	15.8	22.8	100	4			427	27
North West	5.8	20.9	9.3	19.4	18.9	25.9	80	4			855	31
Yorkshire/Humberside	6.8	20.4	11.0	20.0	18.1	23.8	56	4			637	43
West Midlands	8.6	21.3	11.5	19.1	18.8	20.7	50	4			759	63
East Midlands	6.2	25.2	13.3	12.9	18.4	24.1	100	3			600	18
East Anglia	7.1	25.1	13.6	14.0	19.0	21.2	75	4			317	2
South West	5.0	21.7	9.7	19.3	21.2	23.1	86	4			621	13
South East	6.6	20.6	10.3	17.7	22.5	22.3	70	4			1 710	55
Greater London	6.5	13.2	11.0	19.1	17.8	32.3	100	5			1 056	72
Wales	5.4	22.6	11.2	18.6	21.5	20.7	100	4			358	11
Scotland	6.9	21.8	8.7	18.3	17.6	26.6	60	4			681	27
Ethnic group												
White	6.2	20.8	10.5	18.4	19.7	24.4	75	4			7 589	279
Black	12.2	7.9	8.8	12.8	16.7	41.7	72	8			145	16
Asian	14.8	26.5	19.0	22.9	8.0	8.9	50	2			153	45
Other	13.4	12.5	10.7	18.1	19.6	25.7	500	3			111	14
Missing	10.8	31.3	9.9	11.4	23.8	12.8	—	2			22	9
Religious affiliation												
None	6.7	17.1	10.0	18.2	21.0	27.0	80	4.5			4 151	149
Church of England	3.6	24.9	12.5	19.2	19.5	20.4	60	4			1 999	79
Roman Catholic	7.4	17.6	10.2	19.8	17.6	27.4	100	4			688	57
Other Christian	9.4	29.5	8.5	16.6	15.6	20.3	80	3			868	28
Non-Christian	14.8	21.6	12.7	17.6	12.5	20.9	30	1			308	50
Missing	—	—	—	—	—	—	—	—			7†	1

continued on p. 440

Table A5.1A. *Continued*

	0 (%)	1 (%)	2 (%)	3–4 (%)	5–9 (%)	10+ (%)	99th centile	Median	Mean‡	Variance‡	Base	Missing
Education												
Degree	3.4	22.1	11.1	18.2	21.3	24.0	72	4			986	27
A level or other non-degree	5.4	20.8	10.2	18.5	20.1	25.1	70	4			2 679	67
O level/CSE	9.0	20.3	10.6	17.9	19.1	23.2	60	4			2 411	83
Other	4.1	19.3	7.2	20.0	19.8	29.7	200	5			180	14
None	7.0	19.9	11.4	18.8	17.9	25.0	100	4			1 745	158
Missing	15.4	21.3	8.0	31.5	11.1	12.7	—	3			19*	13
Marital status												
Married	0.0	27.1	12.2	18.5	19.2	23.0	75	4			4 554	244
Cohabiting												
Opposite-sex partner	0.4	7.8	7.1	18.3	25.2	41.3	100	7			594	13
Same-sex partner	45.9	19.2	25.6	4.6	0.0	4.7	—	1			20	0
Widowed	0.0	30.8	12.4	18.3	16.1	22.5	70	3			48	1
Divorced, separated	0.2	6.3	6.7	16.1	25.7	45.0	200	8			376	19
Single	21.2	13.4	8.9	18.8	17.7	20.1	50	3			2 426	83
Missing	—	—	—	—	—	—	—	—			3†	3
Smoking												
Non-smoker	12.7	25.4	11.8	18.6	15.4	16.2	50	3			3 176	120
Ex-smoker	1.4	24.3	11.3	18.8	19.8	24.4	75	4			1 729	99
Smokes <15 per day	4.3	13.6	9.7	18.9	23.6	29.9	90	5			1 201	57
Smokes 15+ per day	2.3	13.2	8.6	17.3	23.5	35.1	100	6			1 841	83
Missing	9.1	22.2	9.2	17.1	19.7	22.7	60	3			74	4
Alcohol												
None	18.8	24.1	11.3	16.8	14.8	14.1	100	2			677	65
Low intake	6.2	21.7	11.4	18.4	19.3	22.9	60	4			5 943	247
Moderate intake	2.0	14.3	7.1	18.7	22.4	35.5	100	6			1 112	41
High intake	1.5	13.2	5.4	21.7	20.3	37.9	100	6			275	9
Missing	10.1	15.0	3.2	10.6	32.5	28.6	—	3			13*	0

* Note small base.
† Base <10.
‡ Mean and variance are not given for small subgroups where they are heavily influenced by a few respondents reporting very many partners.

Table A5.1B. Numbers of male partners ever reported by women
[Source: booklet, question 7a]

	0 (%)	1 (%)	2 (%)	3–4 (%)	5–9 (%)	10+ (%)	99th centile	Median	Mean‡	Variance‡	Base	Missing
Total	5.7	39.3	16.9	18.2	13.0	6.8	25	2	3.4	165.3	10 043	447
Not asked											2	
Age												
16–24	20.7	27.0	14.7	18.8	14.1	4.6	20	2	2.8	25.9	2 195	49
25–34	2.1	30.8	18.3	22.5	16.7	9.7	25	3	4.3	315.0	2 795	104
35–44	0.7	40.7	17.7	18.5	13.9	8.5	30	2	3.7	42.2	2 476	100
45–59	1.6	57.7	16.6	12.9	7.4	3.8	20	1	2.6	196.7	2 576	194
Social class												
I	1.3	43.9	13.3	18.5	14.3	8.8	30	2			625	23
II	1.5	41.1	16.8	17.4	13.6	9.5	30	2			2 899	98
III NM	5.3	38.8	16.8	18.5	14.0	6.5	20	2			2 290	91
III M	1.9	47.1	18.9	18.0	10.6	3.5	20	2			1 729	114
IV	5.5	36.3	17.8	21.1	13.7	5.7	21	2			1 038	49
V	2.6	38.6	23.4	19.7	9.1	6.5	20	2			208	9
Other	24.1	25.9	14.8	17.3	12.7	5.1	20	2			1 246	51
Missing	—	—	—	—	—	—	—	—			7†	13
Region												
North	5.9	50.2	18.1	13.4	9.6	2.8	20	1			565	25
North West	5.1	41.6	19.6	18.7	10.7	4.4	20	2			1 163	38
Yorkshire/Humberside	4.8	40.1	17.3	17.7	13.8	6.3	25	2			867	44
West Midlands	7.1	39.4	15.3	20.4	12.8	5.0	20	2			904	80
East Midlands	4.6	39.5	18.9	19.1	12.0	6.0	20	2			674	20
East Anglia	6.5	43.8	16.0	15.5	13.9	4.4	18	2			358	5
South West	3.1	38.1	17.0	18.9	14.8	8.1	25	2			791	19
South East	5.9	37.3	15.7	19.8	13.6	7.8	30	2			1 970	78
Greater London	7.7	28.7	14.7	17.7	17.6	13.7	30	2			1 241	78
Wales	4.0	46.5	17.6	19.3	9.3	3.4	17	2			517	25
Scotland	6.3	42.8	18.3	16.0	11.5	5.2	20	2			993	36
Ethnic group												
White	5.2	39.4	16.9	18.4	13.3	6.9	25	2			9 540	343
Black	11.0	30.7	23.2	20.8	9.9	4.4	20	2			206	17
Asian	25.7	56.3	10.2	5.6	1.8	0.4	6	1			147	56
Other	7.4	29.2	21.4	17.3	13.7	11.0	200	2			120	19
Missing	6.5	31.3	14.4	21.4	18.8	7.7	—	3			30	12
Religious affiliation												
None	6.1	30.4	17.1	20.7	16.1	9.6	30	2			3 755	118
Church of England	3.1	45.8	17.5	17.8	11.4	4.4	20	2			3 301	147
Roman Catholic	5.8	44.6	17.5	16.9	10.4	4.8	20	2			1 142	56
Other Christian	7.6	42.9	16.4	15.5	11.2	6.5	20	2			1 503	53
Non-Christian	17.6	42.9	10.0	12.5	11.2	5.7	30	1			324	73
Missing	16.4	31.0	7.7	5.1	30.6	9.2	—	2			18*	1

continued on p. 442

Table A5.1B. *Continued*

	0 (%)	1 (%)	2 (%)	3–4 (%)	5–9 (%)	10+ (%)	99th centile	Median	Mean‡	Variance‡	Base	Missing
Education												
Degree	3.0	25.6	12.8	20.4	20.4	17.8	40	3			821	18
A level or other non-degree	5.5	35.9	17.6	18.1	14.9	8.0	30	2			2 362	50
O level/CSE	8.0	38.0	16.4	19.1	12.4	6.0	20	2			3 856	127
Other	1.2	38.6	20.8	17.8	13.8	7.9	30	2			149	12
None	3.6	48.0	18.1	16.6	10.2	3.5	17	2			2 845	227
Missing	—	—	—	—	—	—	—	—			9*	12
Marital status												
Married	0.0	51.7	18.4	15.4	9.9	4.6	20	1			6 017	331
Cohabiting												
Opposite-sex partner	0.3	15.5	19.0	29.1	23.0	13.1	32	3			817	17
Same-sex partner	43.7	22.5	28.5	0.0	0.0	5.4	—	1			11	0
Widowed	0.0	53.8	17.7	17.0	8.3	3.2	20	1			191	11
Divorced/separated	0.1	19.3	17.3	27.3	22.8	13.3	30	3			823	37
Single	25.7	20.6	11.8	18.8	14.9	8.3	30	2			2 185	44
Missing	—	—	—	—	—	—	—	—			2†	8
Smoking												
Non-smoker	10.5	46.2	16.4	14.5	9.0	3.5	20	1			4 555	237
Ex-smoker	0.5	37.7	18.5	19.0	15.0	9.3	30	2			1 623	76
Smokes <15 per day	3.1	32.1	16.2	22.8	15.8	10.0	30	3			1 659	42
Smokes 15+ per day	1.0	31.1	17.6	22.7	18.2	9.5	25	3			2 102	78
Missing	13.5	50.6	12.1	9.3	13.1	1.4	15	1			106	15
Alcohol												
None	11.9	46.1	16.9	14.0	7.1	3.8	20	1			1 339	136
Low intake	4.9	39.5	17.4	18.6	13.1	6.4	25	2			7 738	291
Moderate intake	2.9	29.1	13.1	21.6	19.9	13.4	27	3			907	18
High intake	1.4	20.4	16.0	12.5	31.6	18.1	50	3			42	1
Missing	12.9	31.3	9.6	21.2	22.0	3.0	—	3			20	0

* Note small base.
† Base <10.
‡ Mean and variance are not given for small subgroups where they are heavily influenced by a few respondents reporting very many partners.

Table A5.2A. Numbers of female partners reported in the last 5 years by men
[Source: booklet, question 7b]

	0 (%)	1 (%)	2 (%)	3–4 (%)	5–9 (%)	10+ (%)	99th centile	Median	Mean	Variance	Base	Missing
Total	8.7	56.5	10.0	12.0	7.9	4.8	22	1	2.6	37.2	8 047	337
Not asked											0	
Age												
16–24	20.7	20.1	11.8	20.2	16.1	11.2	35	2	4.2	61.6	1 941	43
25–34	4.6	51.7	12.4	15.9	9.6	5.8	30	1	3.1	74.6	2 102	65
35–44	4.5	72.6	9.4	7.5	4.2	1.7	12	1	1.7	5.1	1 973	78
45–59	5.7	80.6	6.4	4.7	1.9	0.7	9	1	1.3	3.9	2 031	151
Social class												
I	5.3	66.2	9.7	9.4	6.2	3.2	16	1	2.1	11.6	559	16
II	3.4	65.7	10.1	11.0	6.5	3.4	20	1	2.2	17.3	2 251	80
III NM	5.1	62.5	10.3	11.1	6.8	4.1	20	1	2.4	21.8	1 513	42
III M	5.9	56.5	10.4	13.4	8.1	5.7	30	1	2.8	81.5	1 917	94
IV	10.6	48.3	9.5	13.3	10.1	8.2	30	1	3.2	35.5	868	49
V	15.6	37.3	10.3	14.8	13.6	8.4	20	1	3.4	27.5	224	22
Other	39.0	23.2	8.8	13.4	11.0	4.6	20	1	2.5	35.2	706	27
Missing	—	—	—	—	—	—	—	—	—	—	8†	8
Region												
North	9.4	63.0	7.8	10.5	4.7	4.6	30	1	2.3	20.7	429	26
North West	8.0	57.0	9.4	12.0	7.3	6.3	20	1	2.8	24.7	857	29
Yorkshire/Humberside	9.4	56.5	10.0	11.5	7.3	5.3	20	1	2.5	15.0	638	41
West Midlands	10.2	59.3	9.8	9.5	6.8	4.5	23	1	2.3	16.8	761	62
East Midlands	7.9	63.8	7.7	8.3	8.2	4.0	20	1	2.2	11.5	603	15
East Anglia	9.2	62.1	9.3	9.6	6.7	3.1	24	1	2.1	13.3	317	2
South West	6.6	55.2	12.8	15.3	6.7	3.5	15	1	2.3	14.7	622	12
South East	7.9	58.0	10.0	13.2	7.4	3.4	20	1	2.3	19.0	1 719	47
Greater London	10.2	44.3	11.6	14.3	11.7	7.9	25	1	3.4	54.2	1 060	68
Wales	6.7	62.4	7.8	11.1	7.7	4.3	30	1	3.0	296.9	357	12
Scotland	10.2	53.0	10.8	11.8	9.2	5.0	30	1	2.8	29.7	684	24
Ethnic group												
White	8.3	56.9	10.0	12.1	7.8	4.9	22	1	2.6	38.2	7 615	253
Black	13.9	39.7	13.6	13.5	8.2	11.1	21	2	3.3	24.9	144	17
Asian	14.7	57.0	10.7	10.8	6.9	0.0	8	1	1.6	3.9	154	44
Other	18.0	50.1	3.6	7.8	18.1	2.5	35	1	2.6	22.0	112	13
Missing	15.6	56.5	4.9	4.2	7.0	1.9	—	1	1.7	4.4	22	9
Religious affiliation												
None	8.6	50.3	10.6	13.8	10.8	6.0	26	1	3.0	54.4	4 165	134
Church of England	6.2	70.0	9.1	8.8	3.3	2.7	17	1	1.8	7.3	2 005	73
Roman Catholic	9.1	53.1	10.3	14.4	6.0	7.0	30	1	3.2	48.6	692	52
Other Christian	12.1	60.0	9.5	9.7	5.9	3.0	20	1	2.1	21.4	869	27
Non-Christian	17.0	51.3	8.4	10.4	9.0	3.8	7	1	1.2	3.6	309	49
Missing	—	—	—	—	—	—	—	—	—	—	7†	1

continued on p. 444

Table A5.2A. *Continued*

	0 (%)	1 (%)	2 (%)	3–4 (%)	5–9 (%)	10+ (%)	99th centile	Median	Mean	Variance	Base	Missing
Education												
Degree	6.0	59.1	12.5	9.8	9.2	3.4	15	1	2.2	8.2	987	26
A level or other non-degree	6.8	55.2	10.7	13.4	8.3	5.7	25	1	2.8	29.5	2 691	56
O level/CSE	10.7	51.8	9.8	13.2	8.9	5.7	25	1	2.7	23.6	2 417	77
Other	6.5	65.5	6.2	8.1	6.0	7.7	30	1	2.9	35.3	182	12
None	10.8	62.6	8.2	10.0	5.5	2.9	20	1	2.2	83.4	1 751	152
Missing	15.4	61.4	8.0	15.2	0.0	0.0	—	1	1.3	1.2	19*	13
Marital status												
Married	0.6	82.8	7.3	5.6	2.2	1.5	10	1	1.5	5.9	4 572	226
Cohabiting												
Opposite-sex partner	0.5	37.0	16.3	23.1	15.7	7.5	27	2	3.7	29.3	597	10
Same-sex partner	90.6	9.4	0.0	0.0	0.0	0.0	—	0	0.1	0.1	19*	1
Widowed	33.3	34.9	12.3	13.4	1.9	4.2	12	1	1.6	3.8	48	1
Divorced, separated	8.6	24.1	18.6	25.0	15.3	8.5	60	2	4.8	223.4	378	18
Single	24.9	17.7	12.2	19.5	15.8	10.0	30	2	3.9	44.9	2 430	79
Missing	—	—	—	—	—	—	—	—	—	—	3†	3
Smoking												
Non-smoker	14.3	53.7	10.5	11.5	6.6	3.4	16	1	2.1	12.3	3 177	118
Ex-smoker	4.1	73.9	7.9	7.8	4.3	2.1	15	1	1.8	9.3	1 734	94
Smokes <15 per day	6.8	43.8	11.5	15.5	13.0	9.5	30	1	3.7	39.5	1 205	52
Smokes 15+ per day	4.6	53.5	10.2	14.9	10.2	6.7	35	1	3.4	100.6	1 855	69
Missing	12.8	55.6	8.1	8.4	8.1	7.0	30	1	3.2	39.4	75	3
Alcohol												
None	22.9	54.4	7.3	7.9	5.7	1.8	15	1	1.6	8.5	679	62
Low intake	8.1	58.8	10.3	11.5	7.3	4.0	20	1	2.3	17.9	5 961	230
Moderate intake	4.0	48.9	10.0	15.8	11.5	10.0	40	1	4.2	153.9	1 117	37
High intake	6.3	43.1	10.6	18.3	11.2	10.5	40	2	4.0	41.6	276	8
Missing	10.1	43.9	21.7	6.9	13.9	3.5	—	1	1.6	7.4	13*	0

* Note small base.
† Base <10.

Table A5.2B. Numbers of male partners reported in the last 5 years by women
[Source: booklet, question 7b]

	0 (%)	1 (%)	2 (%)	3–4 (%)	5–9 (%)	10+ (%)	99th centile	Median	Mean	Variance	Base	Missing
Total	9.1	67.4	11.0	8.1	3.6	0.8	8	1	1.5	4.8	10 057	434
Not asked											2	
Age												
16–24	20.8	33.1	16.3	16.9	10.5	2.5	15	1	2.3	18.4	2 194	50
25–34	3.1	67.6	14.3	10.3	3.8	0.8	8	1	1.7	3.3	2 795	105
35–44	3.3	82.4	9.0	4.3	0.9	0.2	5	1	1.2	0.8	2 484	92
45–59	11.3	81.9	4.9	1.7	0.2	0.0	3	1	1.0	0.3	2 584	187
Social class												
I	2.4	80.8	8.7	5.9	2.0	0.1	6	1	1.3	1.0	625	23
II	3.8	75.7	10.2	7.0	2.6	0.7	8	1	1.5	2.8	2 902	95
III NM	7.9	63.6	12.5	10.0	4.6	1.4	10	1	1.8	10.0	2 294	88
III M	3.9	81.3	7.3	5.3	1.8	0.3	6	1	1.3	4.3	1 734	109
IV	11.0	56.5	14.2	11.4	5.8	1.1	10	1	1.7	3.6	1 039	48
V	12.9	70.4	10.5	4.9	1.1	0.2	6	1	1.2	0.9	208	9
Other	32.0	37.6	13.9	9.6	6.0	0.9	10	1	1.5	3.8	1 249	48
Missing	—	—	—	—	—	—	—	—	—	—	6†	14
Region												
North	10.1	72.2	9.5	5.9	1.9	0.4	6	1	1.3	1.1	565	24
North West	9.7	67.9	13.5	6.1	2.1	0.7	7	1	1.4	2.3	1 164	37
Yorkshire/Humberside	7.6	69.5	9.8	8.9	3.6	0.6	8	1	1.5	2.0	870	42
West Midlands	10.2	68.9	9.7	8.2	2.6	0.5	8	1	1.4	2.2	905	79
East Midlands	7.6	69.3	11.0	7.6	4.0	0.5	7	1	1.5	1.9	674	20
East Anglia	9.3	73.8	9.5	4.8	2.0	0.6	7	1	1.3	1.7	358	5
South West	6.7	68.5	11.9	8.8	3.7	0.4	8	1	1.5	2.2	792	18
South East	8.8	69.4	9.7	7.4	3.9	0.9	10	1	1.5	3.0	1 975	73
Greater London	11.6	54.1	13.8	12.2	6.4	1.9	11	1	1.9	7.4	1 243	76
Wales	7.3	72.9	9.0	8.1	2.4	0.4	6	1	1.4	5.1	519	23
Scotland	9.7	66.1	11.2	7.8	4.3	0.9	8	1	1.7	20.7	991	38
Ethnic group												
White	8.7	67.9	11.0	8.1	3.6	0.8	8	1	1.5	3.4	9 552	331
Black	17.4	55.0	15.2	9.5	1.7	1.2	10	1	1.4	3.2	209	15
Asian	27.4	64.6	6.0	1.6	0.4	0.0	3	1	0.8	0.7	147	56
Other	8.6	54.7	12.5	12.7	9.3	2.2	8	1	3.4	124.8	119	20
Missing	10.3	57.7	14.9	9.0	6.0	2.0	—	1	1.8	6.1	29	13
Religious affiliation												
None	8.3	59.7	13.8	11.6	5.3	1.4	10	1	1.8	9.5	3 763	110
Church of England	7.3	76.5	8.6	5.3	1.9	0.4	6	1	1.3	1.4	3 312	136
Roman Catholic	9.3	67.7	11.0	8.0	3.3	0.7	8	1	1.5	2.5	1 135	63
Other Christian	12.5	68.0	9.7	6.2	3.2	0.6	7	1	1.3	2.1	1 503	53
Non-Christian	20.9	61.5	9.9	4.0	3.2	0.6	7	1	1.2	3.6	326	71
Missing	21.5	32.2	14.4	2.5	29.3	0.0	—	1	2.2	4.3	18*	1

continued on p. 446

Table A5.2B. *Continued*

	0 (%)	1 (%)	2 (%)	3–4 (%)	5–9 (%)	10+ (%)	99th centile	Median	Mean	Variance	Base	Missing
Education												
Degree	5.6	62.2	12.7	12.1	6.2	1.2	11	1	1.9	7.4	822	17
A level or other non-degree	8.7	63.9	12.0	9.4	4.9	1.2	8	1	1.6	3.3	2 361	52
O level/CSE	9.8	64.9	12.2	8.8	3.6	0.8	8	1	1.6	6.3	3 864	119
Other	2.1	71.9	17.5	6.6	1.4	0.4	7	1	1.5	4.5	149	12
None	10.0	74.9	7.9	4.8	2.0	0.4	6	1	1.3	3.3	2 851	220
Missing	—	—	—	—	—	—	—	—	—	—	8†	13
Marital status												
Married	1.0	89.8	6.0	2.5	0.7	0.1	4	1	1.2	0.5	6 027	320
Cohabiting												
Opposite-sex partner	0.7	50.1	22.0	17.7	7.5	2.0	12	1	2.3	7.7	818	16
Same-sex partner	91.6	0.0	8.4	0.0	0.0	0.0	—	0	0.2	0.3	11*	0
Widowed	37.9	49.1	8.2	3.3	1.3	0.2	7	1	0.9	0.8	191	10
Divorced, separated	16.7	38.3	24.8	14.8	4.1	1.3	8	1	1.9	6.5	828	33
Single	29.0	24.8	15.9	17.8	10.2	2.3	12	1	2.2	13.9	2 181	48
Missing	—	—	—	—	—	—	—	—	—	—	2†	8
Smoking												
Non-smoker	13.2	68.6	9.0	6.3	2.6	0.4	7	1	1.3	1.9	4 557	235
Ex-smoker	5.5	78.1	8.3	5.8	1.9	0.4	6	1	1.3	1.6	1 627	71
Smokes <15 per day	6.3	57.1	14.7	13.2	7.0	1.7	10	1	2.1	13.9	1 659	42
Smokes 15+ per day	4.8	64.6	14.8	10.0	4.5	1.4	10	1	1.8	5.9	2 107	73
Missing	19.9	67.0	6.5	2.2	4.4	0.0	6	1	1.1	1.2	108	13
Alcohol												
None	18.6	68.5	7.7	3.2	1.5	0.4	6	1	1.1	1.7	1 340	134
Low intake	8.1	68.8	11.2	7.9	3.4	0.6	7	1	1.5	2.3	7 748	281
Moderate intake	4.3	53.4	14.5	16.3	8.5	3.0	15	1	2.6	28.6	906	19
High intake	4.7	64.1	5.0	16.4	8.5	1.4	30	1	2.1	13.1	44	0
Missing	12.9	64.8	14.9	4.5	0.0	3.0	—	1	1.6	7.4	20	0

* Note small base.
† Base <10.

Table A5.3A. Numbers of female partners reported in the last 2 years by men
[Source: booklet, question 7c]

	0 (%)	1 (%)	2 (%)	3–4 (%)	5+ (%)	99th centile	Median	Mean	Variance	Base	Missing
Total	10.8	67.1	10.0	7.4	4.8	10	1	1.6	11.3	8044	340
Not asked										0	
Age											
16–24	23.0	33.9	15.7	16.1	11.4	18	1	2.3	21.1	1940	44
25–34	6.2	69.0	12.3	7.5	5.0	12	1	1.7	22.0	2102	65
35–44	5.7	81.2	6.8	4.0	2.3	7	1	1.3	1.7	1972	79
45–59	8.7	83.3	5.2	2.3	0.6	4	1	1.1	0.6	2030	152
Social class											
I	8.2	76.1	8.3	5.1	2.3	9	1	1.3	3.1	559	16
II	5.3	75.8	9.9	6.2	2.8	7	1	1.4	2.8	2250	81
III NM	6.2	75.3	8.2	5.9	4.3	8	1	1.4	2.8	1513	42
III M	8.2	67.7	10.7	7.8	5.7	15	1	1.7	27.5	1917	95
IV	12.8	59.6	10.9	8.9	7.7	15	1	1.9	15.5	868	50
V	19.3	45.8	15.9	10.3	8.6	10	1	1.9	11.5	223	22
Other	41.7	29.2	10.1	12.5	6.5	9	1	1.5	13.5	706	27
Missing	—	—	—	—	—	—	—	—	—	8†	8
Region											
North	11.2	71.0	8.6	4.8	4.4	15	1	1.5	5.8	428	26
North West	9.5	68.3	10.1	6.9	5.3	10	1	1.6	6.5	856	30
Yorkshire/Humberside	11.8	67.5	8.2	7.5	5.0	11	1	1.5	4.3	638	41
West Midlands	11.5	70.5	8.4	5.2	4.4	10	1	1.4	4.0	761	62
East Midlands	9.5	70.2	9.0	7.0	4.4	8	1	1.4	1.8	603	15
East Anglia	11.1	71.0	9.5	7.0	1.6	5	1	1.3	2.9	317	2
South West	9.0	68.3	9.9	8.4	4.4	8	1	1.5	2.5	621	13
South East	10.2	66.4	12.5	7.1	3.8	8	1	1.5	5.3	1719	47
Greater London	12.6	58.5	10.0	10.4	8.5	15	1	1.9	15.7	1059	69
Wales	8.2	71.8	9.4	7.3	3.4	10	1	1.8	103.4	357	12
Scotland	12.8	66.5	8.9	7.8	4.0	18	1	1.7	10.1	684	24
Ethnic group											
White	10.4	67.5	10.1	7.4	4.7	10	1	1.6	11.6	7612	256
Black	16.0	56.1	12.8	6.3	8.8	11	1	1.7	4.8	144	17
Asian	18.2	64.2	7.9	8.5	1.2	4	1	1.1	1.2	154	44
Other	18.0	56.7	5.8	8.0	11.6	17	1	1.8	7.2	112	13
Missing	17.9	73.2	0.0	1.9	7.0	—	1	1.1	1.3	22	9
Religious affiliation											
None	10.5	62.8	11.0	9.4	6.3	10	1	1.7	16.8	4163	136
Church of England	8.9	77.3	8.3	3.5	2.1	7	1	1.2	2.0	2005	73
Roman Catholic	10.3	66.0	9.8	7.3	6.5	20	1	1.8	11.3	691	53
Other Christian	13.7	68.5	9.4	6.4	2.1	10	1	1.4	9.0	869	27
Non-Christian	19.3	58.9	8.5	8.1	5.3	5	1	0.9	0.7	309	49
Missing	—	—	—	—	—	—	—	—	—	7†	1

continued on p. 448

Table A5.3A. *Continued*

	0 (%)	1 (%)	2 (%)	3–4 (%)	5+ (%)	99th centile	Median	Mean	Variance	Base	Missing
Education											
Degree	9.5	71.5	9.1	6.2	3.8	7	1	1.3	1.7	987	26
A level or other non-degree	8.3	66.1	12.0	8.4	5.2	10	1	1.7	8.0	2 689	57
O level/CSE	12.5	64.0	9.7	8.2	5.6	11	1	1.6	7.2	2 417	78
Other	8.5	74.7	5.4	4.9	6.6	12	1	1.7	7.7	182	12
None	13.0	69.7	8.2	5.6	3.4	10	1	1.4	27.3	1 751	153
Missing	23.4	61.4	2.9	12.3	0.0	—	1	1.1	1.2	19*	13
Marital status											
Married	1.4	91.4	4.4	2.0	0.7	4	1	1.1	0.8	4 571	227
Cohabiting											
Opposite-sex partner	0.7	67.2	16.4	10.3	5.4	7	1	1.7	2.4	596	11
Same-sex partner	100.0	0.0	0.0	0.0	0.0	—	0	0.0	0.0	19*	1
Widowed	48.7	32.6	12.4	1.1	5.2	7	1	0.9	1.4	48	1
Divorced, separated	14.5	36.3	24.5	15.2	9.5	30	1	2.7	76.9	378	18
Single	28.8	27.4	16.7	15.7	11.5	15	1	2.2	15.2	2 430	79
Missing	—	—	—	—	—	—	—	—	—	3†	3
Smoking											
Non-smoker	15.9	63.7	9.8	6.6	4.0	9	1	1.4	4.7	3 177	118
Ex-smoker	6.3	81.5	6.5	4.1	1.7	6	1	1.2	2.1	1 733	95
Smokes <15 per day	9.8	56.5	12.6	12.1	9.1	15	1	2.0	8.0	1 205	53
Smokes 15+ per day	6.7	66.4	11.9	9.0	6.1	15	1	1.9	32.0	1 854	70
Missing	14.6	68.3	9.3	2.1	5.8	30	1	1.9	19.7	75	3
Alcohol											
None	25.7	60.9	5.6	5.8	2.0	6	1	1.0	1.4	679	62
Low intake	10.0	70.1	9.7	6.4	3.8	10	1	1.4	4.6	5 958	232
Moderate intake	5.9	58.7	13.2	12.2	10.0	20	1	2.4	53.3	1 117	37
High intake	9.6	52.6	13.6	13.4	10.7	15	1	2.1	8.4	276	8
Missing	10.1	47.4	25.1	17.4	0.0	—	1	1.1	1.3	13*	0

* Note small base.
† Base <10.

Table A5.3B. Numbers of male partners reported in the last 2 years by women
[Source: booklet, question 7c]

	0 (%)	1 (%)	2 (%)	3–4 (%)	5+ (%)	99th centile	Median	Mean	Variance	Base	Missing
Total	11.6	76.0	7.9	3.3	1.2	5	1	1.1	1.1	10 050	441
Not asked										2	
Age											
16–24	21.7	49.9	15.4	9.2	3.8	7	1	1.4	4.1	2 194	50
25–34	4.7	82.3	9.0	3.1	0.9	4	1	1.2	0.8	2 794	106
35–44	6.0	87.0	5.5	1.2	0.4	3	1	1.0	0.3	2 483	94
45–59	16.0	80.9	2.7	0.4	0.0	2	1	0.9	0.2	2 580	191
Social class											
I	3.2	90.8	4.7	1.3	0.1	3	1	1.0	0.2	624	25
II	6.0	84.2	7.2	2.0	0.6	4	1	1.1	0.6	2 900	96
III NM	10.6	74.0	8.8	4.7	2.0	5	1	1.2	2.3	2 294	88
III M	5.6	88.4	4.4	1.3	0.3	3	1	1.0	0.4	1 731	112
IV	13.3	68.2	11.2	4.9	2.4	5	1	1.2	1.2	1 039	48
V	17.1	74.7	6.8	0.3	1.1	6	1	1.0	0.5	208	9
Other	36.9	43.3	11.8	6.3	1.7	5	1	1.0	1.4	1 248	49
Missing	—	—	—	—	—	—	—	—	—	6†	14
Region											
North	13.2	78.4	5.2	3.0	0.2	3	1	1.0	0.3	565	25
North West	12.5	76.8	8.1	1.8	0.8	4	1	1.1	0.9	1 164	37
Yorkshire/Humberside	9.6	79.3	6.4	3.8	0.9	4	1	1.1	0.6	870	42
West Midlands	11.9	76.1	8.8	2.7	0.6	4	1	1.1	0.7	905	78
East Midlands	10.1	77.0	7.9	3.7	1.3	5	1	1.1	0.7	674	20
East Anglia	10.7	82.0	4.1	1.7	1.5	7	1	1.1	0.9	356	6
South West	8.5	78.1	8.2	3.7	1.5	5	1	1.1	0.6	792	18
South East	11.9	75.5	8.1	3.7	0.9	5	1	1.1	0.8	1 974	74
Greater London	13.9	68.7	10.1	4.7	2.7	6	1	1.2	1.7	1 241	78
Wales	10.0	79.0	8.7	1.5	0.7	3	1	1.1	1.3	519	23
Scotland	12.6	75.3	7.4	3.5	1.4	5	1	1.2	3.5	991	39
Ethnic group											
White	11.2	76.5	7.9	3.2	1.2	4	1	1.1	0.8	9 545	338
Black	18.8	68.2	8.4	3.7	1.0	4	1	1.0	0.6	209	15
Asian	29.3	64.8	5.1	0.4	0.4	3	1	0.8	0.5	147	56
Other	10.0	64.0	14.4	7.9	3.7	5	1	2.0	26.8	119	20
Missing	10.3	72.3	9.4	6.0	2.0	—	1	1.2	1.1	29	13
Religious affiliation											
None	10.4	72.1	10.9	4.6	2.0	6	1	1.2	2.1	3 762	111
Church of England	10.3	82.0	5.4	1.7	0.6	4	1	1.0	0.4	3 308	140
Roman Catholic	12.2	76.0	7.1	3.7	0.9	5	1	1.1	0.7	1 134	64
Other Christian	14.5	75.1	6.8	3.0	0.6	3	1	1.0	0.5	1 502	54
Non-Christian	23.2	66.1	7.3	3.0	0.5	5	1	0.9	0.7	326	71
Missing	21.5	44.0	2.6	15.5	16.3	—	1	1.9	3.7	18*	1

continued on p. 450

Table A5.4A. *Continued*

	0 (%)	1 (%)	2 (%)	3–4 (%)	5+ (%)	99th centile	Median	Mean	Variance	Base	Missing
Education											
Degree	13.3	73.4	8.8	3.5	1.0	5	1	1.1	0.6	987	26
A level or other non-degree	10.4	73.7	9.7	4.7	1.6	6	1	1.2	2.4	2688	58
O level/CSE	14.4	71.5	7.8	4.4	1.9	6	1	1.2	1.5	2418	77
Other	10.7	74.6	7.2	4.2	3.4	5	1	1.3	2.3	182	12
None	15.6	73.8	6.3	3.1	1.2	5	1	1.1	11.7	1753	150
Missing	33.8	51.0	15.2	0.0	0.0	—	1	0.8	0.5	19*	13
Marital status											
Married	2.1	93.4	3.3	1.0	0.2	3	1	1.1	0.5	4573	224
Cohabiting											
Opposite-sex partner	0.7	84.1	11.0	3.6	0.7	4	1	1.2	0.5	597	10
Same-sex partner	100.0	0.0	0.0	0.0	0.0	—	0	0.0	0.0	19*	1
Widowed	57.4	31.1	6.3	5.3	0.0	4	0	0.6	0.6	48	1
Divorced, separated	21.4	44.5	20.6	10.2	3.2	11	1	1.8	32.6	378	17
Single	34.2	37.5	15.1	9.1	4.1	8	1	1.3	4.0	2428	80
Missing	—	—	—	—	—	—	—	—	—	3†	3
Smoking											
Non-smoker	18.2	69.1	8.1	3.6	1.1	5	1	1.0	1.1	3177	119
Ex-smoker	8.0	84.1	5.0	2.5	0.4	4	1	1.0	0.4	1734	95
Smokes <15 per day	14.0	65.9	9.5	7.5	3.2	7	1	1.3	2.1	1205	52
Smokes 15+ per day	8.7	73.9	10.8	4.2	2.4	8	1	1.4	12.8	1856	68
Missing	15.8	71.5	6.3	2.6	3.9	30	1	1.6	13.3	75	3
Alcohol											
None	29.0	63.2	4.8	2.6	0.6	4	1	0.8	0.6	679	62
Low intake	12.3	75.7	7.5	3.4	1.2	5	1	1.1	1.3	5961	230
Moderate intake	8.4	66.9	13.3	7.8	3.6	10	1	1.6	20.9	1117	37
High intake	11.3	65.2	12.9	7.9	2.7	8	1	1.4	1.9	276	8
Missing	13.7	47.2	21.7	17.4	0.0	—	1	1.0	0.3	13*	0

* Note small base.
† Base <10.

Table A5.4B. Numbers of male partners reported in the last year by women
[Source: booklet, question 7d]

	0 (%)	1 (%)	2 (%)	3–4 (%)	5+ (%)	99th centile	Median	Mean	Variance	Base	Missing
Total	13.9	79.4	4.8	1.6	0.4	3	1	1.0	0.5	10 059	432
Not asked										2	
Age											
16–24	23.9	60.5	10.1	4.5	1.0	4	1	1.0	1.8	2 195	49
25–34	6.7	86.8	4.9	1.3	0.3	3	1	1.0	0.3	2 798	101
35–44	7.4	88.4	3.3	0.8	0.1	2	1	1.0	0.2	2 483	94
45–59	19.3	78.9	1.6	0.2	0.0	2	1	0.8	0.2	2 583	188
Social class											
I	4.7	92.7	2.1	0.5	0.0	2	1	1.0	0.1	625	23
II	7.7	87.1	4.1	0.9	0.2	3	1	1.0	0.2	2 901	96
III NM	12.8	78.0	6.5	2.1	0.7	3	1	1.0	1.1	2 297	85
III M	7.1	90.1	2.1	0.6	0.1	3	1	1.0	0.2	1 732	111
IV	16.1	73.8	6.7	2.9	0.6	3	1	1.0	0.5	1 040	47
V	20.9	76.0	2.4	0.7	0.0	2	1	0.8	0.2	208	9
Other	41.0	48.2	7.3	3.1	0.5	3	1	0.8	0.7	1 249	49
Missing	—	—	—	—	—	—	—	—	—	7†	13
Region											
North	15.3	80.1	4.1	0.6	0.0	2	1	0.9	0.2	565	25
North West	14.3	80.6	3.9	0.7	0.5	3	1	0.9	0.4	1 165	36
Yorkshire/Humberside	11.9	82.2	4.2	1.6	0.2	3	1	1.0	0.3	870	42
West Midlands	14.9	78.9	4.5	1.3	0.4	3	1	0.9	0.4	905	78
East Midlands	11.5	79.7	6.5	1.9	0.4	3	1	1.0	0.3	674	20
East Anglia	12.4	82.9	2.9	1.7	0.1	3	1	1.0	0.3	358	5
South West	10.2	80.9	6.4	2.3	0.2	3	1	1.0	0.3	793	17
South East	14.3	79.1	5.1	1.3	0.2	3	1	0.9	0.3	1 975	73
Greater London	16.4	74.3	5.2	3.2	0.9	4	1	1.0	0.8	1 244	75
Wales	12.0	83.0	3.2	1.5	0.3	3	1	1.0	0.4	519	23
Scotland	15.5	78.0	4.9	1.3	0.4	3	1	1.0	1.7	991	39
Ethnic group											
White	13.4	79.9	4.7	1.6	0.3	3	1	1.0	0.4	9 553	330
Black	23.0	70.5	5.1	1.5	0.0	3	1	0.9	0.3	209	15
Asian	31.8	64.5	3.3	0.0	0.4	2	1	0.7	0.4	147	56
Other	13.2	74.2	10.0	0.4	2.2	4	1	1.5	13.4	119	20
Missing	14.8	78.4	4.8	2.0	0.0	—	1	0.9	0.3	30	12
Religious affiliation											
None	13.0	77.7	6.4	2.3	0.7	3	1	1.0	0.9	3 762	111
Church of England	12.2	83.6	3.2	0.9	0.1	2	1	0.9	0.2	3 310	138
Roman Catholic	14.2	79.4	4.5	1.6	0.4	3	1	1.0	0.3	1 140	58
Other Christian	17.0	76.9	4.7	1.3	0.1	3	1	0.9	0.3	1 503	53
Non-Christian	25.4	70.3	3.4	0.7	0.2	3	1	0.8	0.3	326	71
Missing	25.6	42.6	0.0	31.9	0.0	—	1	1.5	2.1	18*	1

continued on p. 454

Table A6.2. Frequency of sexual intercourse in the last 4 weeks
[Source: booklet, question 2a]

	Men						Women					
	Centiles						Centiles					
	25th	Median 50th	75th	95th	Base‡	Missing	25th	Median 50th	75th	95th	Base‡	Missing
Total (not asked)	0	3	7	16	7 560 0	558	0	3	7	15	9 938 2	820
Age												
16–24	0	1	7	20	1 423	66	0	3	8	20	1 785	103
25–34	1	4	8	18	2 236	132	1	4	8	16	3 058	215
35–44	2	4	8	15	1 997	146	1	4	8	12	2 422	182
45–59	0	2	5	12	1 904	214	0	1	4	10	2 673	320
Social class												
I	1	4	6	15	561	25	2	4	8	12	574	42
II	1	4	8	16	2 198	134	1	4	7	15	2 879	180
III NM	1	4	8	16	1 404	81	0	3	7	15	2 243	159
III M	0	3	7	15	1 801	168	1	4	8	15	1 638	193
IV	0	3	7	15	822	76	0	3	6	15	1 037	98
V	0	1	6	20	214	27	0	3	7	14	218	23
Other	0	0	2	15	551	38	0	0	4	14	1 342	110
Missing	—	—	—	—	9†	9	—	—	—	—	7†	15
Region												
North	0	3	8	12	440	46	0	3	7	14	625	54
North West	0	4	8	15	809	58	0	3	7	14	1 177	90
Yorkshire/Humberside	0	4	8	20	642	62	0.5	4	8	15	876	86
West Midlands	0	3	7	15	722	84	0	3	6	15	876	108
East Midlands	1	3	6	13	585	38	0	3	8	15	713	56
East Anglia	0	3	6	15	309	10	0	4	8	15	373	25
South West	0	3	8	15	615	23	0	3	8	15	837	47
South East	0	3	6	15	1 534	87	0	3	7	15	1 898	129
Greater London	0	3	6	16	833	73	0	2	6	15	998	102
Wales	1	4	8	15	387	27	0	3	6	14	563	50
Scotland	0	3	8	18	684	50	0	3	6	12	1 002	73
Ethnic group												
White	0	3	7	16	7 207	469	0	3	7	15	9 486	702
Black	0	4	8	20	125	24	0	2	6	13	206	33
Asian	0	2	6	14	115	40	0	2	6	15	106	50
Other	0	3	6	16	89	15	0	4	8	16	110	22
Missing	0	1	4.5	14	24	10	0	3	6	14	30	13

continued

Table A6.2. *Continued*

	Men						Women					
	Centiles						Centiles					
	25th	Median 50th	75th	95th	Base‡	Missing	25th	Median 50th	75th	95th	Base‡	Missing
Religious affiliation												
None	0	3	8	16	3 871	250	0	3	8	16	3 706	251
Church of England	0	3	7	15	1 956	135	0	3	6	12	3 362	275
Roman Catholic	0	4	8	16	647	68	0	3	6	14	1 101	105
Other Christian	0	3	6	15	841	58	0	3	6	12	1 485	114
Non-Christian	0	3	6	15	235	45	0	2	6	15	268	73
Missing	—	—	—	—	10†	2	0	0.5	6.5	12	16*	2
Education												
Degree	0	3	6	15	991	43	0	3	7	15	803	33
A level or other non-degree	0	3	8	16	2 538	114	0	3	7	15	2 310	125
O level/CSE	0	4	8	16	2 194	147	0	4	8	15	3 779	252
Other	1	4	8	16	157	16	0	3	6	15	134	14
None	0	3	6	15	1 661	225	0	2	6	12	2 866	382
Missing	0	1	5	22	19*	13	0	0	8	14	9†	13
Marital status												
Married	2	4	8	15	4 090	362	2	4	8	14	5 536	577
Cohabiting												
Opposite-sex partner	4	7	12	20	552	27	3	6	10	20	755	46
Same-sex partner	0	0	0	0	20	1	0	0	0	0	11*	0
Widowed	0	0	0	8	68	3	0	0	0	5	293	17
Divorced, separated	0	1	6	15	584	44	0	0	4	15	1 290	71
Single	0	0	4	15	2 243	116	0	0	5	15	2 051	101
Missing	—	—	—	—	3†	5	—	—	—	—	2†	8
Smoking												
Non-smoker	0	3	7	16	2 971	193	0	3	6	14	4 362	371
Ex-smoker	1	3	6	12	1 668	135	0	3	6	14	1 646	149
Smokes <15 per day	0	3	7	16	1 072	100	0	3	7	15	1 624	117
Smokes 15+ per day	1	4	8	18	1 774	127	0	3	7	16	2 190	167
Missing	0	3	8	20	75	3	0	3	6	15	108	16
Alcohol												
None	0	2	6	15	617	79	0	2	5	12	1 330	180
Low intake	0	3	7	15	5 624	385	0	3	7	15	7 632	592
Moderate intake	0	4	8	16	1 038	75	0	4	8	20	914	47
High intake	0	4	8	20	269	16	0	2.5	8	20	42	1
Missing	0.5	3	7	14	12*	3	0.5	4	5.5	20	20	0

* Note small base.

† Base <10.

‡ Unweighted data.

Table A6.3. Prevalence of different sexual practices in the last year: men
[Source: booklet, question 3a–d]

	Vaginal intercourse			Oral sex			Anal sex			Non-penetrative sex		
	(%)	Base	Missing	(%)	Base	Missing	(%)	Base	Missing	(%)	Base	Missing
Total	85.5	7 870	514	62.1	7 852	532	6.5	7 828	555	65.5	7 490	563
(not asked)		0			0			0			331	
Age												
16–24	71.3	1 901	83	61.9	1 901	83	8.0	1 905	79	73.3	1 637	80
25–34	90.9	2 068	99	76.9	2 061	105	6.7	2 052	114	75.3	2 015	115
35–44	91.4	1 932	119	67.7	1 922	129	6.2	1 913	138	66.6	1 896	137
45–59	87.9	1 969	213	41.3	1 968	214	5.1	1 958	223	47.7	1 942	231
Social class												
I	88.0	549	27	60.1	548	27	3.5	547	28	66.9	532	31
II	92.4	2 208	123	69.6	2 208	123	4.8	2 204	128	68.0	2 178	133
III NM	90.3	1 486	69	67.8	1 478	77	6.6	1 472	83	67.7	1 446	82
III M	87.9	1 860	151	60.7	1 860	151	8.0	1 854	158	64.9	1 811	160
IV	83.3	849	68	57.3	844	73	10.1	840	78	60.8	803	77
V	71.1	217	28	52.5	216	29	10.4	213	32	60.6	201	30
Other	52.9	693	39	40.5	691	42	4.4	692	41	59.0	513	42
Missing	—	7†	9	—	7†	9	—	7†	9	—	6†	9
Region												
North	85.0	410	44	53.7	409	45	5.0	405	49	60.4	389	50
North West	87.6	845	41	65.2	838	48	7.1	839	47	67.1	803	51
Yorkshire/Humberside	84.8	628	52	65.1	625	55	6.9	628	52	67.0	598	54
West Midlands	85.2	737	85	59.0	742	80	5.3	736	86	62.1	706	84
East Midlands	87.6	595	23	62.2	590	28	6.8	590	28	64.6	566	30
East Anglia	82.2	309	10	57.9	309	10	7.0	310	9	64.5	297	9
South West	85.7	611	23	62.1	608	26	7.8	607	27	68.5	584	28
South East	86.1	1 685	80	65.1	1 681	85	5.7	1 683	83	68.4	1 593	28
Greater London	83.5	1 033	94	63.7	1 039	89	8.1	1 031	97	61.9	995	96
Wales	89.2	350	19	62.4	346	24	5.9	345	24	63.3	335	24
Scotland	83.6	665	42	55.6	666	42	5.7	655	53	67.4	625	50
Ethnic group												
White	86.0	7 449	419	63.1	7 435	433	6.5	7 418	450	66.6	7 104	458
Black	82.0	142	19	47.3	141	21	5.3	137	25	51.1	125	24
Asian	75.4	148	50	33.0	148	50	3.5	144	54	36.1	137	53
Other	76.6	109	16	57.3	108	17	10.5	199	16	49.5	105	16
Missing	79.0	21	10	36.6	20	11	9.7	20	11	68.5	19*	11

continued

Table A6.3. *Continued*

	Vaginal intercourse			Oral sex			Anal sex			Non-penetrative sex		
	(%)	Base	Missing	(%)	Base	Missing	(%)	Base	Missing	(%)	Base	Missing
Religious affiliation												
None	85.6	4070	230	66.5	4069	230	7.0	4059	241	68.8	3876	248
Church of England	87.7	1961	45	60.0	1958	120	5.4	1953	125	63.6	786	56
Roman Catholic	86.6	680	65	64.1	674	71	8.3	673	72	65.0	634	75
Other Christian	82.7	851	116	51.3	845	51	4.7	839	57	61.2	1908	123
Non-Christian	75.8	301	57	42.6	300	58	8.0	298	60	46.4	279	60
Missing	—	7†	1	—	7†	1	—	7†	1	—	7†	1
Education												
Degree	85.9	973	40	62.8	972	41	2.8	969	44	66.4	947	45
A level or other non-degree	88.6	2653	94	68.5	2647	99	5.5	2645	102	71.2	2545	107
O level/CSE	83.8	2360	135	63.3	2354	141	6.8	2351	143	67.5	2208	137
Other	88.4	175	19	55.5	174	20	9.1	175	19	53.0	168	19
None	82.8	1691	212	51.0	1687	216	9.5	1670	233	54.9	1604	241
Missing	62.5	18*	14	32.0	18*	15	5.1	18*	15	40.2	17*	15
Marital status												
Married	97.0	4467	331	63.4	4456	342	5.5	4425	372	65.0	4417	378
Cohabiting												
Opposite-sex partner	98.2	588	18	87.9	585	22	9.9	585	21	80.5	584	22
Same-sex partner	0.0	19*	1	0.0	19*	1	0.0	19*	1	0.0	17*	1
Widowed	40.3	46	2	24.0	46	3	5.9	48	1	28.0	46	3
Divorced, separated	75.6	364	32	63.3	366	30	12.0	368	28	55.8	367	29
Single	64.1	2383	126	54.4	2379	130	6.8	2381	127	65.4	2056	126
Missing	—	2†	4	—	2†	4	—	2†	4	—	2†	4
Smoking												
Non-smoker	80.3	3125	170	58.2	3117	178	5.0	3110	185	67.4	2842	194
Ex-smoker	90.7	1693	135	57.4	1682	147	4.8	1684	144	61.1	1669	147
Smokes <15 per day	85.3	1167	91	66.5	1763	95	8.0	1159	99	68.5	1118	101
Smokes 15+ per day	89.9	1812	112	70.1	1818	106	9.4	1802	122	64.6	1792	115
Missing	83.6	72	6	66.8	72	6	13.3	74	4	68.6	68	6
Alcohol												
None	69.6	651	91	40.6	651	90	4.8	647	95	50.4	582	97
Low intake	86.5	5842	348	62.6	5830	360	6.0	5813	377	66.4	5563	381
Moderate intake	89.3	1094	60	69.5	1089	65	8.6	1086	68	68.8	1064	69
High intake	87.7	271	14	73.0	270	15	11.6	271	14	67.2	269	15
Missing	84.2	11*	2	84.2	11*	2	12.6	11*	2	72.4	11*	2

* Note small base.

† Base <10.

Table A6.4. Prevalence of different sexual practices in the last year: women
[Source: booklet, question 3a–d]

	Vaginal intercourse			Oral sex			Anal sex			Non-penetrative sex		
	(%)	Base	Missing	(%)	Base	Missing	(%)	Base	Missing	(%)	Base	Missing
Total	84.7	9 789	701	55.9	9 725	765	5.9	9 721	769	60.2	9 257	825
(not asked)		2			2			2			410	
Age												
16–24	74.9	2 154	89	61.9	2 153	90	7.9	2 155	88	76.5	1 806	90
25–34	92.2	2 747	152	72.9	2 721	178	6.7	2 726	173	68.1	2 666	198
35–44	91.5	2 411	165	58.5	2 393	184	4.8	2 390	187	60.6	2 368	199
45–59	78.4	2 476	294	29.4	2 458	312	4.3	2 450	321	39.0	2 417	338
Social class												
I	94.7	613	35	57.8	604	44	5.2	613	35	64.5	601	43
II	91.2	2 846	150	61.3	2 827	169	4.8	2 832	165	63.5	2 779	186
III NM	85.9	2 248	134	60.0	2 228	154	6.0	2 234	147	63.8	2 135	160
III M	91.4	1 654	189	55.3	1 644	199	7.1	1 633	209	56.1	1 605	221
IV	81.9	1 007	80	51.8	1 003	84	8.0	989	98	57.3	952	99
V	79.3	204	13	43.4	203	13	6.9	201	15	45.7	198	15
Other	56.7	1 212	85	41.6	1 211	87	5.1	1 213	85	53.4	980	88
Missing	—	6†	14	—	6†	14	—	6†	14	—	6†	14
Region												
North	83.3	543	46	48.3	541	48	5.2	539	50	54.7	512	53
North West	84.7	1 131	69	52.1	1 123	78	5.7	1 123	78	57.7	1 075	83
Yorkshire/Humberside	86.2	839	73	55.1	832	79	4.6	835	77	60.1	792	87
West Midlands	83.9	868	115	54.3	869	115	6.3	861	122	56.1	821	126
East Midlands	87.6	657	36	59.8	653	41	6.5	656	38	61.4	624	43
East Anglia	86.1	349	13	54.7	344	18	5.4	344	18	60.5	333	15
South West	87.9	776	34	60.6	770	39	7.0	773	37	63.9	749	44
South East	84.6	1 936	112	59.6	1 921	127	5.6	1 920	128	64.0	1 813	143
Greater London	81.5	1 220	99	59.2	1 208	111	6.9	1 213	106	61.1	1 150	114
Wales	86.4	501	41	50.7	496	46	6.2	495	47	58.3	480	50
Scotland	83.5	968	62	52.2	968	61	5.4	961	69	58.8	906	67
Ethnic group												
White	85.2	9 307	576	56.8	9 247	636	5.8	9 245	637	60.8	8 818	686
Black	75.6	200	24	40.9	199	24	6.8	194	29	50.5	181	31
Asian	65.4	139	64	33.0	135	67	2.8	136	66	39.6	120	69
Other	86.3	117	22	45.6	116	22	12.7	117	22	53.4	112	24
Missing	83.5	27	15	38.0	27	15	5.8	28	14	49.1	26	14

continued

Table A6.4. *Continued*

	Vaginal intercourse			Oral sex			Anal sex			Non-penetrative sex		
	(%)	Base	Missing	(%)	Base	Missing	(%)	Base	Missing	(%)	Base	Missing
Religious affiliation												
None	85.9	3 674	199	63.5	3 665	207	7.2	3 661	212	64.8	3 467	237
Church of England	86.3	3 213	235	53.7	3 179	269	4.6	3 182	266	58.0	3 088	289
Roman Catholic	84.1	1 109	88	51.6	1 098	100	5.6	1 099	99	59.2	1 041	104
Other Christian	87.1	1 469	87	48.3	1 462	94	5.6	1 457	99	57.5	1 369	100
Non-Christian	70.9	307	90	39.6	303	94	4.9	305	92	45.5	275	94
Missing	74.5	18*	1	56.2	18*	1	16.3	18*	1	55.1	16*	1
Education												
Degree	87.4	811	28	65.7	802	37	5.1	806	33	69.2	784	38
A level or other non-degree	85.4	2 325	87	61.7	2 312	101	5.2	2 321	92	66.2	2 207	105
O level/CSE	85.3	3 781	202	60.4	3 764	220	5.5	3 758	225	65.0	3 512	242
Other	90.2	146	15	62.5	146	15	11.0	146	15	58.9	145	15
None	82.4	2 716	355	41.5	2 692	379	7.0	2 680	392	46.2	2 603	412
Missing	—	9†	13	—	9†	13	—	9†	13	—	7†	13
Marital status												
Married	96.3	5 832	515	57.5	5 776	572	5.4	5 764	583	60.9	5 725	622
Cohabiting												
Opposite-sex partner	98.6	802	32	78.3	798	36	9.9	798	36	76.8	787	45
Same-sex partner	0.0	11*	0	0.0	11*	0	0.0	11*	0	0.0	11*	0
Widowed	24.5	184	17	12.0	185	16	0.5	185	17	16.1	185	17
Divorced, separated	62.7	811	50	45.4	807	53	6.1	805	55	41.3	803	57
Single	62.1	2 147	79	51.5	2 146	80	6.0	2 156	70	64.5	1 744	77
Missing	—	2†	8	—	2†	8	—	2†	8	—	2†	8
Smoking												
Non-smoker	81.6	4 448	341	52.0	4 413	376	4.9	4 423	366	61.2	4 054	395
Ex-smoker	88.1	1 570	128	55.2	1 556	143	5.6	1 560	139	58.0	1 539	154
Smokes <15 per day	86.8	1 623	79	62.4	1 611	90	7.9	1 606	95	64.7	1 560	99
Smokes 15+ per day	87.8	2 044	136	60.1	2 040	140	6.6	2 031	149	56.9	2 011	156
Missing	76.4	105	16	51.8	105	15	5.6	101	19	50.5	93	20
Alcohol												
None	74.3	1 296	177	37.5	1 287	187	6.1	1 280	193	46.7	1 194	203
Low intake	85.9	7 540	488	58.0	7 490	538	5.5	7 496	552	61.7	7 138	580
Moderate intake	89.3	891	34	65.6	886	39	8.5	883	42	66.7	866	40
High intake	89.1	43	1	54.7	44	0	10.8	44	0	54.4	43	1
Missing	84.0	19*	1	48.5	19*	1	0.0	18*	2	76.8	16*	1

* Note small base.
† Base <10.

Table A6.5. Multivariate analysis of frequency of intercourse in last 4 weeks
[Source: booklet, question 2a]

	All respondents			All respondents sexually active in last year			All married and cohabiting respondents		
	Coeff.	SE	Sig.	Coeff.	SE	Sig.	Coeff.	SE	Sig.
Intercept	9.40	0.19		10.12	0.23		10.21	0.28	
Age	−0.10	0.004	<0.001	−0.08	0.01	<0.001	−0.03	0.01	<0.02
Men	0.14	0.08	<0.1	0.04	0.10	<0.7	0.06	0.12	<0.6
Marital status									
cohabiting	0.76	0.16	<0.001	0.89	0.17	<0.001	0.56	0.17	<0.002
Widowed/separated/divorced	−2.99	0.12	<0.001	−1.78	0.22	<0.001	—		
Single	−5.21	0.16	<0.001	−4.01	0.16	<0.001	—		
Social class									
III NM	−0.06	0.11	<0.7	−0.06	0.12	<0.7	−0.09	0.13	<0.6
III M	−0.20	0.11	<0.08	−0.20	0.12	<0.2	−0.17	0.13	<0.2
IV, V, other	−0.47	0.11	<0.001	−0.25	0.14	<0.07	−0.07	0.16	<0.7
Heterosexual partners in last 5 years									
2	1.76	0.13	<0.001	1.11	0.16	<0.001	0.89	0.19	<0.001
3–4	2.32	0.14	<0.001	1.42	0.17	<0.001	1.58	0.23	<0.001
5–9	3.09	0.18	<0.001	1.68	0.21	<0.001	3.33	0.33	<0.001
10+	5.94	0.26	<0.001	4.75	0.29	<0.001	6.23	0.49	<0.001
Age of most recent partner	—			−0.04	0.01	<0.001	—		
Age of spouse/cohabitee	—			—			−0.08	0.01	<0.001
Length of marriage/cohabitation	—			—			−0.03	0.01	<0.004
Variance accounted for	16.5%			8.9%			12.4%		
Base	17 495			14 469			10 818		

Coeff., coefficient; Sig., significance.

Table A7.1. Men's sexual experience with men
[Source: booklet, questions 4a; 8a,b]

	Sexual experience with a man			Number of male sexual partners ever						1+ male sexual partner in the last 5 years		
	(%)	Base	Missing	0 (%)	1 (%)	2 (%)	3+ (%)	Base	Missing	(%)	Base	Missing
Total	6.1	8337	47	96.4	1.8	0.5	1.4	8321	62	1.4	8323	61
Age												
16–24	4.3	1978	6	97.4	1.4	0.4	0.8	1977	7	1.7	1977	7
25–34	5.9	2158	9	96.3	1.6	0.4	1.7	2156	11	2.0	2156	11
35–44	8.5	2038	13	95.0	3.0	0.7	1.3	2031	21	1.0	2031	20
45–59	5.7	2163	19	96.8	1.2	0.3	1.6	2158	24	0.9	2160	22
Social class												
I	13.9	575	1	91.7	3.8	1.2	3.4	573	2	2.7	574	2
II	8.4	2323	8	94.9	2.4	0.7	2.0	2318	13	1.6	2319	12
III NM	5.2	1551	4	96.9	1.6	0.2	1.3	1547	8	1.4	1547	8
III M	3.2	2002	10	98.3	1.1	0.1	0.5	2000	11	0.7	2000	11
IV	5.3	909	8	96.2	1.3	0.9	1.7	907	10	2.2	906	11
V	7.4	241	4	98.0	1.8	0.0	0.2	240	5	0.2	240	5
Other	3.0	722	10	98.3	1.4	0.3	0.1	722	10	1.2	722	10
Missing	12.6	14*	2	87.4	0.0	0.0	12.6	14*	2	12.6	14*	2
Region												
North	3.2	450	4	97.7	0.9	0.3	1.1	449	5	1.5	449	5
North West	4.6	880	6	96.9	1.7	0.4	1.0	879	7	1.1	880	6
Yorkshire/Humberside	4.6	674	5	98.0	1.1	0.2	0.8	673	6	0.9	673	6
West Midlands	3.7	814	8	97.8	1.2	0.2	0.8	812	10	0.6	812	10
East Midlands	6.2	615	4	95.8	1.9	0.2	2.0	615	4	0.5	615	4
East Anglia	6.3	319	0	96.0	3.0	0.1	0.9	317	2	0.7	317	2
South West	5.6	634	0	97.4	1.5	0.7	0.4	633	1	0.6	633	1
South East	7.0	1757	9	96.8	1.7	0.3	1.2	1756	10	1.2	1756	10
Greater London	11.9	1125	2	91.5	3.4	1.1	4.0	1120	7	4.6	1121	6
Wales	3.3	368	1	98.0	0.7	0.5	0.8	368	1	0.5	367	2
Scotland	4.4	700	7	97.4	1.6	0.5	0.5	698	10	1.0	698	10
Ethnic group												
White	6.1	7837	31	96.3	1.8	0.5	1.4	7824	44	1.4	7826	42
Black	6.6	160	1	96.3	2.4	0.6	0.7	159	2	1.0	159	2
Asian	2.4	188	10	99.4	0.0	0.6	0.0	187	12	0.6	187	12
Other	9.8	124	1	96.5	1.7	0.0	1.8	123	2	1.8	123	2
Missing	14.4	28	2	94.3	0.0	0.0	5.7	28	2	2.0	28	2

continued on p. 464

Table A7.1. *Continued*

	Sexual experience with a man			Number of male sexual partners ever						1+ male sexual partner in the last 5 years		
	(%)	Base	Missing	0 (%)	1 (%)	2 (%)	3+ (%)	Base	Missing	(%)	Base	Missing
Religious affiliation												
None	6.4	4284	15	96.1	1.8	0.5	1.5	4273	26	1.5	4274	25
Church of England	5.0	2069	9	97.0	1.3	0.2	1.4	2067	11	1.2	2068	10
Roman Catholic	3.7	741	4	97.7	1.7	0.1	0.5	740	4	0.7	740	4
Other Christian	7.4	888	8	96.4	2.1	0.2	1.3	887	9	1.3	887	9
Non-Christian	11.4	348	10	92.9	3.6	1.9	1.5	346	12	3.2	346	12
Missing	—	8†	0	—	—	—	—	8†	0	—	8†	0
Education												
Degree	16.7	1008	5	89.9	5.1	1.2	3.8	1003	10	3.4	1005	8
A level or other non-degree	6.5	2741	6	96.1	1.8	0.7	1.4	2737	10	1.3	2737	10
O level/CSE	4.2	2484	10	97.5	1.2	0.2	1.1	2481	13	1.4	2481	14
Other	6.0	193	1	99.0	0.3	0.0	0.8	190	4	1.0	191	3
None	2.6	1882	21	98.5	1.0	0.1	0.4	1880	23	0.6	1880	23
Missing	0.0	29	3	100.0	0.0	0.0	0.0	29	3	0.0	29	3
Marital status												
Married												
Cohabiting	5.0	4770	28	97.5	1.5	0.4	0.6	4760	37	0.4	4760	38
Opposite-sex partner	7.0	606	1	96.0	2.6	0.7	0.8	606	1	0.0	606	1
Same-sex partner	100.0	20	0	0.0	5.1	4.4	90.5	19*	1	100.0	20	0
Widowed	4.4	49	0	97.1	0.0	0.9	1.9	49	0	0.0	49	0
Divorced, separated	8.3	393	2	95.5	3.5	0.2	0.8	391	4	1.0	392	4
Single	6.9	2494	15	95.2	1.9	0.6	2.4	2491	18	3.1	2492	17
Missing	—	5†	1	—	—	—	—	5†	1	—	5†	1
Smoking												
Non-smoker	5.0	3272	23	97.0	1.5	0.5	1.1	3266	29	1.2	3267	28
Ex-smoker	7.4	1815	13	95.9	2.1	0.3	1.7	1812	17	1.1	1812	16
Smokes <15 per day	6.1	1256	2	96.6	1.6	0.5	1.4	1253	5	1.6	1253	5
Smokes 15+ per day	6.7	1916	8	95.6	2.2	0.5	1.7	1915	9	2.0	1915	9
Missing	6.6	77	1	98.8	1.2	0.0	0.0	76	2	0.0	76	2
Alcohol												
None	7.2	730	11	96.7	2.2	0.3	0.9	727	14	0.7	727	14
Low intake	6.0	6158	33	96.3	1.6	0.5	1.6	6147	43	1.5	6149	42
Moderate intake	5.7	1152	2	96.7	1.9	0.3	1.1	1150	4	1.2	1150	4
High intake	6.9	284	0	95.6	4.0	0.3	0.2	284	1	2.8	284	1
Missing	7.3	13*	0	96.0	4.0	0.0	0.0	13*	0	0.0	13*	0

* Note small base.
† Base <10.

Table A7.2. Women's sexual experience with women
[Source: booklet, questions 4a; 8a,b]

	Sexual experience with a woman			Number of female sexual partners ever						1+ female sexual partner in the last 5 years		
	(%)	Base	Missing	0 (%)	1 (%)	2 (%)	3+ (%)	Base	Missing	(%)	Base	Missing
Total	3.4	10 421	71	98.3	1.2	0.3	0.3	10 411	81	0.6	10 412	80
Age												
16–24	3.0	2 234	12	98.6	0.9	0.3	0.2	2 233	13	1.2	2 233	13
25–34	3.9	2 880	19	98.0	1.2	0.4	0.4	2 878	21	0.8	2 879	20
35–44	4.2	2 559	18	97.9	1.5	0.4	0.2	2 558	19	0.5	2 558	19
45–59	2.6	2 748	23	98.7	1.1	0.1	0.2	2 743	28	0.1	2 743	28
Social class												
I	6.5	642	6	96.3	3.1	0.3	0.3	642	6	0.3	642	6
II	4.6	2 976	20	97.8	1.6	0.5	0.1	2 975	22	0.5	2 975	22
III NM	3.0	2 371	11	98.6	0.9	0.3	0.2	2 370	12	0.8	2 370	12
III M	1.3	1 829	14	99.2	0.6	0.1	0.2	1 828	15	0.2	1 828	15
IV	3.1	1 079	8	98.5	0.6	0.2	0.7	1 075	12	1.0	1 076	11
V	3.9	214	2	99.0	1.0	0.0	0.0	214	2	0.0	214	2
Other	3.2	1 294	6	98.3	1.1	0.3	0.4	1 292	8	1.0	1 292	8
Missing	6.1	16*	4	96.8	0.0	0.0	3.2	15*	5	3.2	15*	5
Region												
North	1.9	586	4	99.2	0.5	0.1	0.2	586	4	0.6	586	4
North West	2.6	1 193	8	98.3	1.1	0.3	0.2	1 192	9	0.4	1 193	8
Yorkshire/ Humberside	2.7	907	4	99.0	1.0	0.0	0.0	907	4	0.1	907	4
West Midlands	2.2	973	12	99.1	0.5	0.1	0.3	972	14	0.1	972	14
East Midlands	3.1	691	3	98.3	1.3	0.3	0.1	691	3	0.7	691	3
East Anglia	3.2	362	0	99.3	0.5	0.0	0.3	362	0	0.7	362	0
South West	3.9	804	6	98.5	0.6	0.8	0.1	802	8	0.2	802	8
South East	3.7	2 034	14	98.4	1.1	0.2	0.4	2 032	16	0.6	2 032	16
Greater London	5.6	1 308	12	96.5	2.6	0.3	0.7	1 307	13	1.2	1 307	13
Wales	3.5	541	0	98.2	1.1	0.4	0.3	541	0	0.9	541	0
Scotland	3.9	1 022	8	97.8	1.4	0.8	0.0	1 020	10	1.2	1 020	10
Ethnic group												
White	3.5	9 833	53	98.3	1.2	0.3	0.3	9 824	61	0.6	9 825	60
Black	1.4	221	2	99.5	0.5	0.0	0.0	221	2	0.0	221	2
Asian	1.3	189	14	100.0	0.0	0.0	0.0	188	15	0.0	188	15
Other	3.3	139	0	96.7	1.4	1.9	0.0	139	0	1.9	139	0
Missing	5.7	39	3	94.3	1.2	4.5	0.0	39	3	4.5	39	3

continued on p. 466

Table A7.2. *Continued*

	Sexual experience with a woman			Number of female sexual partners ever						1+ female sexual partner in the last 5 years		
	(%)	Base	Missing	0 (%)	1 (%)	2 (%)	3+ (%)	Base	Missing	(%)	Base	Missing
Religious affiliation												
None	4.7	3 864	11	97.7	1.4	0.5	0.5	3 860	15	1.0	3 861	14
Church of England	2.3	3 423	25	98.9	0.9	0.1	0.1	3 422	26	0.2	3 422	26
Roman Catholic	2.1	1 183	14	98.9	0.9	0.1	0.1	1 183	15	0.7	1 183	15
Other Christian	3.9	1 549	7	98.2	1.4	0.3	0.2	1 546	10	0.6	1 546	10
Non-Christian	3.3	384	13	97.5	1.7	0.7	0.1	382	15	0.3	382	15
Missing	0.0	19*	0	100.0	0.0	0.0	0.0	19*	0	0.0	19*	0
Education												
Degree	10.7	837	2	94.4	3.9	1.1	0.6	836	3	1.2	836	3
A level or other non-degree	4.3	2 398	15	98.0	1.3	0.5	0.2	2 396	16	0.9	2 396	16
O level/CSE	2.6	3 967	17	98.7	0.9	0.2	0.2	3 965	19	0.6	3 966	18
Other	7.6	158	3	95.3	4.5	0.0	0.3	156	5	1.0	156	5
None	1.7	3 042	30	99.2	0.6	0.1	0.2	3 039	33	0.3	3 039	33
Missing	0.0	18*	4	100.0	0.0	0.0	0.0	18*	4	0.0	18*	4
Marital status												
Married												
Cohabiting	2.6	6 299	48	98.8	0.9	0.2	0.1	6 294	53	0.2	6 295	52
Opposite-sex partner	4.9	829	5	97.6	1.5	0.6	0.3	829	5	0.8	829	5
Same-sex partner	100.0	11*	0	13.6	10.8	29.9	45.7	11*	0	86.4	11*	0
Widowed	1.9	200	1	99.1	0.2	0.7	0.0	200	1	0.0	200	1
Divorced, separated	4.9	855	5	97.1	2.4	0.1	0.5	854	6	0.6	854	6
Single	4.5	2 220	9	97.8	1.3	0.4	0.5	2 217	12	1.5	2 117	12
Missing	—	6†	3	—	—	—	—	6†	3	—	6†	3
Smoking												
Non-smoker	2.6	4 755	37	99.0	0.7	0.2	0.1	4 749	42	0.5	4 749	42
Ex-smoker	4.1	1 688	10	97.9	1.4	0.6	0.2	1 687	11	0.4	1 687	11
Smokes <15 per day	4.2	1 696	5	97.9	1.6	0.5	0.1	1 696	6	0.9	1 696	6
Smokes 15+ per day	4.5	2 168	12	97.3	1.8	0.2	0.7	2 165	15	1.0	2 166	14
Missing	0.0	114	7	100.0	0.0	0.0	0.0	114	7	0.0	114	7
Alcohol												
None	1.9	1 452	23	99.1	0.7	0.2	0.1	1 450	25	0.3	1 450	25
Low intake	3.3	7 981	47	98.5	1.1	0.3	0.2	7 974	55	0.5	7 975	54
Moderate intake	6.4	924	1	95.5	2.8	0.8	0.9	924	1	2.5	924	1
High intake	12.3	44	0	93.0	0.0	2.3	4.7	44	0	1.4	44	0
Missing	4.8	20	0	95.2	4.8	0.0	0.0	20	0	0.0	20	0

* Note small base.
† Base <10.

Table A8.1. Age below which young people ought not to start having sexual intercourse
[Source: interview, question 34a,b]

	Boys						Girls					
	<16 (%)	16+ (%)	Indi-viduals vary (%)	Not before marriage (%)	Base	Missing	<16 (%)	16+ (%)	Indi-viduals vary (%)	Not before marriage (%)	Base	Missing
Men												
Total	16.9	64.6	15.2	3.3	7961	422	14.4	68.1	13.9	3.6	8005	379
Age												
16–24	25.7	55.2	17.3	1.8	1842	142	22.2	60.3	15.6	1.9	1847	136
25–34	19.9	65.5	12.8	1.8	2067	100	16.4	70.0	11.9	1.9	2077	89
35–44	13.1	68.3	12.5	3.2	1967	84	11.7	70.7	14.2	3.4	1980	71
45–59	9.9	68.4	15.6	6.2	2085	96	8.1	70.7	14.0	7.1	2100	82
Social class												
I	11.2	67.8	15.2	5.8	555	21	12.2	66.9	15.0	6.0	555	20
II	14.7	64.8	17.2	3.3	2256	75	13.1	67.0	16.2	3.7	2263	69
III NM	17.5	66.4	13.0	3.1	1488	69	14.4	70.2	11.7	3.7	1503	52
III M	18.1	64.8	14.2	2.8	1918	94	14.7	69.4	12.6	3.2	1933	79
IV	20.3	61.8	13.9	4.0	849	69	16.0	68.1	11.9	4.0	849	69
V	17.2	63.9	16.7	2.3	226	19	14.9	68.6	14.1	2.4	228	18
Other	20.2	60.0	17.3	2.5	664	68	17.2	64.5	15.9	2.5	669	64
Missing	—	—	—	—	6†	9	—	—	—	—	6†	9
Region												
North	13.1	74.7	10.1	2.2	422	33	9.8	78.9	8.9	2.4	424	30
North West	16.2	64.9	16.5	2.4	838	48	13.2	68.7	15.7	2.4	841	45
Yorkshire/Humberside	17.8	64.0	14.9	3.3	650	30	13.3	70.1	13.1	3.5	651	29
West Midlands	16.5	61.6	14.6	7.3	779	43	14.4	66.2	12.2	7.2	785	38
East Midlands	15.1	69.2	12.5	3.2	587	31	12.9	71.7	12.0	3.4	591	27
East Anglia	15.7	66.4	15.7	2.2	305	14	12.5	71.0	14.0	2.5	306	13
South West	21.0	62.4	12.7	3.9	598	36	20.2	63.9	12.0	4.0	607	27
South East	18.1	64.1	15.0	2.7	1692	74	16.1	67.4	13.4	3.1	1699	67
Greater London	17.7	60.9	18.5	3.0	1075	52	16.1	62.6	17.0	4.3	1079	49
Wales	12.9	65.2	18.7	3.3	356	13	8.7	70.1	17.7	3.6	359	10
Scotland	16.3	65.5	15.8	2.4	660	47	12.6	70.0	14.8	2.6	663	44
Ethnic group												
White	17.4	64.8	15.4	2.5	7474	394	14.8	68.5	14.0	2.8	7517	351
Black	19.7	67.1	10.5	2.8	154	7	12.5	75.1	8.9	3.4	155	6
Asian	2.9	56.0	9.9	31.3	193	6	4.4	53.6	10.6	31.5	191	7
Other	11.0	63.5	18.7	6.9	120	5	12.2	60.0	18.6	9.2	121	4
Missing	2.9	47.6	28.9	20.6	20	11	2.9	47.6	28.9	20.6	20	11

continued on p. 468

Table A8.1. *Continued*

	Boys						Girls					
	<16 (%)	16+ (%)	Individuals vary (%)	Not before marriage (%)	Base	Missing	<16 (%)	16+ (%)	Individuals vary (%)	Not before marriage (%)	Base	Missing
Religious affiliation												
None	20.2	61.8	17.4	0.6	4 040	259	17.3	66.2	15.6	0.8	4 071	228
Church of England	14.3	70.9	12.1	2.7	2 003	75	12.5	74.0	10.6	2.9	2 005	73
Roman Catholic	14.7	65.0	15.0	5.4	711	33	9.7	69.4	14.8	6.2	712	32
Other Christian	12.5	65.4	13.7	8.5	851	45	10.8	66.6	13.3	9.3	858	38
Non-Christian	10.0	57.3	11.8	20.9	348	10	9.6	57.1	12.3	21.0	352	7
Missing	—	—	—	—	8†	0	—	—	—	—	8†	0
Education												
Degree	14.5	62.9	17.7	4.8	975	38	15.0	62.4	17.9	4.8	978	35
A level or other non-degree	16.8	65.3	15.1	2.9	2 648	99	14.3	68.9	13.8	2.9	2 655	91
O level/CSE	20.0	62.5	15.1	2.6	2 374	121	16.6	66.8	13.6	3.1	2 391	104
Other	13.7	70.6	12.9	2.8	188	6	11.0	72.2	10.7	6.0	191	2
None	15.0	66.7	14.4	3.9	1 758	145	11.7	71.6	12.5	4.3	1 772	131
Missing	7.9	51.8	18.4	21.9	18*	14	7.9	49.3	13.1	29.8	18*	14
Marital status												
Married												
Cohabiting	13.4	68.3	13.8	4.6	4 617	180	10.8	71.6	12.5	5.1	4 641	157
Opposite-sex partner	21.2	61.0	17.3	0.6	591	16	19.8	64.0	15.4	0.8	597	8
Same-sex partner	24.9	55.6	19.5	0.0	18*	2	24.9	55.6	19.5	0.0	18*	2
Widowed	4.2	78.0	16.6	1.9	47	2	4.2	76.1	18.5	1.2	47	1
Divorced, separated	18.2	63.8	16.0	1.9	368	28	15.4	68.1	14.5	2.0	370	25
Single	22.9	58.1	17.3	1.7	2 319	190	20.1	62.2	16.0	1.8	2 328	181
Missing	—	—	—	—	1†	5	—	—	—	—	1†	5
Smoking												
Non-smoker	16.0	66.2	13.9	4.0	3 134	161	13.5	69.6	12.8	4.2	3 145	150
Ex-smoker	14.6	65.4	16.2	3.9	1 760	69	13.2	67.6	14.8	4.4	1 765	63
Smokes <15 per day	20.0	60.4	17.1	2.5	1 171	87	18.3	63.2	15.8	2.7	1 181	77
Smokes 15+ per day	19.3	63.9	15.0	1.9	1 825	99	14.9	69.3	13.5	2.4	1 842	83
Missing	6.4	59.7	26.0	7.8	72	6	7.7	67.1	17.5	7.8	72	6
Alcohol												
None	12.1	61.5	13.6	12.8	685	56	9.7	64.5	12.8	13.0	686	55
Low intake	16.7	65.5	15.2	2.6	5 905	285	14.3	68.9	13.9	3.0	5 937	254
Moderate intake	20.5	62.8	15.3	1.5	1 091	63	17.3	67.1	13.8	1.8	1 099	55
High intake	20.1	59.7	19.4	0.9	267	17	18.0	63.3	16.7	2.0	270	14
Missing	0.0	71.6	28.4	0.0	13*	0	0.0	71.6	28.4	0.0	13*	0
Women												
Total	10.2	71.6	13.8	4.4	10 019	473	8.9	73.8	12.4	5.0	10 153	339

continued

Table A8.1. *Continued*

	Boys						Girls					
	<16 (%)	16+ (%)	Indi-viduals vary (%)	Not before marriage (%)	Base	Missing	<16 (%)	16+ (%)	Indi-viduals vary (%)	Not before marriage (%)	Base	Missing
Age												
16–24	16.8	63.6	17.2	2.4	2 128	118	14.7	67.7	15.1	2.5	2 164	82
25–34	10.9	74.8	12.0	2.3	2 776	123	9.4	77.4	10.5	2.7	2 806	94
35–44	7.8	73.8	14.0	4.4	2 460	117	6.7	75.8	12.7	4.9	2 490	87
45–59	6.4	72.5	12.9	8.3	2 655	115	5.6	73.3	11.9	9.3	2 693	77
Social class												
I	6.4	75.0	13.9	4.8	625	23	7.5	75.4	11.8	5.4	632	16
II	8.6	71.9	15.0	4.5	2 875	122	8.0	73.3	13.9	4.9	2 902	95
III NM	10.4	71.2	14.9	3.6	2 278	104	8.5	74.3	13.2	4.0	2 311	71
III M	10.2	74.1	11.6	4.2	1 770	73	8.2	76.7	10.2	4.9	1 791	51
IV	11.2	71.7	11.4	5.7	1 031	56	9.6	74.2	9.6	6.7	1 052	35
V	11.7	78.6	6.2	3.5	209	8	9.6	80.0	6.0	4.5	211	5
Other	14.5	64.8	15.7	5.0	1 223	76	12.6	67.7	14.3	5.5	1 247	53
Missing	—	—	—	—	8†	12	—	—	—	—	8†	12
Region												
North	8.7	75.1	12.1	4.1	567	23	7.4	77.3	10.8	4.5	569	20
North West	10.0	72.8	13.6	3.5	1 159	42	9.1	75.1	11.7	4.1	1 173	28
Yorkshire/Humberside	9.3	73.1	14.4	3.3	865	47	8.4	75.0	13.1	3.5	882	30
West Midlands	9.2	65.6	15.4	9.8	936	50	8.7	67.8	13.7	9.8	948	38
East Midlands	12.0	73.9	10.3	3.8	670	24	10.8	75.5	8.7	5.0	677	17
East Anglia	8.8	73.2	13.8	4.2	342	21	6.8	75.2	13.1	5.0	349	14
South West	11.1	73.4	11.5	4.1	775	35	10.4	74.5	10.7	4.3	798	21
South East	11.6	69.4	15.1	4.0	1 976	77	9.9	71.7	13.9	4.5	1 995	54
Greater London	11.3	69.0	15.8	4.0	1 250	70	9.6	72.0	13.8	4.6	1 273	46
Wales	7.9	75.4	12.5	4.1	527	14	6.1	77.7	11.6	4.6	531	11
Scotland	8.5	74.6	13.0	4.0	953	76	6.6	77.4	11.3	4.7	969	61
Ethnic group												
White	10.2	72.2	14.1	3.6	9 457	428	8.9	74.5	12.6	4.1	9 580	305
Black	18.6	67.1	9.1	5.3	213	10	16.9	68.8	8.9	5.4	216	7
Asian	3.8	53.8	6.0	36.4	190	13	1.8	54.8	4.5	38.9	193	10
Other	8.4	63.0	15.7	12.9	129	10	8.5	65.8	10.3	15.5	132	7
Missing	10.3	57.8	16.1	15.9	30	12	3.7	60.7	20.7	15.0	32	10
Religious affiliation												
None	13.7	69.4	16.0	1.0	3 980	195	12.4	71.8	14.3	1.5	3 739	136
Church of England	7.9	75.6	13.2	3.3	3 304	144	6.6	77.7	11.9	3.8	3 347	101
Roman Catholic	8.2	75.4	12.0	4.4	1 160	38	7.1	78.0	10.0	5.0	1 169	29
Other Christian	9.2	68.6	12.1	10.1	1 484	72	7.7	70.8	11.2	10.3	1 499	57
Non-Christian	4.7	58.7	10.3	26.3	373	24	3.6	59.3	9.3	27.8	380	17
Missing	21.0	49.0	24.9	5.1	18*	1	20.6	59.5	14.8	5.0	19*	0

continued on p. 470

Table A8.1. *Continued*

	Boys						Girls					
	<16 (%)	16+ (%)	Indi-viduals vary (%)	Not before marriage (%)	Base	Missing	<16 (%)	16+ (%)	Indi-viduals vary (%)	Not before marriage (%)	Base	Missing
Education												
Degree	10.2	68.9	17.4	3.5	796	43	11.8	68.2	16.3	3.7	802	37
A level or other non-degree	10.1	68.7	17.0	4.2	2 327	86	9.2	70.7	15.5	4.6	2 351	62
O level/CSE	11.3	72.4	13.0	3.4	3 803	181	9.5	75.2	11.6	3.7	3 850	134
Other	5.7	73.3	16.6	4.3	151	10	7.0	73.2	15.3	4.6	156	5
None	9.0	73.6	11.3	6.1	2 933	139	7.1	76.1	9.7	7.1	2 984	88
Missing	—	—	—	—	9†	14	—	—	—	—	9†	14
Marital status												
Married	8.1	73.8	12.8	5.4	6 104	244	7.0	75.4	11.6	6.1	6 166	82
Cohabiting												
Opposite-sex partner	15.1	71.0	13.6	0.3	799	35	12.6	74.9	11.9	0.6	808	26
Same-sex partner	14.4	43.7	41.9	0.0	11*	0	22.8	57.3	19.9	0.0	11*	0
Widowed	4.9	72.3	13.8	9.1	193	8	3.6	73.5	12.8	10.1	195	7
Divorced, separated	10.8	73.4	12.0	3.8	817	43	9.0	75.7	10.9	4.4	842	19
Single	14.8	64.6	17.6	3.0	2 093	136	13.1	68.2	15.4	3.2	2 130	99
Missing	—	—	—	—	2†	8	—	—	—	—	2†	8
Smoking												
Non-smoker	9.3	69.9	13.9	6.8	4 556	236	8.5	71.9	12.6	7.1	4 612	180
Ex-smoker	9.0	72.1	15.2	3.7	1 640	59	7.9	74.2	13.5	4.4	1 659	39
Smokes <15 per day	13.1	71.7	13.5	1.6	1 621	81	11.1	75.1	11.7	2.1	1 646	55
Smokes 15+ per day	10.9	74.7	12.8	1.5	2 089	91	8.9	77.0	11.6	2.5	2 121	59
Missing	6.6	70.0	12.8	10.9	114	7	7.3	69.2	11.9	11.6	115	6
Alcohol												
None	8.0	68.4	11.3	12.3	1 381	94	6.7	69.6	10.5	13.2	1 406	69
Low intake	10.0	72.0	14.6	3.4	7 698	331	8.9	74.2	13.0	3.9	7 783	246
Moderate intake	15.3	73.3	10.4	1.0	879	46	12.2	76.9	9.5	1.4	900	25
High intake	13.5	69.1	14.6	2.8	41	3	13.5	72.4	11.4	2.7	43	0
Missing	12.0	55.8	32.2	0.0	20	0	7.5	65.7	26.9	0.0	20	0

* Note small base.
† Base <10.

Table A8.2A. Proportions of men and women who consider particular sexual behaviour to be mostly or always wrong
[Source: interview, question 39a–d]

	Sex before marriage			Sex outside marriage			Sex outside live-in partnership			Sex outside regular partnership		
	(%)	Base	Not answd/ not known	(%)	Base	Not answd/ not known	(%)	Base	Not answd/ not known	(%)	Base	Not answd/ not known
Men												
Total	8.2	8 242	142	78.7	8 155	228	68.5	8 083	301	59.4	8 082	301
Age												
16–24	5.1	1 962	22	81.5	1 960	24	66.2	1 954	30	61.0	1 950	34
25–34	5.2	2 140	27	76.8	2 110	57	69.2	2 085	81	61.0	2 102	65
35–44	7.8	2 017	34	74.7	1 987	64	65.7	1 969	82	56.0	1 975	76
45–59	14.4	2 123	59	82.0	2 099	83	72.5	2 074	108	60.0	2 055	127
Social class												
I	13.2	563	12	83.0	562	13	77.2	550	25	63.1	554	22
II	7.6	2 297	34	74.3	2 259	73	66.7	2 240	92	56.0	2 247	84
III NM	6.9	1 529	26	79.1	1 522	33	67.9	1 511	44	59.4	1 507	48
III M	7.6	1 983	29	79.4	1 955	56	68.9	1 944	68	60.7	1 942	69
IV	9.6	903	15	82.4	902	16	69.9	892	26	62.4	889	28
V	8.1	241	4	79.7	235	10	71.5	234	11	62.9	234	11
Other	8.4	719	13	81.9	715	18	64.9	706	26	59.0	703	29
Missing	—	6†	9	—	6†	9	—	6†	9	—	6†	9
Region												
North	8.9	443	11	85.0	437	18	70.8	433	21	54.9	432	22
North West	7.3	872	14	78.8	860	25	67.2	860	26	60.7	854	31
Yorkshire/Humberside	8.9	669	10	80.3	655	25	71.3	650	30	64.1	656	24
West Midlands	11.4	800	22	78.4	806	16	68.7	797	26	60.2	798	24
East Midlands	9.3	606	13	76.8	603	15	65.5	594	24	56.5	598	20
East Anglia	6.9	316	4	81.2	312	7	66.1	311	8	62.4	312	7
South West	7.9	630	4	77.1	624	10	68.7	618	16	62.0	623	11
South East	6.9	1 742	24	76.8	1 714	52	68.9	1 703	63	57.0	1 700	66
Greater London	9.1	1 112	16	75.9	1 097	31	66.5	1 081	47	58.1	1 076	51
Wales	6.6	362	7	78.9	353	16	67.1	347	22	58.3	351	19
Scotland	7.0	690	18	84.8	695	13	72.0	689	18	63.0	681	26
Ethnic group												
White	6.4	7 747	121	78.5	7 659	209	68.3	7 593	275	59.0	7 598	270
Black	15.1	160	1	71.0	156	5	63.9	153	8	52.1	151	11
Asian	62.8	190	8	93.5	195	3	80.9	191	7	80.7	189	10
Other	21.3	122	3	80.1	124	1	68.9	124	1	64.1	123	2
Missing	22.9	23	8	81.6	21	10	72.1	22	9	58.9	23	8

continued on p. 472

Table A8.2A. *Continued*

	Sex before marriage			Sex outside marriage			Sex outside live-in partnership			Sex outside regular partnership		
	(%)	Base	Not answd/ not known	(%)	Base	Not answd/ not known	(%)	Base	Not answd/ not known	(%)	Base	Not answd/ not known
Religious affiliation												
None	2.6	4 245	54	73.6	4 177	123	64.4	4 141	158	54.5	4 143	156
Church of England	7.7	2 048	29	82.8	2 017	61	71.5	2 005	73	61.4	2 010	68
Roman Catholic	9.4	729	15	82.9	727	17	69.6	722	22	64.4	717	27
Other Christian	20.3	865	31	87.0	877	19	77.3	863	33	68.9	862	34
Non-Christian	46.2	346	12	88.1	350	8	76.5	345	13	73.1	343	15
Missing	—	8†	0	—	7†	1	—	7†	1	—	7†	1
Education												
Degree	11.6	997	16	74.9	973	39	67.8	961	52	56.0	962	51
A level or other non-degree	6.8	2 711	36	76.8	2 681	66	68.4	2 662	85	58.4	2 667	80
O level/CSE	6.0	2 467	28	80.6	2 445	50	67.6	2 418	76	60.0	2 427	68
Other	15.0	190	4	82.6	187	7	74.0	185	8	64.2	181	13
None	10.3	1 857	46	80.6	1 849	54	69.4	1 836	67	61.3	1 827	76
Missing	27.1	19*	13	100.0	19*	13	92.7	19*	13	75.6	18*	14
Marital status												
Married	10.5	4 704	94	80.5	4 663	135	70.1	4 605	193	59.4	4 614	184
Cohabiting												
Opposite-sex partner	1.3	604	2	68.8	591	16	68.5	588	19	60.8	582	25
Same-sex partner	0.0	19*	1	68.9	18*	3	67.3	19*	1	57.0	19*	1
Widowed	10.9	49	0	88.2	47	1	85.5	48	1	68.8	47	2
Divorced, separated	5.0	393	2	73.7	383	12	67.0	385	11	58.6	382	13
Single	6.0	2 471	38	78.5	2 452	56	65.3	2 437	71	59.2	2 437	71
Missing	—	1†	5	—	1†	5	—	1†	5	—	1†	5
Smoking												
Non-smoker	10.6	3 232	63	80.2	3 219	77	69.3	3 184	111	61.2	3 181	114
Ex-smoker	8.1	1 796	33	79.4	1 765	64	70.0	1 756	72	58.7	1 757	71
Smokes <15 per day	6.5	1 244	14	79.1	1 222	35	67.2	1 219	39	60.2	1 214	44
Smokes 15+ per day	5.0	1 894	31	75.2	1 872	52	66.2	1 849	75	56.2	1 858	66
Missing	12.4	76	2	86.0	78	0	76.8	74	4	68.6	72	6
Alcohol												
None	26.5	723	18	83.6	721	20	73.9	716	26	70.4	709	32
Low intake	7.0	6 086	105	79.6	6 020	171	69.5	5 962	229	59.9	5 983	208
Moderate intake	3.9	1 139	15	74.4	1 127	27	62.2	1 121	33	52.9	1 110	44
High intake	3.1	280	4	65.4	275	9	58.7	272	13	46.4	267	17
Missing	6.7	13*	1	73.9	13*	1	64.8	13*	1	50.6	13*	1

continued

Table A8.2A. *Continued*

	Sex before marriage			Sex outside marriage			Sex outside live-in partnership			Sex outside regular partnership		
	(%)	Base	Not answd/ not known	(%)	Base	Not answd/ not known	(%)	Base	Not answd/ not known	(%)	Base	Not answd/ not known
Women												
Total	10.8	10 191	301	84.3	10 258	234	79.6	10 210	283	69.9	10 178	314
Age												
16–24	5.2	2 225	21	84.8	2 219	27	77.7	2 208	38	71.6	2 206	40
25–34	6.0	2 851	49	84.5	2 848	52	80.8	2 848	52	72.9	2 838	62
35–44	9.5	2 497	80	80.5	2 513	64	76.5	2 497	79	65.5	2 485	92
45–59	22.1	2 619	152	87.2	2 680	91	82.9	2 657	114	69.6	2 649	122
Social class												
I	13.0	624	24	82.0	634	14	75.3	625	23	66.0	619	30
II	10.2	2 906	91	82.1	2 926	71	79.0	2 908	89	67.6	2 898	99
III NM	8.9	2 327	55	83.5	2 341	41	78.5	2 330	53	70.1	2 332	50
III M	11.4	1 780	62	87.3	1 803	39	82.7	1 802	40	71.5	1 796	47
IV	12.9	1 064	23	84.3	1 064	23	79.5	1 062	26	70.0	1 056	31
V	11.8	212	4	91.5	209	8	86.7	208	8	75.8	208	8
Other	11.7	1 270	30	86.5	1 275	25	79.9	1 268	31	73.7	1 264	36
Missing	—	7†	13	—	7†	13	—	7†	13	—	7†	13
Region												
North	11.3	566	23	87.6	574	15	76.0	574	16	67.0	569	20
North West	10.0	1 160	41	84.9	1 185	16	81.2	1 180	21	73.2	1 169	32
Yorkshire/Humberside	8.5	886	25	84.5	884	27	76.8	880	31	66.6	881	31
West Midlands	16.1	960	25	85.9	966	20	82.8	955	31	76.3	955	31
East Midlands	11.4	674	19	83.2	677	16	81.4	674	20	71.1	674	20
East Anglia	10.4	354	8	83.9	356	6	76.3	356	6	67.8	356	6
South West	11.0	792	18	82.1	799	11	77.4	786	24	66.3	786	23
South East	8.6	1 984	64	83.8	1 999	49	80.8	1 991	58	68.2	1 985	64
Greater London	10.9	1 288	31	80.4	1 266	53	76.9	1 272	48	67.6	1 265	55
Wales	9.9	526	16	88.6	535	7	81.1	536	5	75.0	534	7
Scotland	12.8	1 000	29	86.1	1 017	13	81.6	1 007	23	71.4	1 004	26
Ethnic group												
White	9.5	9 610	275	84.1	9 681	204	79.4	9 636	249	69.9	9 608	278
Black	18.7	218	6	86.1	213	10	82.2	220	3	71.1	219	5
Asian	56.2	198	5	93.4	199	3	87.6	193	10	85.0	190	13
Other	23.8	132	7	82.7	133	6	80.7	129	10	74.7	130	9
Missing	16.4	32	10	77.8	31	11	68.7	31	11	61.8	32	10

continued on p. 474

Table A8.2A. *Continued*

	Sex before marriage			Sex outside marriage			Sex outside live-in partnership			Sex outside regular partnership		
	(%)	Base	Not answd/ not known	(%)	Base	Not answd/ not known	(%)	Base	Not answd/ not known	(%)	Base	Not answd/ not known
Religious affiliation												
None	3.8	3 795	80	79.8	3 778	97	75.5	3 760	115	65.9	3 748	127
Church of England	9.8	3 330	118	86.0	3 367	81	80.9	3 352	96	69.8	3 340	108
Roman Catholic	12.3	1 156	41	88.0	1 173	25	82.6	1 174	24	73.9	1 171	26
Other Christian	22.0	1 508	48	87.1	1 531	25	82.6	1 526	30	73.6	1 519	37
Non-Christian	41.3	383	14	92.1	390	7	89.4	380	17	84.5	381	16
Missing	2.5	19*	0	66.6	19*	0	72.1	19*	0	60.6	19*	0
Education												
Degree	8.3	817	22	75.6	810	29	71.0	807	32	61.3	801	38
A level or other non-degree	9.1	2 361	51	83.6	2 375	38	79.0	2 360	52	69.2	2 355	58
O level/CSE	8.3	3 903	82	83.7	3 912	72	79.8	3 910	75	70.2	3 904	80
Other	16.1	161	0	84.1	153	8	80.1	150	11	66.0	145	17
None	15.8	2 941	131	87.9	3 001	71	82.3	2 975	97	72.7	2 966	106
Missing	—	7†	16	—	7†	16	—	7†	16	—	7†	16
Marital status												
Married	13.0	6 126	222	85.7	6 210	138	79.8	6 160	187	68.7	6 142	206
Cohabiting												
Opposite-sex partner	1.6	826	8	76.3	817	17	80.2	818	16	70.5	814	20
Same-sex partner	0.0	11*	0	72.1	11*	0	46.5	11*	0	54.3	11*	0
Widowed	23.9	193	8	88.2	193	8	88.7	193	8	74.7	193	9
Divorced, separated	8.2	840	20	82.8	836	24	82.0	834	26	72.2	831	29
Single	8.0	2 193	36	83.5	2 189	40	77.3	2 191	38	71.9	2 185	44
Missing	—	2†	8	—	2†	8	—	2†	8	—	2†	8
Smoking												
Non-smoker	14.7	4 637	155	85.7	4 691	101	80.8	4 665	126	71.9	4 650	142
Ex-smoker	9.7	1 644	55	84.2	1 644	54	79.1	1 642	57	68.2	1 635	63
Smokes <15 per day	6.3	1 674	27	81.5	1 671	31	77.7	1 668	33	67.9	1 667	34
Smokes 15+ per day	6.5	2 122	58	83.1	2 134	46	78.8	2 124	56	69.1	2 112	68
Missing	16.4	115	6	91.6	119	2	86.0	110	10	62.0	113	8
Alcohol												
None	26.4	1 402	73	90.2	1 436	39	83.0	1 419	56	75.2	1 419	56
Low intake	8.9	7 815	214	83.6	7 850	179	79.2	7 812	217	69.0	7 790	239
Moderate intake	3.7	911	14	81.4	909	16	78.6	916	9	70.1	908	17
High intake	5.8	44	0	83.6	44	0	77.3	44	0	70.3	42	1
Missing	0.0	20	0	76.4	19*	1	53.6	19*	1	52.4	19*	1

* Note small base.

† Base <10.

Table A8.2B. Proportions of men and women who consider particular sexual behaviour to be mostly or always wrong
[Source: interview question 39e–h]

	One-night stands			Sex between two men			Sex between two women			Abortion		
	(%)	Base	Not answd/ not known	(%)	Base	Not answd/ not known	(%)	Base	Not answd/ not known	(%)	Base	Not answd/ not known
Men												
Total	57.5	8 067	316	70.2	8 022	362	64.5	7 951	432	33.1	7 642	741
Age												
16–24	48.5	1 942	42	68.6	1 930	54	63.2	1 916	68	36.5	1 837	147
25–34	50.4	2 096	71	64.7	2 069	98	58.6	2 055	112	33.1	2 018	148
35–44	60.8	1 963	88	67.9	1 952	99	62.0	1 937	114	33.0	1 869	182
45–59	70.1	2 067	115	79.3	2 072	110	74.1	2 043	139	30.1	1 918	263
Social class												
I	60.5	559	16	55.8	552	23	51.5	547	28	25.1	537	38
II	58.4	2 232	99	62.4	2 211	121	56.7	2 192	139	26.0	2 145	186
III NM	58.6	1 504	51	72.6	1 500	55	65.7	1 484	71	29.8	1 412	143
III M	57.9	1 934	78	79.6	1 949	63	73.5	1 929	83	39.1	1 821	190
IV	58.6	894	24	75.5	874	44	70.1	871	46	42.2	843	75
V	49.6	238	7	82.7	233	12	74.8	232	13	53.1	207	38
Other	49.9	701	32	64.3	698	34	61.8	691	41	35.5	671	62
Missing	—	5†	10	—	6†	9	—	5†	10	—	6†	9
Region												
North	58.4	426	29	80.7	442	12	75.3	436	18	41.9	399	55
North West	54.3	853	33	70.3	856	30	65.9	851	35	36.2	817	69
Yorkshire/Humberside	58.1	654	26	72.1	637	42	67.1	628	51	33.1	607	72
West Midlands	63.0	783	39	74.9	792	30	69.8	786	36	35.4	735	87
East Midlands	58.1	599	19	71.7	592	26	65.9	585	34	31.9	557	62
East Anglia	57.6	311	8	72.9	311	8	68.0	310	9	34.9	301	18
South West	58.2	610	24	72.5	608	26	65.4	606	28	31.8	595	39
South East	57.7	1 716	50	66.6	1 685	81	59.4	1 671	95	28.2	1 614	152
Greater London	53.8	1 084	44	61.4	1 089	39	55.1	1 084	43	30.9	1 055	73
Wales	65.6	349	20	78.6	349	21	74.7	343	27	32.0	342	27
Scotland	54.3	683	25	70.0	661	47	66.4	652	56	39.6	620	88
Ethnic group												
White	56.6	7 582	286	69.5	7 534	334	63.6	7 467	401	31.9	7 188	680
Black	62.0	155	7	78.4	151	10	73.4	149	12	49.0	142	19
Asian	84.6	189	9	88.2	192	6	87.1	192	7	60.1	180	18
Other	65.7	121	5	75.7	122	3	75.8	121	4	42.9	115	10
Missing	71.5	21	10	74.5	22	9	72.6	22	9	55.1	17*	14

continued on p. 476

Table A8.2B. *Continued*

	One-night stands			Sex between two men			Sex between two women			Abortion		
	(%)	Base	Not answd/ not known	(%)	Base	Not answd/ not known	(%)	Base	Not answd/ not known	(%)	Base	Not answd/ not known
Religious affiliation												
None	50.6	4 147	153	64.1	4 105	194	57.5	4 082	217	28.0	3 942	357
Church of England	64.4	1 995	83	77.4	2 000	78	71.9	1 977	101	29.3	1 891	187
Roman Catholic	56.9	712	32	74.3	712	33	68.3	699	45	58.8	680	65
Other Christian	67.9	861	35	78.0	853	43	74.3	843	53	38.8	797	99
Non-Christian	76.4	345	13	73.3	344	14	73.9	342	16	50.4	326	33
Missing	—	8†	0	—	8†	0	—	8†	0	—	7†	1
Education												
Degree	55.9	962	51	43.2	960	53	40.8	958	55	23.4	950	63
A level or other non-degree	56.5	2 665	82	66.6	2 649	98	60.1	2 617	130	29.2	2 524	223
O level/CSE	55.5	2 419	75	74.6	2 391	104	68.3	2 371	123	34.0	2 282	213
Other	57.4	184	10	71.2	186	8	64.5	185	9	37.2	173	21
None	62.3	1 822	81	83.7	1 820	84	78.5	1 803	100	42.6	1 696	207
Missing	75.9	15*	17	78.2	17*	15	78.2	17*	15	54.9	17*	15
Marital status												
Married	62.8	4 598	200	74.1	4 586	212	68.5	4 546	252	33.3	4 344	454
Cohabiting												
Opposite-sex partner	53.5	589	17	63.5	578	28	54.8	575	32	25.7	559	47
Same-sex partner	20.2	19*	1	0.0	20	0	0.0	20	0	21.1	19*	2
Widowed	70.9	49	0	84.7	47	2	82.2	46	2	29.5	42	7
Divorced, separated	56.2	382	14	69.7	376	20	63.3	372	24	35.5	359	37
Single	48.8	2 429	79	64.7	2 414	94	60.0	2 392	117	34.3	2 318	191
Missing	—	1†	5	—	1†	5	—	1†	5	—	1†	5
Smoking												
Non-smoker	59.0	3 180	116	69.1	3 159	137	64.6	3 139	156	31.8	3 021	274
Ex-smoker	61.7	1 741	88	70.3	1 738	90	64.9	1 730	98	28.0	1 639	189
Smokes <15 per day	54.5	1 215	43	68.1	1 210	47	62.1	1 197	61	35.9	1 157	101
Smokes 15+ per day	52.8	1 856	69	73.4	1 840	85	65.9	1 812	112	38.5	1 756	168
Missing	60.7	77	1	67.1	75	3	58.5	73	5	31.7	69	9
Alcohol												
None	73.2	702	39	81.0	708	33	78.6	701	40	48.9	672	69
Low intake	59.0	5 962	229	69.0	5 910	280	63.3	5 860	330	32.2	5 646	544
Moderate intake	43.9	1 113	41	68.5	1 112	42	61.8	1 102	52	29.6	1 052	102
High intake	41.3	278	6	74.6	279	5	64.1	276	8	28.6	259	25
Missing	28.4	11*	2	92.5	12*	1	84.2	12*	1	14.8	12*	1

continued

Table A8.2B. *Continued*

	One-night stands			Sex between two men			Sex between two women			Abortion		
	(%)	Base	Not answd/ not known	(%)	Base	Not answd/ not known	(%)	Base	Not answd/ not known	(%)	Base	Not answd/ not known
Women												
Total	82.7	10 251	241	57.9	9 629	863	58.8	9 667	826	37.7	9 458	1 034
Age												
16–24	76.1	2 193	53	52.4	2 104	141	54.0	2 115	130	39.9	2 089	157
25–34	75.5	2 834	65	52.7	2 682	218	53.5	2 685	214	36.7	2 654	246
35–44	85.2	2 512	64	56.6	2 361	216	57.0	2 363	214	36.0	2 299	278
45–59	93.3	2 711	59	69.6	2 482	288	70.4	2 503	267	38.5	2 417	354
Social class												
I	80.9	625	23	45.8	587	61	46.4	587	62	28.8	592	57
II	82.9	2 920	77	50.1	2 716	281	50.8	2 725	272	32.5	2 700	297
III NM	82.8	2 345	37	59.2	2 198	184	61.0	2 219	163	35.5	2 166	216
III M	86.1	1 806	36	69.2	1 708	134	70.0	1 709	134	43.6	1 652	191
IV	80.9	1 068	19	63.2	1 002	85	64.3	1 009	78	46.0	976	111
V	84.8	210	6	69.9	201	15	70.0	201	15	52.5	191	26
Other	79.1	1 269	30	56.7	1 208	91	56.7	1 210	90	40.4	1 175	125
Missing	—	7†	13	—	7†	13	—	7†	13	—	7†	13
Region												
North	83.9	567	23	68.5	548	42	69.5	548	42	43.6	521	69
North West	84.2	1 173	27	59.4	1 116	85	60.3	1 119	81	44.0	1 094	107
Yorkshire/Humberside	83.8	888	23	55.9	821	90	57.4	828	83	38.6	804	108
West Midlands	86.7	972	14	65.5	902	84	66.0	908	77	43.1	889	97
East Midlands	81.8	681	13	59.7	642	52	59.1	645	49	37.1	615	79
East Anglia	83.6	355	8	59.9	347	16	60.6	347	15	36.0	351	11
South West	81.2	792	18	60.5	754	56	61.1	756	53	37.4	735	75
South East	81.4	1 998	50	53.4	1 873	175	54.3	1 883	165	34.1	1 857	192
Greater London	78.3	1 285	34	47.0	1 213	107	48.8	1 214	105	29.9	1 221	98
Wales	90.0	528	14	70.7	486	56	71.3	485	56	39.5	472	70
Scotland	81.1	1 012	17	57.3	928	102	58.1	931	98	38.6	900	130
Ethnic group												
White	82.6	9 668	217	57.0	9 073	812	57.9	9 111	775	37.1	8 921	965
Black	83.6	222	1	77.1	210	13	77.1	210	14	37.6	200	23
Asian	87.5	196	7	79.3	189	14	81.2	190	13	59.5	183	20
Other	79.8	136	3	59.5	131	9	61.1	131	9	46.3	128	11
Missing	84.3	30	12	53.9	26	16	53.9	26	16	45.7	26	16

continued on p. 478

Table A8.2B. *Continued*

	One-night stands			Sex between two men			Sex between two women			Abortion		
	(%)	Base	Not answd/ not known	(%)	Base	Not answd/ not known	(%)	Base	Not answd/ not known	(%)	Base	Not answd/ not known
Religious affiliation												
None	77.0	3 780	95	49.8	3 574	301	50.8	3 581	294	31.7	3 485	390
Church of England	86.1	3 364	84	61.8	3 153	295	62.7	3 175	273	33.7	3 088	359
Roman Catholic	86.2	1 175	23	61.7	1 086	112	63.5	1 088	110	58.9	1 096	102
Other Christian	85.9	1 530	26	64.5	1 429	127	65.0	1 435	121	41.8	1 405	151
Non-Christian	87.1	383	14	67.5	369	28	67.0	369	28	49.0	366	31
Missing	69.1	19*	0	51.7	19*	0	49.2	19*	0	48.4	17*	2
Education												
Degree	68.3	807	32	26.9	769	70	26.9	768	71	24.1	766	73
A level or other non-degree	80.3	2 361	52	48.0	2 199	214	49.1	2 208	204	31.9	2 202	210
O level/CSE	83.6	3 907	77	58.1	3 669	315	59.5	3 685	300	37.2	3 625	359
Other	84.6	156	5	58.7	144	17	60.7	147	14	39.2	143	18
None	87.3	3 013	59	73.7	2 840	232	73.9	2 851	221	46.8	2 714	358
Missing	—	7†	16	—	7†	16	—	7†	16	—	7†	16
Marital status												
Married	85.8	6 205	142	62.1	5 805	543	62.9	5 827	521	38.9	5 671	677
Cohabiting												
Opposite-sex partner	75.7	820	14	48.1	768	66	47.6	769	66	34.0	774	60
Same-sex partner	58.3	10*	1	22.7	11*	0	0.0	11*	0	50.8	11*	0
Widowed	93.6	198	3	69.0	179	22	68.9	182	19	41.1	176	26
Divorced, separated	81.1	838	23	55.8	779	81	56.4	785	76	35.5	769	91
Single	76.2	2 178	51	50.0	2 085	144	51.9	2 092	137	36.2	2 056	173
Missing	—	2†	8	—	2†	8	—	2†	8	—	2†	8
Smoking												
Non-smoker	83.4	4 687	105	59.3	4 420	372	60.0	4 436	356	38.3	4 331	461
Ex-smoker	83.4	1 655	44	55.6	1 540	158	56.5	1 549	149	32.4	1 525	174
Smokes <15 per day	79.3	1 666	35	55.1	1 577	125	56.2	1 579	122	38.5	1 563	138
Smokes 15+ per day	83.3	2 134	46	58.8	1 991	189	59.9	2 000	180	40.1	1 937	243
Missing	81.2	109	12	64.1	101	20	64.6	103	18	30.1	102	19
Alcohol												
None	87.8	1 423	52	71.7	1 365	110	72.4	1 365	110	50.9	1 303	172
Low intake	82.8	7 854	174	55.7	7 345	684	56.6	7 375	654	35.6	7 257	772
Moderate intake	75.4	912	13	55.6	860	65	57.2	867	58	35.1	839	86
High intake	72.8	43	0	56.7	40	4	56.2	39	4	43.8	41	3
Missing	51.0	19*	1	45.3	19*	1	46.7	20	0	40.5	19*	1

* Note small base.
† Base <10.

Table A9.1. Reported state of health and STD clinic attendance in the last 5 years
[Source: interview, question 2a; booklet, question 16]

	State of health							STD clinic attendance in last 5 years		
	Very good (%)	Fairly good (%)	Average (%)	Rather poor (%)	Very poor (%)	Base	Missing	(%)	Base	Missing
Men										
Total	39.7	34.4	21.8	3.2	0.9	8 382	2	3.4	7 632	437
Not asked						0			315	
Age										
16–24	37.2	40.4	20.4	1.7	0.4	1 984	0	4.9	1 644	76
25–34	39.5	35.3	22.7	2.2	0.3	2 166	1	5.4	2 072	75
35–44	40.3	33.8	22.4	2.9	0.7	2 050	1	2.7	1 939	96
45–59	41.6	28.6	21.8	5.9	2.0	2 181	0	0.9	1 977	190
Social class										
I	49.8	32.6	16.5	0.8	0.4	575	0	3.3	550	19
II	44.5	34.4	18.5	2.2	0.4	2 330	1	3.3	2 230	91
III NM	40.4	34.6	22.3	2.5	0.2	1 555	0	4.0	1 469	56
III M	35.5	34.0	25.4	4.1	1.0	2 011	0	2.8	1 856	127
IV	31.5	35.0	27.2	4.3	2.0	917	0	3.9	814	64
V	33.0	32.0	25.4	6.4	3.3	245	0	4.7	210	28
Other	39.4	36.0	17.9	5.2	1.5	733	0	3.5	496	42
Missing	22.2	54.9	15.6	0.0	7.3	15*	1	—	6†	9
Region										
North	35.5	30.9	26.0	5.4	2.1	454	0	1.3	402	35
North West	38.6	34.0	21.5	4.5	1.4	886	0	2.8	813	44
Yorkshire/Humberside	39.1	34.8	22.1	2.6	1.3	679	0	3.6	603	50
West Midlands	35.3	35.0	25.3	3.8	0.6	822	0	1.8	703	74
East Midlands	36.6	36.2	22.9	3.5	0.8	618	0	3.0	580	18
East Anglia	36.8	40.2	20.9	1.4	0.7	319	0	1.9	297	5
South West	41.6	31.8	23.0	2.9	0.8	634	0	3.4	598	15
South East	39.1	37.1	21.5	1.5	0.7	1 765	1	3.3	1 648	64
Greater London	48.9	31.4	16.7	2.7	0.4	1 128	0	7.4	1 001	84
Wales	45.9	29.7	17.9	5.3	1.2	369	0	3.0	341	15
Scotland	35.4	34.7	24.7	4.8	0.4	707	1	2.7	645	33
Ethnic group										
White	39.0	34.7	22.4	3.1	0.9	7 866	2	3.4	7 250	343
Black	50.2	28.4	16.0	4.4	0.9	161	0	6.8	133	21
Asian	51.4	27.8	14.0	6.3	0.5	198	0	1.6	131	49
Other	49.6	34.8	12.0	2.6	1.0	125	0	4.1	98	14
Missing	59.0	30.9	7.8	1.5	0.7	31	0	3.0	19*	10

continued on p. 480

Table A9.I. *Continued*

	State of health							STD clinic attendance in last 5 years		
	Very good (%)	Fairly good (%)	Average (%)	Rather poor (%)	Very poor (%)	Base	Missing	(%)	Base	Missing
Religious affiliation										
None	37.2	35.7	23.7	2.6	0.8	4 298	1	3.8	3 946	181
Church of England	41.4	33.5	20.9	3.3	0.9	2 078	0	2.9	1 951	93
Roman Catholic	42.7	30.5	20.4	5.1	1.4	744	1	2.5	648	72
Other Christian	41.4	35.4	18.9	3.5	0.9	896	0	3.0	808	36
Non-Christian	49.8	29.2	14.9	5.7	0.4	358	0	6.2	272	53
Missing	—	—	—	—	—	8†	0	—	7†	1
Education										
Degree	50.4	33.5	14.0	1.7	0.5	1 013	0	5.1	974	30
A level or other non-degree	41.5	33.8	20.6	1.9	0.2	2 744	2	4.2	2 618	76
O level/CSE	38.5	36.0	22.5	2.5	0.5	2 495	0	3.4	2 234	108
Other	36.8	33.1	19.0	8.5	2.6	194	0	0.6	176	16
None	33.3	30.8	27.3	6.3	2.4	1 903	0	1.7	1 614	192
Missing	35.2	41.9	16.4	5.8	0.7	32	0	0.0	15*	15
Marital status										
Married	41.9	32.4	21.6	3.2	0.9	4 797	1	1.5	4 526	271
Cohabiting										
Opposite-sex partner	35.6	34.7	26.1	3.4	0.3	606	0	5.0	592	13
Same-sex partner	42.2	23.7	34.1	0.0	0.0	20	0	37.4	20	0
Widowed	26.2	45.6	11.8	12.3	4.1	49	0	3.0	48	1
Divorced, separated	39.6	27.5	24.5	6.7	1.8	395	1	5.8	370	25
Single	36.8	39.1	21.0	2.4	0.8	2 509	0	6.5	2 073	122
Missing	—	—	—	—	—	6†	0	—	2†	4
Smoking										
Non-smoker	45.9	35.0	17.1	1.6	0.3	3 295	1	2.6	2 892	144
Ex-smoker	42.4	33.4	19.1	4.0	1.2	1 827	1	2.4	1 706	115
Smokes <15 per day	34.2	37.6	23.8	3.3	1.1	1 258	0	5.2	1 153	77
Smokes 15+ per day	29.7	32.5	31.4	5.1	1.4	1 924	0	4.6	1 818	92
Missing	50.3	27.7	16.6	5.4	0.0	78	0	1.3	64	9
Alcohol										
None	42.2	29.4	19.8	6.7	1.9	741	0	2.1	574	76
Low intake	40.8	34.9	20.9	2.7	0.8	6 189	2	3.3	5 677	294
Moderate intake	34.7	36.1	25.3	3.2	0.7	1 154	0	4.8	1 096	56
High intake	30.3	29.1	34.3	5.1	1.2	284	0	4.1	273	9
Missing	28.6	48.7	22.8	0.0	0.0	13*	0	0.0	12*	0

continued

Table A9.1. *Continued*

	State of health							STD clinic attendance in last 5 years		
	Very good (%)	Fairly good (%)	Average (%)	Rather poor (%)	Very poor (%)	Base	Missing	(%)	Base	Missing
Women										
Total	43.2	31.8	20.6	3.7	0.8	10 488	5	2.6	9 584	543
Not asked									365	
Age										
16–24	38.0	37.1	23.2	1.7	0.1	2 244	2	4.7	1 867	64
25–34	46.2	31.8	19.3	2.2	0.5	2 899	0	4.2	2 756	123
35–44	47.6	30.6	18.0	3.2	0.7	2 576	1	1.3	2 461	108
45–59	40.3	28.6	22.2	7.3	1.6	2 769	2	0.6	2 499	249
Social class										
I	55.9	30.0	12.1	2.0	0.0	648	0	1.5	618	26
II	52.1	29.6	15.4	2.3	0.6	2 995	2	2.9	2 866	120
III NM	44.3	33.5	19.2	2.7	0.4	2 380	2	3.4	2 221	105
III M	35.6	33.1	25.3	5.3	0.7	1 842	0	1.8	1 682	142
IV	35.2	33.0	27.2	3.7	0.9	1 087	0	2.3	991	59
V	26.1	31.9	30.9	9.4	1.7	216	0	1.6	200	12
Other	34.8	31.8	25.5	6.1	1.9	1 299	1	2.8	1 001	65
Missing	55.2	25.1	12.6	7.1	0.0	20	0	—	5*	14
Region										
North	37.7	35.4	20.3	5.3	1.5	589	1	0.8	535	33
North West	42.4	32.1	21.1	3.9	0.5	1 201	0	1.9	1 105	51
Yorkshire/Humberside	40.0	30.0	25.4	4.0	0.7	911	1	2.7	832	55
West Midlands	40.0	34.5	20.3	4.5	0.8	986	0	2.0	852	92
East Midlands	42.1	33.4	20.8	3.5	0.2	693	0	2.1	646	28
East Anglia	43.9	31.6	20.0	3.9	0.7	362	0	1.9	338	6
South West	43.0	32.9	20.5	3.1	0.5	810	0	2.1	773	24
South East	46.6	30.6	19.1	2.9	0.8	2 046	3	2.3	1 880	89
Greater London	47.1	31.8	17.2	3.3	0.6	1 319	0	6.7	1 167	86
Wales	46.4	29.9	16.6	5.3	1.9	542	0	0.5	500	28
Scotland	40.8	29.6	25.8	3.1	0.7	1 030	0	2.7	956	51
Ethnic group										
White	42.9	32.0	20.7	3.6	0.8	9 881	4	2.5	9 141	431
Black	47.0	30.0	19.4	2.8	0.8	223	0	9.0	187	20
Asian	49.2	29.3	14.5	6.8	0.3	203	0	0.0	117	58
Other	53.0	24.6	18.6	2.7	1.1	139	0	5.9	111	21
Missing	39.8	32.7	21.4	6.1	0.0	42	0	3.9	28	13

continued on p. 482

Table A9.1. *Continued*

	State of health							STD clinic attendance in last 5 years		
	Very good (%)	Fairly good (%)	Average (%)	Rather poor (%)	Very poor (%)	Base	Missing	(%)	Base	Missing
Religious affiliation										
None	40.2	33.3	22.9	3.0	0.7	3 873	2	4.1	3 563	148
Church of England	45.4	30.6	19.4	3.8	0.8	3 446	2	1.3	3 206	172
Roman Catholic	46.5	29.4	18.9	4.1	1.1	1 198	0	2.5	1 086	72
Other Christian	43.2	33.3	19.1	4.0	0.4	1 555	1	2.0	1 434	70
Non-Christian	45.2	27.8	19.4	6.6	1.0	397	0	2.1	278	80
Missing	29.3	53.9	16.8	0.0	0.0	19*	0	0.0	16*	1
Education										
Degree	56.1	32.0	9.9	1.7	0.3	839	0	6.1	811	21
A level or other non-degree	50.3	30.3	15.9	2.7	0.7	2 410	3	3.3	2 304	67
O level/CSE	43.3	33.3	20.6	2.5	0.3	3 984	0	2.3	3 615	144
Other	47.7	25.5	23.0	3.6	0.3	161	0	4.0	148	12
None	33.8	31.3	27.0	6.5	1.5	3 070	1	1.4	2 699	286
Missing	49.9	26.9	16.8	6.4	0.0	22	0	—	7†	13
Marital status										
Married	45.2	30.7	19.6	3.7	0.8	6 344	3	1.1	5 957	390
Cohabiting										
Opposite-sex partner	41.2	33.9	21.4	2.9	0.7	834	0	6.3	812	20
Same-sex partner	63.0	19.6	8.9	0.0	8.4	11*	0	0.0	11*	0
Widowed	34.9	27.6	27.7	8.0	1.9	201	0	0.8	186	15
Divorced, separated	41.1	28.2	22.6	6.5	1.7	860	0	4.3	819	40
Single	39.9	35.8	21.8	2.3	0.3	2 227	2	5.4	1 797	70
Missing	43.5	40.3	16.2	0.0	0.0	10*	0	—	2†	8
Smoking										
Non-smoker	49.0	31.1	16.6	2.8	0.5	4 790	2	1.9	4 203	289
Ex-smoker	47.5	29.4	18.2	4.0	0.9	1 697	2	2.8	1 616	80
Smokes <15 per day	39.1	34.7	22.3	3.4	0.6	1 701	0	3.1	1 599	64
Smokes 15+ per day	30.4	33.0	30.0	5.4	1.2	2 180	0	3.5	2 076	93
Missing	46.7	31.6	17.7	3.5	0.5	121	0	3.5	91	17
Alcohol										
None	38.6	29.6	21.4	7.5	2.9	1 474	0	2.6	1 180	166
Low intake	45.2	31.7	19.6	3.1	0.4	8 027	2	2.6	7 456	354
Moderate intake	34.8	35.2	27.5	2.4	0.2	924	2	2.9	888	21
High intake	26.0	42.2	22.9	7.7	1.3	44	0	1.1	43	1
Missing	33.6	32.4	23.9	10.1	0.0	20	0	3.4	17*	1

* Note small base.
† Base <10.

Table A9.2. Abortion and stillbirth or miscarriage (women)
[Source: booklet, questions 13;14]

	Abortion						Stillbirth or miscarriage					
	Ever (%)	Base	Missing	Last 5 years (%)	Base	Missing	Ever (%)	Base	Missing	Last 5 years (%)	Base	Missing
Total	12.5	9 841	648	4.5	9 818	672	20.9	9 914	576	5.8	9 882	608
Not asked		2			2			2			2	
Age												
16–24	9.4	2 164	79	7.9	2 161	82	5.7	2 184	60	5.4	2 184	60
25–34	14.8	2 758	141	6.3	2 752	147	18.2	2 778	121	10.9	2 772	127
35–44	15.7	2 432	144	3.6	2 424	152	27.0	2 464	113	5.6	2 450	126
45–59	9.7	2 487	284	0.3	2 480	290	31.3	2 488	282	0.7	2 477	294
Social class												
I	15.2	620	28	5.3	619	29	24.6	617	31	6.8	617	31
II	13.6	2 845	152	3.9	2 841	156	22.6	2 863	134	5.8	2 861	135
III NM	11.6	2 252	130	5.1	2 246	136	17.4	2 270	112	5.1	2 269	113
III M	12.0	1 677	165	3.7	1 671	171	24.8	1 690	152	7.2	1 672	170
IV	12.5	1 016	71	5.0	1 012	75	21.4	1 031	56	6.1	1 028	59
V	12.6	196	20	4.3	195	22	24.5	205	11	7.3	205	11
Other	10.8	1 230	68	5.0	1 228	70	15.3	1 231	66	4.4	1 224	74
Missing	—	6†	14	—	6†	14	—	6†	14	—	6†	14
Region												
North	6.6	553	36	1.8	553	36	18.1	556	33	5.8	554	36
North West	9.3	1 123	77	2.4	1 120	81	21.5	1 143	57	5.8	1 139	62
Yorkshire/Humberside	9.9	858	54	3.9	857	55	20.7	862	49	5.0	860	51
West Midlands	12.7	876	108	4.5	873	111	20.4	891	93	5.4	889	95
East Midlands	12.3	655	39	4.7	653	40	23.1	662	31	6.3	662	31
East Anglia	11.5	348	14	4.3	348	14	22.6	350	12	4.6	350	13
South West	14.3	778	32	3.3	776	34	21.3	781	29	7.1	780	29
South East	13.9	1 945	103	4.9	1 940	108	22.4	1 954	94	6.2	1 944	105
Greater London	21.2	1 226	93	8.7	1 224	95	18.3	1 227	92	5.4	1 225	94
Wales	9.2	508	34	4.2	507	35	21.8	511	30	5.7	508	33
Scotland	8.7	971	59	3.5	967	63	19.9	976	54	5.6	971	59
Ethnic group												
White	12.1	9 349	534	4.1	9 327	556	21.0	9 419	464	5.7	9 390	493
Black	26.2	202	21	14.0	201	22	18.4	204	19	7.6	203	20
Asian	18.5	144	58	9.9	144	58	19.6	142	61	7.6	140	62
Other	16.0	118	21	8.2	117	22	15.6	120	19	6.7	120	19
Missing	15.3	28	14	5.4	28	14	23.3	29	13	2.0	29	13

continued on p. 484

Table A9.2. *Continued*

	Abortion						Stillbirth or miscarriage					
	Ever (%)	Base	Missing	Last 5 years (%)	Base	Missing	Ever (%)	Base	Missing	Last 5 years (%)	Base	Missing
Religious affiliation												
None	14.7	3698	175	6.5	3687	186	17.6	3716	156	6.2	3703	170
Church of England	11.4	3233	215	2.6	3230	218	24.4	3253	195	5.5	3244	204
Roman Catholic	10.3	1107	91	3.6	1101	97	21.3	1125	72	7.4	1122	76
Other Christian	9.9	1469	87	3.4	1466	90	21.1	1482	74	4.1	1479	77
Non-Christian	18.4	318	79	8.3	318	79	21.6	320	77	6.8	318	79
Missing	2.7	17*	1	2.7	17*	1	19.7	17*	1	6.9	17*	1
Education												
Degree	17.5	812	27	6.5	811	28	17.1	815	24	7.0	815	24
A level or other non-degree	12.8	2322	91	5.3	2318	94	19.8	2346	66	6.0	2345	68
O level/CSE	11.5	3803	180	4.4	3791	192	17.8	3826	157	6.5	3818	165
Other	19.9	149	12	5.9	149	12	26.0	149	12	5.2	146	15
None	11.7	2747	325	3.1	2740	332	27.1	2768	303	4.3	2749	322
Missing	—	9†	13	—	9†	13	—	9†	13	—	9†	13
Marital status												
Married	11.1	5875	473	2.6	5863	485	26.4	5916	431	6.9	5890	457
Cohabiting												
Opposite-sex partner	20.2	805	29	10.2	804	30	14.4	812	22	6.6	810	24
Same-sex partner	0.0	11*	0	0.0	11*	0	17.6	11*	0	0.0	11*	0
Widowed	9.2	182	19	1.3	181	20	31.5	185	17	0.3	184	17
Divorced, separated	21.6	812	48	5.4	806	55	29.9	813	48	5.7	810	50
Single	10.3	2155	72	7.3	2152	75	4.1	2176	51	3.0	2175	51
Missing	—	2†	8	—	2†	8	—	2†	8	—	2†	8
Smoking												
Non-smoker	8.6	4469	320	3.5	4464	325	17.6	4497	293	5.2	4484	305
Ex-smoker	13.5	1601	97	3.1	1599	100	25.3	1602	97	6.0	1597	101
Smokes <15 per day	15.1	1605	96	7.2	1599	103	19.1	1634	67	6.9	1633	69
Smokes 15+ per day	18.2	2062	118	5.6	2053	127	26.0	2074	106	6.1	2061	119
Missing	10.4	104	17	2.8	103	18	23.0	107	14	8.4	107	14
Alcohol												
None	12.1	1297	177	4.3	1292	182	23.0	1311	162	7.2	1304	170
Low intake	12.1	7597	431	4.2	7580	448	21.0	7646	382	5.8	7628	400
Moderate intake	16.2	886	39	7.0	884	42	17.0	894	32	4.2	887	38
High intake	13.1	42	1	1.4	42	1	30.3	44	0	2.5	44	0
Missing	17.8	20	0	3.0	20	0	21.5	20	0	0.0	20	0

* Note small base.
† Base <10.

Table A9.3. Reported HIV testing
[Source: booklet, question 2o]

	Men						Women					
	HIV test			HIV test for other reason‡			HIV test			HIV test for other reason‡		
	(%)	Base	Missing	(%)	Base	Missing	(%)	Base	Missing	(%)	Base	Missing
Total	13.1	7577	492	4.3	7548	521	13.7	9463	664	2.9	9419	709
Not asked		315			315			365			365	
Age												
16–24	12.7	1650	70	4.5	1645	75	15.9	1852	79	3.6	1850	81
25–34	15.5	2067	79	5.5	2060	87	18.9	2732	147	3.3	2723	156
35–44	14.9	1920	115	4.2	1914	121	12.8	2440	129	2.7	2427	142
45–59	8.9	1939	228	2.7	1928	238	7.0	2438	310	2.1	2418	330
Social class												
I	16.7	546	23	3.9	546	23	16.6	615	30	1.9	615	30
II	16.0	2217	104	4.7	2214	107	15.0	2846	140	3.0	2829	157
III NM	12.0	1462	64	3.8	1457	68	12.8	2195	131	2.7	2186	140
III M	10.7	1849	134	3.1	1835	148	11.8	1646	178	2.5	1642	182
IV	11.3	801	77	6.5	796	82	13.3	973	76	3.2	966	83
V	8.8	205	33	4.8	205	34	12.5	193	19	1.7	191	21
Other	11.8	490	47	4.2	487	50	13.6	991	76	4.1	985	82
Missing	—	6†	9	—	6†	9	—	5†	14	—	5†	14
Region												
North	8.2	395	41	3.4	393	43	7.1	526	41	2.3	525	43
North West	10.4	802	56	3.2	800	58	10.2	1091	65	1.8	1081	76
Yorkshire/Humberside	14.1	601	52	4.7	599	54	16.2	825	62	3.7	822	65
West Midlands	10.3	693	83	2.6	689	88	11.9	832	111	2.8	830	113
East Midlands	12.5	576	22	3.9	573	25	12.0	646	27	2.4	646	28
East Anglia	11.1	300	3	3.5	299	3	10.1	335	9	2.4	332	11
South West	11.1	595	18	4.0	591	22	9.7	766	32	2.1	763	34
South East	13.8	1642	70	4.0	1639	73	15.6	1860	109	3.2	1854	115
Greater London	16.6	995	90	7.6	989	95	16.8	1158	95	4.4	1152	101
Wales	11.4	337	19	4.6	337	19	14.3	491	38	2.5	486	43
Scotland	18.0	640	38	3.8	637	41	18.2	933	75	2.8	928	80
Ethnic group												
White	13.2	7197	396	4.2	7173	420	13.6	9021	551	2.8	8981	592
Black	15.1	134	20	8.7	132	22	15.7	186	20	3.8	185	22
Asian	12.9	129	51	5.3	126	54	13.9	119	57	2.6	117	59
Other	5.3	98	15	2.5	98	15	15.6	109	23	7.1	109	23
Missing	5.7	19*	10	3.0	19*	10	14.1	28	13	3.3	28	13

continued on p. 486

Table A9.3. *Continued*

	Men						Women					
	HIV test			HIV test for other reason‡			HIV test			HIV test for other reason‡		
	(%)	Base	Missing	(%)	Base	Missing	(%)	Base	Missing	(%)	Base	Missing
Religious affiliation												
None	12.8	3 924	203	4.3	3 910	217	15.9	3 519	192	3.3	3 506	205
Church of England	12.8	1 935	110	3.1	1 928	116	11.3	3 165	213	2.4	3 153	225
Roman Catholic	13.5	639	80	6.1	637	82	13.1	1 066	92	2.6	1 056	103
Other Christian	15.7	802	43	5.3	798	46	14.0	1 420	84	3.0	1 413	91
Non-Christian	9.7	270	55	4.7	267	59	12.7	276	82	4.0	274	84
Missing	—	7†	1	—	7†	1	19.5	16*	1	0.0	16*	1
Education												
Degree	18.4	970	35	6.1	969	36	18.7	807	26	2.9	806	27
A level or other non-degree	16.2	2 608	86	4.7	2 601	93	16.6	2 289	81	3.0	2 279	92
O level/CSE	10.1	2 234	108	3.2	2 225	117	13.9	3 596	162	2.5	3 581	177
Other	19.6	175	17	9.0	172	19	14.2	143	18	7.6	142	18
None	8.2	1 576	230	3.4	1 565	242	9.3	2 622	364	3.1	2 604	381
Missing	3.4	15*	15	0.0	15*	15	—	6†	13	—	6†	13
Marital status												
Married	12.1	4 475	323	3.2	4 457	341	12.7	5 875	473	2.1	5 845	503
Cohabiting												
Opposite-sex partner	13.8	589	16	4.4	589	16	19.8	808	24	3.5	802	30
Same-sex partner	56.2	20	0	43.3	20	0	17.4	11*	0	17.4	11*	0
Widowed	5.0	46	2	3.1	46	2	6.6	182	19	1.5	180	21
Divorced, separated	15.4	371	24	6.1	369	27	14.4	807	52	5.4	804	55
Single	14.3	2 074	122	5.8	2 065	131	14.3	1 779	88	4.0	1 775	92
Missing	—	2†	4	—	2†	4	—	2†	8	—	2†	8
Smoking												
Non-smoker	14.0	2 872	164	3.9	2 866	170	12.6	4 149	343	2.0	4 134	358
Ex-smoker	11.5	1 695	125	3.5	1 691	130	12.9	1 594	102	3.1	1 590	107
Smokes <15 per day	13.3	1 125	76	3.9	1 119	83	15.8	1 588	69	3.1	1 574	83
Smokes 15+ per day	12.7	1 819	118	5.8	1 810	128	14.6	2 041	134	4.4	2 031	144
Missing	19.6	65	8	0.0	63	10	12.8	91	17	1.6	91	17
Alcohol												
None	12.5	559	92	6.4	558	93	11.2	1 155	191	3.4	1 147	198
Low intake	13.2	5 638	333	4.0	5 614	357	14.1	7 373	437	2.7	7 339	471
Moderate intake	12.4	1 096	56	4.0	1 092	60	13.5	875	34	3.9	872	38
High intake	14.8	271	11	5.6	271	11	2.0	43	1	1.0	43	1
Missing	0.0	12*	0	0.0	12*	0	10.8	17*	1	5.3	17*	1

* Note small base.

† Base <10.

‡ Reason for testing other than blood donation, pregnancy, insurance, mortgage or travel.

Table A10.1. Contraception used in the last year
[Source: interview, question 30b; booklet, question 7d]

	Pill (%)	IUD (%)	Condom (%)	Female sterilization (%)	Vas-ectomy (%)	Natural method* (%)	Other method† (%)	None (%)	Abstin-ence (%)	Base‡	Miss-ing
Men											
Total	30.4	4.9	36.9	9.0	12.8	7.9	2.9	17.6	1.5	7 154	165
Age											
16–24	53.1	2.2	60.8	0.5	0.1	11.1	3.2	9.0	2.6	1 439	18
25–34	49.4	5.0	44.4	4.8	4.7	9.3	3.2	11.2	1.6	1 955	30
35–44	18.7	7.8	28.1	14.2	22.1	6.6	3.0	14.7	1.1	1 875	41
45–59	4.9	3.8	19.6	14.8	21.6	5.5	2.3	33.7	1.0	1 886	75
Social class											
I	28.9	4.9	40.1	7.7	13.9	10.7	5.7	14.1	2.6	505	7
II	27.9	5.3	35.4	11.2	16.4	7.5	4.5	14.2	1.5	2 163	40
III NM	32.3	5.4	33.8	9.6	14.7	7.4	1.8	15.9	1.5	1 393	34
III M	30.4	5.1	34.3	8.6	11.5	7.7	1.3	21.7	0.9	1 771	45
IV	30.5	4.0	36.1	9.0	8.4	7.5	2.4	22.7	1.6	764	19
V	27.6	5.4	34.5	4.8	6.5	10.0	2.8	29.9	2.4	182	6
Other	39.8	1.4	65.3	2.1	1.8	8.9	2.6	12.6	1.7	402	12
Missing	—	—	—	—	—	—	—	—	—	9**	2
Region											
North	29.9	3.6	19.3	9.0	16.7	7.8	2.0	25.6	0.5	386	15
North West	26.5	3.9	39.6	8.6	13.1	11.3	2.5	17.3	2.2	776	11
Yorkshire/Humberside	34.3	3.0	34.6	7.4	14.2	6.9	2.2	17.6	0.3	580	12
West Midlands	28.0	5.3	39.2	7.2	10.6	8.6	3.0	19.7	0.7	702	22
East Midlands	26.6	4.8	37.6	10.7	13.7	7.3	3.0	17.8	2.5	542	7
East Anglia	30.3	3.1	35.5	12.7	15.8	6.8	3.4	14.9	1.7	267	3
South West	33.5	5.3	36.9	12.5	13.9	4.8	1.6	12.7	0.9	547	9
South East	30.0	5.1	36.8	9.2	15.4	7.5	3.0	16.0	1.8	1 502	45
Greater London	34.4	6.2	44.4	5.4	6.7	8.6	4.7	18.6	1.7	936	21
Wales	29.2	5.7	30.7	7.9	16.5	10.6	2.5	17.6	1.5	325	6
Scotland	30.6	5.6	35.5	13.3	8.6	6.4	2.5	18.5	1.9	589	13
Ethnic group											
White	30.6	4.8	36.6	9.2	13.3	7.9	2.9	17.1	1.5	6 745	143
Black	30.3	4.5	36.0	11.1	4.1	5.8	4.8	23.4	1.3	133	2
Asian	21.1	7.4	44.0	3.9	1.7	7.1	1.0	30.3	0.3	158	11
Other	33.5	7.1	43.2	5.8	5.8	12.9	3.4	18.9	0.0	95	4
Missing	27.6	5.0	36.3	8.4	8.6	0.0	4.3	24.8	8.4	23	4
Religious affiliation											
None	36.0	4.5	39.9	8.4	10.8	8.6	3.0	15.1	1.8	3 676	67
Church of England	23.9	5.0	35.3	10.5	14.4	5.7	3.3	19.7	0.9	736	17
Roman Catholic	28.5	5.5	35.4	7.5	9.0	10.0	2.1	22.5	1.6	639	21
Other Christian	23.3	5.0	31.2	10.9	18.6	7.0	2.7	18.7	1.9	1 823	40
Non-Christian	23.1	6.8	42.8	4.6	4.5	6.8	3.1	26.5	0.4	274	19
Missing	—	—	—	—	—	—	—	—	—	7**	1

continued on p. 488

Table A10.1. *Continued*

	Pill (%)	IUD (%)	Condom (%)	Female sterilization (%)	Vasectomy (%)	Natural method* (%)	Other method† (%)	None (%)	Abstinence (%)	Base‡	Missing
Education											
Degree	29.0	5.9	44.7	7.4	11.8	9.8	7.4	12.9	2.7	863	17
A level or other non-degree	34.4	4.3	41.3	8.5	13.6	9.1	3.6	12.3	1.4	2422	41
O level/CSE	35.3	5.1	38.7	8.6	11.6	7.5	1.7	14.8	1.4	2096	49
Other	16.5	7.7	30.4	11.8	14.7	7.1	2.2	21.9	2.8	167	7
None	19.9	4.6	24.2	11.2	13.2	5.9	1.0	31.4	1.0	1583	47
Missing	30.5	0.0	28.3	0.0	22.3	4.6	0.0	29.2	0.0	22	4
Marital status											
Married	21.3	5.6	27.9	11.9	18.2	6.6	2.6	20.4	1.0	4584	116
Cohabiting											
Opposite-sex partner	51.9	5.7	31.0	7.8	7.5	11.8	4.5	11.4	2.5	597	5
Same-sex partner	—	—	—	—	—	—	—	—	—	1**	0
Widowed	15.7	5.0	32.4	0.0	6.8	4.4	0.0	40.1	0.0	21	0
Divorced, separated	27.7	5.8	37.1	12.6	9.2	7.9	3.3	24.9	1.7	307	8
Single	48.7	2.5	64.3	1.1	0.1	9.9	3.1	10.2	2.4	1638	36
Missing	—	—	—	—	—	—	—	—	—	5**	0
Smoking											
Non-smoker	34.3	4.5	42.9	5.8	11.5	8.3	2.9	14.2	1.5	2655	58
Ex-smoker	18.5	4.6	28.8	12.4	19.4	6.6	2.8	21.9	1.3	1635	56
Smokes <15 per day	39.1	4.4	44.0	6.6	9.1	8.8	3.3	15.2	1.3	1065	24
Smokes 15+ per day	30.7	6.1	30.6	12.4	10.8	7.8	2.7	20.1	1.8	1735	25
Missing	18.9	2.8	44.4	6.3	13.0	12.1	4.4	17.5	0.0	64	2
Alcohol											
None	21.6	3.6	30.3	9.7	9.0	6.4	2.4	29.6	1.8	522	23
Low intake	30.5	5.1	38.0	8.6	13.2	7.7	3.0	16.6	1.5	5328	122
Moderate intake	34.0	4.0	36.5	9.5	12.7	9.3	2.6	16.4	1.5	1043	17
High intake	30.4	6.1	27.9	16.2	11.4	9.7	2.4	19.9	0.2	251	2
Missing	36.8	10.1	48.7	0.0	15.8	16.3	0.0	8.6	0.0	11§	0
Women											
Total	28.8	6.6	25.9	11.0	12.6	5.2	3.6	21.1	1.0	8911	181
Age											
16–24	64.1	3.1	41.8	0.4	1.1	7.7	2.5	9.5	1.7	1692	24
25–34	43.6	8.9	31.0	6.2	7.4	5.8	5.6	12.7	1.6	2667	44
35–44	11.3	9.3	20.7	17.8	24.3	4.8	3.4	16.2	0.6	2344	49
45–59	2.5	3.7	12.8	17.9	15.0	3.1	2.2	45.3	0.1	2208	63

continued

Table A10.1. *Continued*

	Pill (%)	IUD (%)	Condom (%)	Female sterilization (%)	Vas-ectomy (%)	Natural method* (%)	Other method† (%)	None (%)	Abstin-ence (%)	Base‡	Miss-ing
Social class											
I	21.9	6.7	28.6	8.2	15.0	7.4	7.3	19.2	1.4	607	12
II	23.7	7.0	27.0	12.1	15.8	4.7	4.1	19.4	1.0	2 730	42
III NM	36.0	6.4	27.3	9.6	11.5	5.4	3.0	18.6	0.6	2 044	44
III M	24.2	6.6	19.5	13.1	14.9	4.9	2.5	24.7	0.7	1 683	35
IV	33.4	7.0	23.1	11.3	7.7	5.4	2.1	24.2	1.0	899	21
V	27.8	7.0	15.5	15.3	8.6	2.4	1.9	29.7	0.0	170	2
Other	38.6	5.8	35.4	7.5	3.2	5.4	5.0	21.5	2.4	764	20
Missing	41.0	0.0	14.8	0.0	16.3	0.0	3.2	31.3	0.0	14§	4
Region											
North	27.2	6.2	22.3	11.5	14.3	3.3	2.7	23.9	0.2	491	11
North West	26.2	7.0	23.4	11.1	12.1	5.6	2.4	23.8	0.7	1 015	19
Yorkshire/Humberside	30.1	4.6	23.8	10.4	13.3	4.3	2.0	23.6	1.4	786	21
West Midlands	27.6	6.8	27.0	9.7	13.0	6.1	1.5	21.6	0.7	820	31
East Midlands	28.1	7.1	24.3	11.7	15.9	5.7	1.8	20.0	1.0	611	6
East Anglia	25.6	5.6	26.6	18.8	14.3	5.8	4.5	18.7	0.5	317	1
South West	29.2	7.2	21.9	13.7	15.2	4.2	2.8	19.3	0.8	718	11
South East	29.6	5.1	28.9	11.7	13.5	4.6	5.1	17.7	1.1	1 721	43
Greater London	32.6	9.8	32.4	5.1	6.9	8.0	7.2	18.9	1.9	1 092	23
Wales	27.6	6.6	23.6	9.9	15.1	5.4	2.7	21.7	1.0	474	6
Scotland	28.6	6.9	22.4	13.8	9.8	3.1	3.5	25.9	0.7	868	8
Ethnic group											
White	28.7	6.6	25.7	11.3	13.0	5.1	3.6	20.7	1.0	8 443	157
Black	36.8	6.9	26.5	9.4	3.6	7.1	5.8	27.3	2.3	169	6
Asian	21.1	7.1	26.1	6.7	4.4	6.3	1.7	37.5	0.0	142	14
Other	31.6	11.5	32.8	2.9	7.0	5.4	3.8	21.6	0.4	122	1
Missing	38.1	1.3	22.2	13.1	7.7	5.1	0.0	18.8	2.4	35	3
Religious affiliation											
None	37.7	6.9	27.7	9.4	10.3	5.4	3.8	16.9	1.0	3 339	45
Church of England	24.0	5.8	25.6	13.7	13.8	4.5	3.6	23.0	0.8	1 277	22
Roman Catholic	31.0	7.1	25.8	7.0	8.8	6.5	3.8	24.3	1.7	1 004	32
Other Christian	21.4	6.3	23.8	13.4	16.4	4.7	3.1	22.6	0.8	2 978	66
Non-Christian	17.0	8.8	27.6	8.6	7.0	6.1	5.7	32.1	1.8	299	16
Missing	37.0	3.1	19.8	0.0	0.0	3.0	0.0	53.3	3.2	14§	0
Education											
Degree	34.1	6.2	38.4	5.5	9.8	6.7	9.5	13.2	3.9	740	9
A level or other non-degree	33.5	6.6	32.3	9.7	11.1	6.0	4.4	16.2	1.0	2 059	37
O level/CSE	35.4	7.2	27.4	9.3	13.0	5.6	2.9	15.9	0.9	3 391	60
Other	22.7	8.1	24.4	11.1	15.2	6.5	4.6	22.3	0.0	142	7
None	15.2	6.0	15.2	16.2	13.8	3.5	2.1	34.0	0.2	2 564	65
Missing	31.2	6.8	21.5	0.0	14.9	0.0	0.0	31.7	0.0	15§	4

continued on p. 490

Table A10.1. *Continued*

	Pill (%)	IUD (%)	Condom (%)	Female sterilization (%)	Vas-ectomy (%)	Natural method* (%)	Other method† (%)	None (%)	Abstin-ence (%)	Base‡	Miss-ing
Marital status											
Married	19.7	7.1	21.8	13.1	17.1	4.7	3.2	0.6	23.9	6053	131
Cohabiting											
opposite-sex partner	48.7	5.7	26.2	9.8	4.9	6.4	5.1	1.8	12.4	816	7
Same-sex partner	—	—	—	—	—	—	—	—	—	0	0
Widowed	4.6	4.4	2.2	16.8	3.5	0.2	0.8	0.7	67.7	64	1
Divorced, separated	24.5	12.0	19.1	16.7	5.7	3.0	5.3	0.8	26.7	544	17
Single	59.0	3.2	46.7	0.5	0.6	8.1	3.9	2.4	9.9	1429	22
Missing	—	—	—	—	—	—	—	—	—	6**	3
Smoking											
Non-smoker	30.3	5.6	30.3	8.9	12.8	5.4	4.1	1.1	19.3	3923	92
Ex-smoker	21.4	8.0	21.2	12.9	16.3	4.7	3.4	0.8	22.7	1493	30
Smokes <15 per day	36.6	7.4	28.1	9.4	7.6	7.2	3.5	1.8	18.6	1495	19
Smokes 15+ per day	25.5	7.2	18.5	15.5	12.7	3.6	2.8	0.4	25.6	1911	33
Missing	29.4	4.9	28.7	7.4	19.0	3.6	3.1	0.5	19.5	29	6
Alcohol											
None	21.1	6.5	21.7	12.0	8.8	4.6	3.0	0.7	31.1	1119	36
Low intake	28.5	6.6	26.9	10.8	13.7	5.4	3.7	1.1	19.9	6909	129
Moderate intake	41.5	6.9	23.3	11.4	8.2	3.9	3.2	0.7	17.9	829	15
High intake	41.0	7.6	14.8	14.3	11.8	2.4	3.9	2.7	20.7	38	0
Missing	20.2	5.5	34.6	5.4	22.9	5.8	0.0	0.0	17.3	17§	0

* Safe period, withdrawal.
† Cap, pessaries, sponge, douche, other.
‡ Respondents with at least one heterosexual partner in the last year.
§ Note small base.
** Base <10.

Table A10.2. Condom use, lifestyle change and 'unsafe' sex in the last year
[Source: booklet, questions 1c; 7d; interview, questions 30b; 44a]

	Condom use at the last occasion of heterosexual sex			Sexual lifestyle change because of AIDS			'Unsafe' sex in the last year		
	(%)	Base	Missing	(%)	Base	Missing	(%)	Base	Missing
Men									
Total	23.2	7384	472	19.5	8352	31	6.0	7490	361
Not asked		528			0			533	
Age									
16–24	38.9	1523	66	36.2	1983	1	9.7	1539	43
25–34	24.0	2000	100	22.9	2154	13	5.8	2030	72
35–44	19.6	1895	119	13.9	2043	9	5.7	1926	88
45–59	13.6	1966	187	6.2	2173	9	3.7	1995	159
Social class									
I	24.0	529	24	13.4	574	1	4.3	534	17
II	20.9	2172	123	16.6	2323	8	5.8	2209	84
III NM	22.1	1436	66	16.8	1553	2	5.0	1452	50
III M	21.6	1816	128	19.1	2011	1	7.6	1839	104
IV	23.9	790	59	23.8	916	1	5.1	802	48
V	22.6	198	28	19.9	243	2	8.5	204	23
Other	42.4	435	36	34.7	725	7	6.1	443	27
Missing	—	7†	8	—	6†	9	—	7†	8
Region									
North	13.8	393	31	13.1	452	3	7.6	397	28
North West	25.0	795	42	17.7	883	3	6.4	808	29
Yorkshire/Humberside	21.1	587	49	14.7	678	1	5.4	592	45
West Midlands	25.1	688	69	15.9	821	1	4.5	695	62
East Midlands	25.5	555	27	16.7	617	2	5.9	566	16
East Anglia	28.5	291	6	20.4	318	1	3.5	294	2
South West	23.3	583	20	18.7	631	3	6.0	589	11
South East	21.8	1570	83	19.8	1760	5	6.7	1589	61
Greater London	27.3	969	89	31.4	1121	7	6.0	987	70
Wales	22.4	331	19	15.8	369	0	6.3	337	13
Scotland	19.4	622	38	19.9	702	6	6.0	637	24
Ethnic group									
White	22.9	7018	380	19.1	7849	19	6.0	7114	278
Black	17.9	124	20	38.5	160	1	9.8	127	17
Asian	36.7	130	46	15.5	197	2	3.9	131	44
Other	29.4	95	15	32.3	124	1	4.0	97	13
Missing	33.9	18*	11	11.5	22	9	5.0	20	9

continued on p. 492

Table A10.2. *Continued*

	Condom use at the last occasion of heterosexual sex			Sexual lifestyle change because of AIDS			'Unsafe' sex in the last year		
	(%)	Base	Missing	(%)	Base	Missing	(%)	Base	Missing
Religious affiliation									
None	24.6	3 809	212	23.0	4 288	12	7.0	3 871	146
Church of England	20.4	1 904	103	12.5	2 071	7	4.1	1 934	75
Roman Catholic	20.8	635	59	21.0	742	2	8.1	635	57
Other Christian	22.8	771	44	16.9	889	6	5.3	783	29
Non-Christian	29.3	259	52	21.2	354	4	7.4	260	53
Missing	—	7†	1	—	8†	0	—	7†	1
Education									
Degree	27.9	940	40	24.0	1 011	2	4.1	950	27
A level or other non-degree	25.9	2 507	96	21.4	2 744	3	6.3	2 534	65
O level/CSE	23.9	2 146	131	21.1	2 491	3	6.6	2 191	85
Other	19.3	172	14	12.5	193	1	4.6	173	14
None	15.5	1 603	176	13.1	1 896	7	6.0	1 625	157
Missing	31.5	16*	14	19.6	18*	15*	5.8	16*	13
Marital status									
Married	16.7	4 491	306	6.3	4 783	14	3.0	4 553	243
Cohabiting									
Opposite-sex partner	12.6	587	17	20.9	604	2	10.4	593	11
Same-sex partner	—	9†	2	66.2	20	0	0.0	10*	1
Widowed	15.5	47	2	20.5	49	0	4.0	48	1
Divorced, separated	20.5	368	27	37.8	396	0	17.0	378	18
Single	42.8	1 880	115	41.1	2 499	10	9.7	1 906	84
Missing	—	3†	3	—	1†	5	—	3†	3
Smoking									
Non-smoker	28.3	2 732	160	21.4	3 284	11	5.0	2 766	119
Ex-smoker	18.7	1 678	127	11.8	1 820	8	4.1	1 701	105
Smokes <15 per day	27.5	1 129	76	25.6	1 257	1	7.4	1 147	59
Smokes 15+ per day	16.3	1 778	105	19.9	1 914	10	8.6	1 809	73
Missing	34.7	68	3	12.9	78	0	2.9	67	5
Alcohol									
None	24.9	540	73	14.9	740	2	4.8	549	65
Low intake	23.8	5 482	338	18.9	6 164	27	4.8	5 663	249
Moderate intake	21.0	1 080	51	25.9	1 151	3	11.1	1 094	39
High intake	14.7	270	11	19.7	284	0	11.8	271	8
Missing	30.7	12*	0	6.6	13*	0	7.9	12*	0

continued

Table A10.2. *Continued*

	Condom use at the last occasion of heterosexual sex			Sexual lifestyle change because of AIDS			'Unsafe' sex in the last year		
	(%)	Base	Missing	(%)	Base	Missing	(%)	Base	Missing
Women									
Total	17.5	9 292	627	14.2	10 458	34	4.0	9 453	460
Not asked		573			0			580	
Age									
16–24	24.3	1 708	79	29.7	2 236	9	9.2	1 732	52
25–34	18.9	2 700	142	15.7	2 891	8	3.8	2 731	108
35–44	16.2	2 404	155	9.4	2 572	5	3.1	2 454	104
45–59	12.4	2 479	252	4.5	2 758	13	1.6	2 536	195
Social class									
I	19.1	604	36	8.4	648	0	2.0	617	24
II	18.3	2 798	154	11.7	2 991	6	2.7	2 843	105
III NM	18.4	2 139	122	16.2	2 380	2	5.4	2 165	95
III M	13.3	1 660	150	6.1	1 841	1	1.7	1 696	114
IV	14.9	963	67	15.4	1 082	5	7.0	979	52
V	9.1	195	15	7.4	215	1	1.8	202	9
Other	23.3	927	70	30.7	1 295	5	7.2	945	49
Missing	—	5†	13	—	6†	14	—	6†	13
Region									
North	16.1	517	39	10.3	588	1	2.4	530	25
North West	16.3	1 084	58	12.6	1 199	2	3.4	1 101	40
Yorkshire/Humberside	15.5	806	63	11.2	909	3	3.4	820	49
West Midlands	18.5	819	101	10.9	984	1	4.3	839	83
East Midlands	15.5	633	30	14.1	686	7	5.6	640	23
East Anglia	17.7	327	13	10.9	362	0	2.6	334	5
South West	14.5	755	31	13.7	806	4	6.2	766	19
South East	18.8	1 820	112	15.1	2 041	7	3.6	1 850	80
Greater London	22.5	1 129	95	24.0	1 315	4	4.3	1 145	96
Wales	17.3	492	29	10.1	542	0	2.4	498	23
Scotland	15.2	911	57	13.5	1 025	4	4.5	928	39
Ethnic group									
White	17.3	8 868	516	13.9	9 865	20	4.0	9 022	357
Black	18.2	185	16	25.3	223	0	5.0	184	15
Asian	22.6	105	60	7.6	200	3	1.8	109	56
Other	23.1	107	23	23.6	138	1	7.5	110	20
Missing	22.3	28	12	17.0	32	10	3.7	28	12

continued on p. 494

Table A10.2. *Continued*

	Condom use at the last occasion of heterosexual sex			Sexual lifestyle change because of AIDS			'Unsafe' sex in the last year		
	(%)	Base	Missing	(%)	Base	Missing	(%)	Base	Missing
Religious affiliation									
None	17.2	3 472	172	19.2	3 863	12	5.1	3 519	121
Church of England	16.9	3 137	209	9.6	3 438	10	2.9	3 193	151
Roman Catholic	17.6	1 045	87	14.7	1 195	3	3.8	1 071	61
Other Christian	18.2	1 360	82	11.5	1 549	7	3.8	1 387	55
Non-Christian	22.7	263	76	14.7	395	2	3.7	268	71
Missing	26.7	15*	1	19.9	19*	0	22.6	15*	1
Education									
Degree	23.8	784	30	21.4	838	1	3.5	797	18
A level or other non-degree	21.2	2 189	93	18.5	2 410	2	4.3	2 211	59
O level/CSE	17.9	3 489	184	14.7	3 980	5	4.2	3 545	126
Other	15.6	144	16	11.4	160	1	2.4	147	12
None	12.1	2 678	291	8.4	3 064	8	3.6	2 735	233
Missing	—	8†	12	—	6†	17	—	8†	12
Marital status									
Married	15.1	5 902	444	3.3	6 331	16	1.3	6 005	342
Cohabiting									
Opposite-sex partner	12.4	806	25	21.6	834	0	5.7	815	17
Same-sex partner	—	6†	0	8.8	11*	0	—	5†	1
Widowed	16.4	188	14	11.0	201	0	4.0	191	11
Divorced, separated	14.8	796	63	30.7	859	1	9.0	824	35
Single	30.3	1 591	74	36.3	2 221	8	10.6	1 611	47
Missing	—	2†	8	—	0	9	—	2†	8
Smoking									
Non-smoker	21.4	3 988	325	12.9	4 768	23	3.1	4 063	244
Ex-smoker	14.5	1 584	107	9.8	1 696	3	1.8	1 616	95
Smokes <15 per day	17.7	1 583	66	20.9	1 698	4	6.8	1 600	49
Smokes 15+ per day	12.0	2 047	113	15.4	2 177	3	5.4	2 081	78
Missing	14.9	90	16	10.4	119	1	3.2	93	14
Alcohol									
None	15.8	1 152	161	7.7	1 464	11	2.0	1 178	137
Low intake	18.3	7 212	434	14.4	8 006	23	3.6	7 338	300
Moderate intake	13.1	868	32	23.1	925	0	10.0	876	23
High intake	2.7	43	0	8.5	44	0	2.4	43	0
Missing	27.9	17*	0	4.8	20	0	3.4	17*	0

* Note small base.
† Base <10.

Index

Abortion 288–92, 483–4
  number of sexual partners 290–2
  validity of data 61–2
  views on 243–4, 475–8
Acquired immune deficiency syndrome
    (AIDS) 5–6
  behaviour changes 326–34, 491–4
    influences 332–4
  public education 320
Age
  changing importance of sex 253–4
  condom use 336–7
  distribution in survey 57
  first heterosexual intercourse
    69–80, 435–8
    views on 228–35, 467–70
  frequency of heterosexual sex
    148–50
  heterosexual partnerships 114–19
  homosexual behaviour 197–203
  sexual practices 163–9
  unsafe sex 323
AIDS see Acquired immune deficiency
    syndrome
Alcohol
  consumption and sexual behaviour
    265–7
  first heterosexual intercourse 101
All-Party Parliamentary Group on
    AIDS 16
Anal intercourse 161–3, 178, 458–61
  and age 166–7
  homosexual 216–20
  marital status 170–2

Bisexuality 208–12
Boarding schools and homosexual
    behaviour 205–6
Body mass index
  and sexual behaviour 267–9

validity of data 60–1

Casual sex, views on 240–1, 475–8
Cervical cancer
  first heterosexual intercourse 82
  smoking 263–5
Circumcision 283–4
Commercial sex, male experience
    135–40
Complex standard errors and design
    factors 431–4
Condoms 304
  first heterosexual intercourse 88–9
  use 487–90, 491–4
    risk reduction strategy 332,
      334–40
    with other contraceptive methods
      319
  see also contraception
Contraception 296–319, 487–90
  first heterosexual intercourse
    86–90, 101
    nature of relationship 99
  gender differences in reporting 316
  methods used 297–316
    children, numbers 310–11
    multivariate analysis 312–16
    number of partners 310–12
    religion 308–10
    social class 306–8
    trends 316–19
    users and non-users 297
Cunnilingus 159–61

Data
  collection, method 21–2
  editing and coding 53–4
  internal consistency 62–3
  preparation 53–6
  statistical presentation 64–5

Data *Cont.*
  validity, external checks   60–2
  weighting   54–5, 429–30
Demographic variables   435–94
  complex standard errors and design
    factors   431–2
Department of Health (DoH, DHSS)
    13–15

Economic and Social Research Council
    13–16
Education and first heterosexual
    intercourse   80–3
Electoral register   38–9
Entryphones and survey response
    51–2
Ethnic groups
  distribution in survey   57–8
  first heterosexual intercourse   83–6
Extra-marital sex, views on   238–40,
    471–4

Fellatio   159–61
First heterosexual intercourse
  age at   69–80, 435–8
    biological effects   76–8
    cultural influences   79–80
    decline   69–73
    gender differences   76
  age of partner   91–5
  before the age of 16   73–5
  context   95–7
  contraception   87–90
  experience   90–106
  factors associated with   99–101
  feelings about   102–3
  ideal age and actual age   231–3
    reasons for choice   233–5
  influence of social class and
    education   80–3
  multivariate analysis   103–6
  number of sexual partners   126–7
  questions asked   68–9
  recommended minimum age
    compared with legal age
    228–30
  relationship with first partner   95–9
  views on age   228–35, 467–70
First sexual experience, age at   72–3

Gallup International, pilot survey
    12–13

Gender
  distribution in survey   57
  number of reported partners
    119–20
Health, reported   260–2, 479–82
  and sexual behaviour   259
  question format   260
Health Education Authority (HEA)
    13–16
Health service use and sexual
    behaviour   273–92
Health-related behaviour   263–73
  relationship with sexual behaviour
    266–70
Height, validity of data   60–1
Heterosexual partnerships   110–42
  age at first intercourse   126–7
  age difference between partners
    133–5, 455
  concurrent   130–3
  definition   111–12
  gender differences   119–20
  generational changes   116–19
  influence of marital/partnership
    status   120–3
  item non-response and coding
    assumptions   112
  length and frequency of sex   154–6
  measurement precision   112–13
  numbers
    frequency of sex   156–7
    in different time intervals   113–14
    men   439–40, 443–4, 447–8,
      451–2
    sexual practices   117–8
    women   441–2, 445–6, 449–50,
      453–4
  pattern   130–3
  question format   111–12
  respondent's current age   114–19
  social class   123–6
  travel   140–1
Heterosexual practices   145–79,
    458–61
  age   163–9
  marital status   169–74
  methodological aspects   146–7
  number of partners   177–8
  question format   146–7
  repertoire   158–63

factors influencing   163
response assumptions   147
secular trends   169
social class   175–7
Heterosexual sex, frequency   148,
    455–7
  age and   148–50
  and health   262
  length of relationship   154–6
  marital status   151
  number of partners   156–7
  social class   151–4
HIV *see* Human immunodeficiency
    virus
Homosexual acceptance scale   246–50
Homosexual behaviour   183–223
  age-related variations   197–203
  attitudes, implications for research
    184–5
  exclusivity   208–12
  facultative   205
  number of partners   212–16,
    463–6
  prevalence   189–93
    sociodemographic variation
    193–203
  question formulation   185–6
  regions   195–7
  social class   194–5
Homosexual experience   189–93
  men   463–4
  women   465–6
Homosexual partnerships   190–216,
    463–6
  number of partners   212–6, 463–6
Homosexual practices   216–21
Homosexuality, views on   241–3,
    475–8
Housing type and survey response   51
Human immunodeficiency virus (HIV)
  antibody testing   278–82, 485–6
    sexual behaviour   280–1
  transmission
    heterosexual anal intercourse   167
    homosexual sex   189
    injecting drug use   271
    perceived risk   322
    prostitutes   135–6

Infertility   284–8
  and sexual behaviour   284–6

Injecting drug use   271–3
Intrauterine device (IUD)   305
  see also contraception

Law and sexual attitudes   225

Marital status
  distribution in survey   59
  extra-marital sex, views on   238–40
  frequency of heterosexual sex   151
  health and sexual behaviour   260–2
  miscarriage, stillbirth and abortion
    288–9
  numbers of sexual partners   120–3
  pattern of sexual relationships   132
  sexual practices   169–74
  STD clinic attendance   275
  unsafe sex   323–4
Marriage
  importance of sex   250–3
  suitable age for   233–5
Masturbation   146
Medical research council (MRC)
    14–16
Memory error   32–3
Menarche and first heterosexual
    intercourse   76–8
Miscarriage   288–92, 483–4
  number of sexual partners   290–2
Monogamy   130–3
  gender and attitudes   241
  importance, views on   254–5

National Survey of Sexual Attitudes
    and Lifestyles
  characteristics of responders and
    non-responders   51–3
  confidentiality   31–2
  emergency   12–17
  feasibility study   15, 23
  fieldwork
    organization and procedures
    43–4
    quality control   45–6
    timing   44–5
  internal and external validity   36–7,
    60–3
  interviewers   44–5
    gender   49–50
    training and briefing   425–6
  interviews   21–2

National Survey *Cont.*
  item non-response   55–6
  measurement objectives   19–21
  rationale for   5–10
  reliability and validity   30–7
  research variables   20–1
  response
    rates   46–9
    regional   50
  selection of respondent   425
  statistical considerations   63–5
  technical details   423–6
  theoretical framework   8–10
  wards, stratification for selection
    423–5
  see also Data; Questionnaire;
    Sampling
Non-penetrative sex   159, 458–61
  age and   167–9

Odds ratio adjusted   65
Oral contraception   300–3, 487–90
  first heterosexual intercourse
    79–80, 89–90
  smoking   263
Oral sex   159–61, 458–61
  age and   163–6
  homosexual   216–20
Orgasm, views on role in sexual
    satisfaction   255–6

Permissiveness scale   246–50
Post Office Postcode Address File
    (PAF)   15, 38–9
Pre-marital sex   95
  views on   236–8, 471–4
Prostitutes   135–40
  first heterosexual intercourse with
    95

Questionnaire
  choice of language   25–6
  designing   22–5
  encouraging reliable responses
    31–2
  format   23–5
  order effect   34–6
  problem of understanding   27–9
  question wording   29–30
  respondents' preference for
    terminology   26–7

single occurrences vs habits   36

Recall, aiding process   33
Regions
  attitudes towards homosexuality
    243
  first heterosexual intercourse   86
  homosexual behaviour   195–7
  injecting drug use   272–3
  STD clinic attendance   274–5
Religion
  contraceptive use   310
  early heterosexual intercourse
    84–6
Response rates   46–9
  comparison with other studies
    47–9, 428
  regional   50

Safer sex   319–22
Sampling
  demographic representativeness of
    sample   57–60
  details of sample design   42–3
  errors   63–4
  frame   38–9
  population coverage   37–8
  sample size and type   37
Serial monogamy   130–3
Sex
  abstinence, risk reduction strategy
    331
  changing importance
    with age   253–4
    with length of relationship   254
  importance within marriage   250–3
  opinions on significance   250–6
  safer   319–22
    meaning   320–2
  unsafe, prevalence and distribution
    322–5, 491–4
Sexual attitudes   225–7
  beliefs and knowledge   227–8
  methodological note   226–7
  relationship with behaviour   244–6
Sexual attraction   186–9
Sexual behaviour
  biological determinants   9
  changes because of AIDS   326–34,
    491–4
    influences   332–4

response rates in different surveys 428

studies of the AIDS era 10–12

variations, complex standard errors and design factors 433–4

Sexual consent 229–31

knowledge of law 230–1

Sexual lifestyles, absence of existing data 3–5

Sexual orientation 183–222

attitudes, implications for research 184–5

question formulation 185–6

stability 203–6

Sexual partners

change, pattern 6–7

numbers and risk reduction strategy 328–30

see also Heterosexual partnerships; Homosexual partnerships

Sexual practices

avoiding as risk reduction strategy 332

prevalence

men 458–9

women 460–1

see also Heterosexual practices; Homosexual practices

Sexual relationships

non-exclusive, views on 238–40

views on 235–43

Sexual satisfaction, views on role of orgasm 255–6

Sexuality, diversity 9

Sexually transmitted diseases

age difference between partners 133

clinic attendance 273–8, 479–82

multivariate analysis 276–8

sexual behaviour 276

partner change 111, 114

prostitutes 135

Smoking and sexual behaviour 263–5

Social class

allocation 64–5

contraceptive use 306–8

first heterosexual intercourse 80–3

frequency of heterosexual sex 151–4

heterosexual partnerships 123–6

heterosexual practices 175–7

homosexual behaviour 194–5

Social pressure and first heterosexual intercourse 101

Socioeconomic groups, distribution in

statistical methods 63–5

survey 59–60

STD see sexually transmitted diseases

Sterilization 303–4, 487–91

trends 316

variation with social class 308

Stillbirth 288–92, 483–4

number of sexual partners 290–2

Surveys 3–4

Teenagers, sexual behaviour 4–5

Travel and sexual partnership 140–1

Vaginal intercourse 159, 458–61

and marital status 169–172

Weight, validity of data 60–1

Weighting 54–5, 429–30

Wolfendon Committee's Report on Homosexuality, impact 199–202